# Equine Sc Health and Performance

Sarah Pilliner
and
Zoe Davies

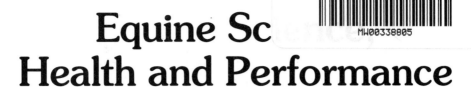

**b**

Blackwell
Science

© 1996 by
Blackwell Science Ltd
Editorial Offices:
Osney Mead, Oxford OX2 0EL
25 John Street, London WC1N 2BL
23 Ainslie Place, Edinburgh EH3 6AJ
350 Main Street, Malden
  MA 02148 5018, USA
54 University Street, Carlton
  Victoria 3053, Australia
10, rue Casimir Delavigne
  75006 Paris, France

Other Editorial Offices:

Blackwell Wissenschafts-Verlag GmbH
Kurfürstendamm 57
10707 Berlin, Germany

Blackwell Science KK
MG Kodenmacho Building
7–10 Kodenmacho Nihombashi
Chuo-ku, Tokyo 104, Japan

Iowa State University Press
A Blackwell Science Company
2121 S. State Avenue
Ames, Iowa 50014-8300, USA

First published 1991
Reprinted 1997, 1998, 2001

Set in 10/11.5 pt Souvenir
by DP Photosetting, Aylesbury, Bucks
Printed and bound in Great Britain
at the Alden Press Limited, Oxford and Northampton

DISTRIBUTORS

Marston Book Services Ltd
PO Box 269
Abingdon
Oxon OX14 4YN
(*Orders*: Tel: 01235 465500
         Fax: 01235 465555

USA and Canada
  Iowa State University Press
  A Blackwell Science Company
  2121 S. State Avenue
  Ames, Iowa 50014-8300
  (*Orders*: Tel: 800-862-6657
           Fax: 515-292-3348
           Web: www.isupress.com
           email: orders@isupress.com)

Australia
  Blackwell Science Pty Ltd
  54 University Street
  Carlton, Victoria 3053
  (*Orders*: Tel: 03 9347 0300
           Fax: 03 9349 5001)

A catalogue record for this title is available
from the British Library

ISBN 0–632–03913–2

Library of Congress
Cataloging-in-Publication Data
Pilliner, Sarah.
    Equine science, performance, and health/Sarah
  Pilliner and Zoe Davies.
      p.    cm.
    Includes index.
    ISBN 0-632-03913-2 (alk. paper)
    1. Horses.   2. Horses–Health.   I. Davies, Zoe.
  II. Title.
  SF 285.3.P54   1996
  636.1′089—dc20                          96-11750
                                              CIP

For further information on
Blackwell Science, visit our website:
www.blackwell-science.com

# Contents

# Preface

Equine welfare is becoming an increasingly important aspect of the care and management of the horse, both on a day-to-day basis and during competition. In order for horses to fit into our lives they are kept in an unnatural situation; they are stabled, transported all over the country, pushed to the limit in competition and fed a potentially lethal diet. The horse owners of today are increasingly aware of their responsibilities towards their animals and seek more knowledge and understanding of how the horse functions in order to be able to care for their animals more efficiently.

*Equine Science, Health and Performance* gives an insight into the way the horse's mind and body works; clear explanation of the structure and function of the body systems fosters understanding and thus better horse care and management. The authors explain the science behind practical horse husbandry.

All horse owners and riders recognise that prevention is always better than cure – yet it is difficult to prevent ill-health, injury or disease if the causes of the problem are not properly understood. A study of the way the horse's body works in health will help keep the horse fit and well by recognising the management and environment that will predispose to ill-health. Unfortunately no animal can avoid problems at some point in its life; here a knowledge of anatomy and physiology will facilitate effective recognition, treatment and recovery.

*Equine Science, Health and Performance* will be invaluable to students on National and Higher National Diploma Courses, Equine Studies Degree programmes, Advanced National Certificate and BHS Stage IV students, and will be of great interest to all horse owners.

# Part I
# The Systems of the Horse

# Chapter 1
# The Skeleton

## Points of the horse

It is important to be familiar with the surface anatomy of the horse in order to be able to identify the underlying structures (Fig. 1.1).

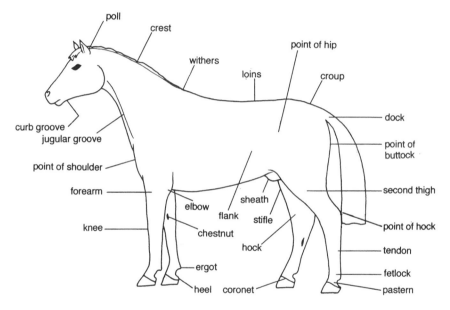

**Fig. 1.1**   Points of the horse.

# Bone

## Functions of bone

Bone has several functions including:

- giving support and rigidity;
- acting as levers for the muscles to work against;
- protecting the internal organs;
- storing calcium, phosphorus and magnesium.

## Classification, development and growth of bone

Bone has two important properties. It is both *rigid*, giving strength, and *elastic*, allowing some flexibility, without which bone would be brittle and easily broken.

Living, organic, fibrous tissue consisting mainly of the protein collagen makes up about 30% of an adult horse's bone, and this provides the flexibility. The remaining 70% is made up of inorganic bone salts of which the most important is hydroxy-apatite $(Ca_{10}(PO_4)_6(OH)_2)$. Calcium and phosphorus are thus essential in the diet to maintain bone structure, but sodium, magnesium, potassium, chloride, fluoride, bicarbonate and citrate ions are all present in variable amounts. Essentially bone consists of a matrix encrusted with mineral salts which impart strength.

The proportion of organic and inorganic material in bone varies with age. Thus young horses have 'soft' bones containing up to 60% fibrous tissue, while old horses develop 'brittle' bones with a fibrous content as low as 35%.

While bone may look inelastic and almost lifeless it is a highly dynamic structure – the entire calcium content of the skeleton is replaced every 200 days. This ability to mobilise minerals allows the skeleton to act as a mineral reservoir in times of stress. A lactating mare, for example, can make up the required calcium for milk from her body should her diet lack calcium. No tissue in the body is capable of as much overgrowth and as much absorption as bone.

There are two types of bone:

## Classification of bone

- dense or compact
- spongy or cancellous.

Spongy bone is made up of slender, irregular trabeculae or bars which branch and unite to form a network. Compact bone is solid except for microscopic spaces. Both contain the same histological elements. With few exceptions both spongy and compact types are present in every bone, but the amount and distribution of each type can vary considerably. Spongy bone is associated with red bone marrow and the synthesis of red blood cells. Both types are penetrated by tiny blood and lymph vessels as well as nerves.

Each bone has a characteristic shape which is determined by its function within the skeleton. There are four main types:

- long bones
- flat bones
- short bones
- irregular bones.

*Long bones* act as supporting columns and levers, for example the cannon bone. They consist of a shaft (diaphysis) and two ends (epiphyses). Compact bone makes up the shaft and is organised in a tube-like form surrounding yellow bone marrow (the medullary cavity). Each end of the long bone is spongy bone covered by a thin shell of compact bone. Long bones are characteristic of limbs and have terminal enlargements which are associated with joints, for example the end of the femur and tibia. This is for two reasons:

- to spread the pressure over a larger articular surface and thus reduce the wear and tear on the joint surfaces;
- the joint is more stable and less likely to move out of alignment, i.e. to become dislocated.

*Flat bones*, for example the skull, act as protection. In flat bones, two plates of compact bone enclose a middle layer of spongy bone.

*Short bones*, for example the carpal bones of the knee and the tarsal bones of the hock, act as shock absorbers.

*Irregular bones* generally have a specialist function, such as the vertebrae. Most irregular bones consist of spongy bone covered by a thin shell of compact bone.

Regardless of their shape the composition of these bones is similar. A cross-section of long bone (Fig. 1.2) shows an outer layer of compact bone for strength and then an inner layer of spongy bone. The compact bone is thickest where stress is the greatest. Surrounding the compact bone is a dense connective tissue membrane called the periosteum which acts as an attachment point for tendons and ligaments. The periosteum is lined with cells called osteoblasts which secrete new bone matrix. The bone is laid down in bands called lamellae supplied with capillaries which run from the arterioles in the Haversian canal. This structure facilitates the passage of nutrients and waste to and from the bone cells. The canal also carries lymph and nerve fibres. The lamellar structure means that bone can withstand high compressive and tensile forces.

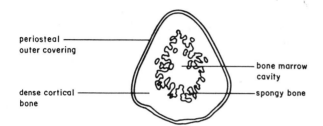

periosteal outer covering

bone marrow cavity

dense cortical bone

spongy bone

**Fig. 1.2**   Cross-section through a long bone.

## Bone formation and growth

In the unborn foal there are two main types of bone formation or ossification:

- intramembranous bone formation
- endochondral ossification.

Intramembranous bone formation gives rise to flat bones such as the skull, jaws and pectoral girdle and involves ossification of the dermis. Mesenchyma cells become differentiated into rows of osteoblasts which begin to lay down bony plates. The osteoblasts also increase in number and lay down bone salts onto the plates resulting in an increase in size.

The best example of endochondral ossification is in the long bones (Fig. 1.3). In the embryo bone begins as cartilage, then osteoblasts invade the cartilage and lay down bone matrix. Mineral salts are then deposited in the matrix, a process called calcification, resulting in bone. By the time the foal is born, calcification is complete in most bones.

Once the bone is formed it grows; growth involves an increase in diameter as well as in length. The increase in length takes place at two narrow bands of cartilage called the epiphyseal growth plates. Cartilage grows continuously on the side of the growth plate nearest the end of the bone, meanwhile the cartilage on the shaft side of the growth plate is invaded by osteoblasts and converted to bone. Gradually the osteoblasts 'catch up' on the cartilage so that when the bone is the correct length the growth plate 'closes'. The growth plates close at different times:

- lower end of the radius, i.e. just above knee – 2.5 years
- lower end of cannon bone – 9–12 months
- fetlock – 8–9 months.

The closure of the plates is affected by the sex hormones. Colts and fillies grow at a similar rate until they reach puberty when testosterone, the male sex hormone, stops

1. The early cartilagenous template

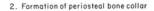

calcified cartilage

periosteum

bone collar

2. Formation of periosteal bone collar

epiphyseal plate {

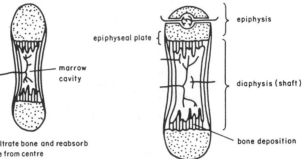

marrow cavity

epiphysis

diaphysis (shaft)

bone deposition

3. Blood vessels infiltrate bone and reabsorb calcified cartilage from centre

4. Blood vessels invade epiphysis, resorbing cartilage and forming a growth centre at the bone's end. Osteoblasts deposit bone in the epiphyseal plate

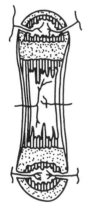

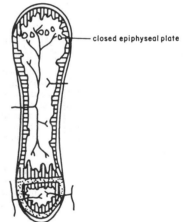

closed epiphyseal plate

5. In epiphysis cartilage replaced by bone. At other end same transformation. Shaft lengthened by bone deposited at epiphyseal plate

6. At bone's upper end all cartilage (except joint cartilage) replaced by bone. Bone has grown upward across epiphyseal plate and the marrow of the epiphysis is continuous with that of the shaft. Growth at that end of bone is ceased

**Fig. 1.3**   Growth and development of a long bone.

the closure of the plates, so that colts continue to grow. Oestrogen promotes the closure of the plates and the growth rate of fillies slows down. Anabolic steroids tend to hasten the closure of the plates and if given to the young animal will stunt the growth of the skeleton while enhancing muscle development.

Growth-related problems or developmental orthopaedic diseases can occur when the correct nutrients for bone growth are not supplied in the correct amounts and proportions. Growth must take place so that the horse's athletic ability is not compromised. Using horses before the closure of the plates can also lead to growth-related problems. The distal radial plates do not close until well into the racing career of the flat racehorse. The cartilage of the open epiphysis is very sensitive to jarring which can give rise to large lumpy swellings immediately above the knee.

The increase in diameter is brought about by osteoblasts which line the periosteum (Fig. 1.4). In simple terms the osteoblasts lay down new layers of bone over the old in a similar way to the growth of a tree which gives rise to rings which can be seen when the tree is felled. Simultaneously the old bone lining the marrow cavity is eaten away by osteoclasts, cells which reabsorb bone. This means that the bone marrow cavity will enlarge but the wall of the shaft does not become too thick and heavy.

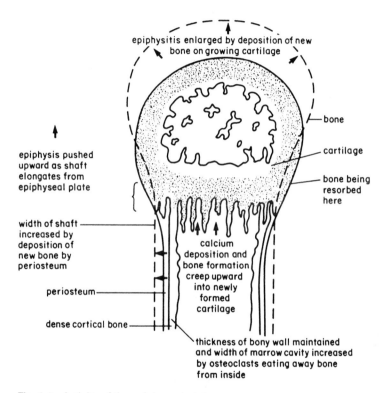

**Fig. 1.4** Activity of the epiphyseal plate.

## Adaptation of bone to stress

Throughout the horse's life bone undergoes a remodelling process which is a balance between the breakdown of old bone and the formation of new bone. Remodelling occurs to allow the bone to act as a mineral store and also to let the bone adapt to stress such as exercise.

Remodelling starts when the foal is about three-months-old, when the newly formed bone begins to rearrange itself into Haversian systems. These systems consist of a series of vertically aligned tubules through which the blood vessels travel. If the Haversian systems are formed too quickly with too little mineral content, the bone becomes porous and not as strong as dense bone. It is essential that there are adequate and balanced amounts of calcium and phosphorus in the diet to allow effective remodelling to take place.

## Mineral storage in bone

Bone acts as a store of calcium and phosphorus which can be readily called upon, for example, during pregnancy or lactation.

## Blood cell production

The soft red bone marrow found in the ribs, sternum and long bones of young foals produces red blood cells. As the animal matures the red bone marrow in the long bones is replaced by yellow bone marrow and the red cell production is taken over mainly by the spleen.

# The skeleton (Fig. 1.5)

The skeleton consists of bones, cartilage and joints and can be divided into two parts:

- the appendicular skeleton consisting of the limbs;
- the axial skeleton consisting of the skull, vertebrae, ribs and sternum.

## The axial skeleton

### The spine

The spine provides longitudinal support for the body and the necessary strength for suspending the enormous weight of the gut. It is relatively rigid and incompressible compared to cats, for example. The vertebrae themselves are wholly incompressible; bending is allowed by the joints between the vertebrae while the cartilaginous discs between each vertebra allow slight compression. The spine can be divided into five regions:

- the neck – 7 cervical vertebrae
- upper back – 18 thoracic vertebrae
- loins – 6 lumbar vertebrae
- croup – 5 fused sacral vertebrae
- tail – 15–20 coccygeal vertebrae.

The vertebrae make up a long bony chain housing and protecting the spinal cord. At each vertebra a pair of spinal nerves branch off from the spinal cord to penetrate *every* part of the body. Each vertebra has the same basic shape:

- the vertebral body or centrum;
- an arch surmounted by the dorsal spine;
- a pair of transverse processes of very variable size and shape;
- two pairs of articular surfaces.

The spinal, lateral and articular processes allow for the attachment of muscles and ligaments and the body and arch protect the spinal cord.

### Cervical vertebrae (Fig. 1.6)

The horse's neck consists of seven cervical vertebrae; the first is the atlas which consists of a short tube with large wings, it articulates with the skull at the occiput, allowing the horse's head to nod. The wings of the atlas can be felt on either side of the horse's neck below the poll and behind the jawbone. The second is the axis united to the atlas by a tooth-like projection, the odontoid process which allows the head to

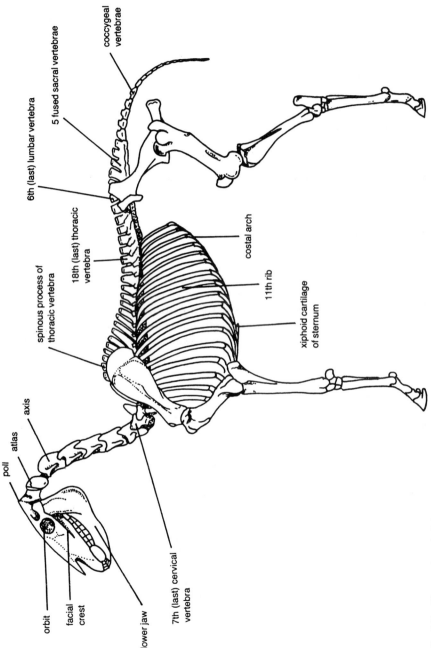

**Fig. 1.5**  The equine skeleton.

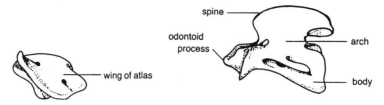

**Fig. 1.6**   Atlas (left) and axis (right) vertebrae.

move from side to side. The long, strong ligament of the neck, the nuchal ligament, attaches to the axis; it helps hold up the horse's very heavy head and neck, and allows the head and neck to be raised and lowered. The joints between the other cervical vertebrae enable the horse to bend its neck sideways and to arch its neck. The curves formed by the vertebrae are deep in the neck and do not follow the crest.

**Thoracic vertebrae** (Fig. 1.7)

The back consists of eighteen thoracic vertebrae, five or six lumbar vertebrae, the sacrum and the coccygeal vertebrae. The thoracic vertebrae are typical vertebrae linked by cartilaginous pads called discs; the spinous processes are very large giving the horse its pronounced withers and allowing extensive muscle and ligament attachment. The withers are the highest point of the thoracic spine and are formed by the spinous processes of the third to tenth thoracic vertebrae. The withers are held firmly in place by ligaments between the spines and other muscles and ligaments attached to the spines, including the funicular portion of the nuchal ligament. The way the spinous processes are directed is of great importance to the athletic horse; there are two articulations, one between the discs and the bodies of the vertebrae, and the lateral articulations on each side of the vertebrae. The movement between the horse's thoracic vertebrae is strictly defined and limited in comparison to many other animals.

**Lumbar vertebrae** (Fig. 1.8)

The lumbar vertebrae make up the loin region and, as with the thoracic vertebrae, have a strictly defined and very limited degree of movement. In fact, apart from the neck and tail, the horse's back shows very little movement; some movement is seen between the last thoracic and first lumbar vertebrae and between the first three lumbar

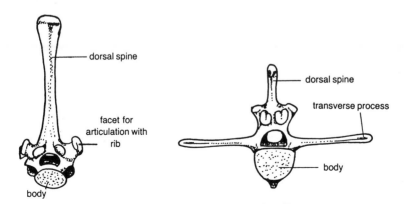

**Fig. 1.7**   Thoracic vertebra.      **Fig. 1.8**   Lumbar vertebra.

vertebrae. The degree of movement depends on the thickness of the intervertebral discs, which are firmly attached to the vertebrae, almost like part of the bone that has not yet become calcified or bony. Indeed, as the horse ages it is common to find that the discs do become calcified thus joining the vertebrae together. There may even be further outgrowths of bone acting as bridges across neighbouring vertebrae; two adjacent lumbar vertebrae may be joined by the transverse process on one side and not the other, and this will cause pain until both sides become fused.

### Sacrum (Fig. 1.9)

The sacrum is a composite bone made up of five vertebrae, situated beneath the loins in the croup region. The pelvic bones are attached to either side of it by the sacro-iliac joint.

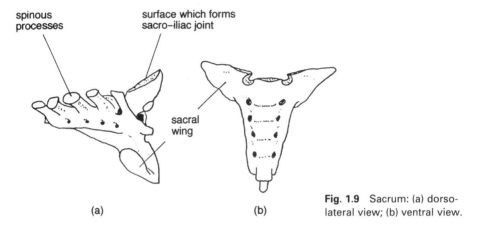

(a)  (b)

**Fig. 1.9** Sacrum: (a) dorso-lateral view; (b) ventral view.

### Coccygeal vertebrae

There are usually 18 coccygeal or tail vertebrae but the number can vary from 15 to 21 in number and they decrease in size and complexity from first to last.

The total length of the spine is a series of curves, so that it is slightly arched at the upper end of the neck and concave above in the lower third of the neck (Fig. 1.10). At the junction of the neck and the chest there is a marked change in direction, followed by a gentle curve, concave below, through the thoracic and lumbar region, which helps to support the body weight. The dorsal spines of the thoracic vertebrae are held in

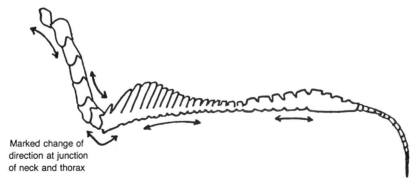

**Fig. 1.10** The spine is a series of curves.

position by strong ligaments. The horse's spine is designed like a suspension bridge and these curves give it the strength needed to carry the enormous weight of its gut – up to 200 kg in a 16.2 hh horse – and in the mare, to carry the foetus and the associated fluid and membranes. The horse is not designed to carry a rider's weight on top of its back.

At walk the spine can be seen to move sideways but at faster paces there is increased muscular resistance which minimises any movement. Above the spine the longissimus dorsi muscle and below the spine, the psoas minor muscle, contract to stop the horse flexing its back; when this synchronisation fails, for example if the horse falls, then the back is vulnerable to damage.

The ligaments associated with the vertebrae include the supra-spinous ligament, which runs along the top of the spines of the vertebrae and unites the summits of all lumbar and thoracic vertebrae. It divides to go up either side of the neck, becoming the nuchal ligament. The nuchal ligament consists of two parts:

- the funicular part is a rope-like ligament which supports the head and runs along the top of the neck;
- the lamellar part is a band attaching to the cervical vertebrae which restrains the movement of the dorsal spines and supports the weight of the head.

## The ribs

Each thoracic vertebra carries a pair of ribs, thus there are 18 pairs of ribs. Eight true ribs are attached to the sternum, ten pairs of false ribs are connected to each other and form the costal arch.

## The sternum

The sternum or breastbone forms the floor of the chest and supports the true ribs. The rear of the sternum is drawn out into the xiphoid cartilage.

# The appendicular skeleton

The appendicular skeleton is attached to the axial skeleton by the pelvic girdle and the pectoral girdle. However the horse has no collar bone so that the pectoral girdle is attached only by muscles and ligaments to the spine, ribs and sternum. This means that the forehand of the horse is designed to support the body and absorb concussion, not to propel the horse forwards.

# The forelimb (Fig. 1.11)

The forelimb consists of the following:

- scapula
- humerus
- radius and ulna
- carpus or knee
- three metacarpals (cannon and splint bones)
- three phalanges (long and pastern bones and the pedal bone)
- three sesamoid bones (the 'sesamoids' and the navicular bone).

## Scapula

The scapula is a triangular, flattened bone which glides back and forth over the rib

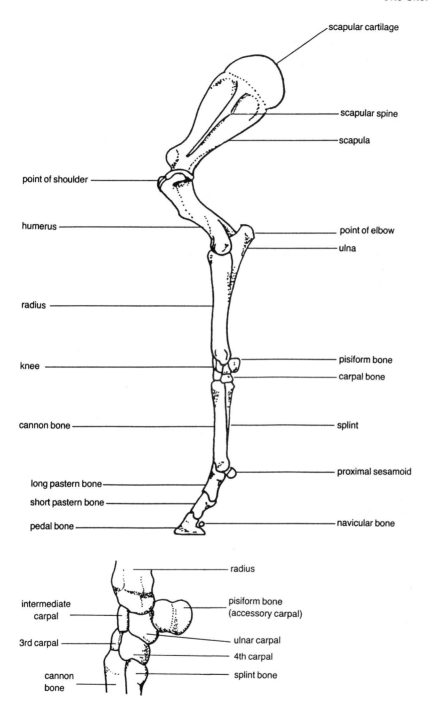

**Fig. 1.11** Forelimb and knee.

cage. There is no bony attachment between the scapula and the spine so that the thorax is slung between the two scapulae, allowing the horse freedom of movement and compensating for the lack of flexibility of the spine. The length of the scapula will determine the slope of the shoulder and hence the length of stride of the horse. The scapula is divided lengthways by a prominent ridge called the scapular spine which can be felt through the skin. The supraspinatus muscle lies in front of the ridge and the infraspinatus muscle behind the ridge. The trapezius muscle and deltoid muscle also are attached to the scapular spine.

## Humerus

The shoulder joint is formed between the scapula and the humerus. The humerus is one of the strongest bones in the body. The angulation of the humerus allows for shock absorption, and it is also the site of attachment for many muscles.

## Radius and ulna

Unlike the human, the radius and ulna of the horse (equivalent to our lower arm) are fused together to prevent any twisting of the horse's forearm. The ulna has become very small except for the olecranon process which forms the point of the elbow. The elbow joint itself is a hinge (ginglymus) joint which allows movement in one direction only.

## The carpus (knee)

The horse's knee is equivalent to the human wrist and consists of seven or eight small carpal bones; in the upper row are the radial, intermediate and ulnar carpals, with the pisiform bone or accessory carpal bone at the back of the knee. The lower row consists of the first, second, third and fourth carpal bones. The knee is a hinge joint allowing movement in only one direction and the arrangement of the small carpal bones is designed to absorb shock.

## The metacarpals

The three metacarpal bones are better known as the cannon-bone and the two splint bones. The splint bones are a legacy from when the horse's ancestors had several toes but while they do support the knee they are no longer weight-bearing. The cannon-bone is capable of carrying substantial weight, having little spongy or cancellous bone surrounded by solid bone. The amount of 'bone' a horse has is the circumference of the leg just below the knee and indicates the weight-carrying capacity of the horse.

## The phalanges

The three phalanges are known as the long pastern, short pastern and pedal bone and are equivalent to the human finger. The tendons from the muscles of the forearm attach to these bones, giving increased leverage and a powerful stride. The joint between the cannon-bone and the long pastern bone is the fetlock joint and is another hinge joint. It is subjected to large amounts of stress and has a great deal of movement. The pastern joint is between the long and short pastern bones and has limited movement. The coffin joint is between the short pastern and the pedal bone and has a great deal of movement.

## The sesamoid bones

The horse has three sesamoid bones; the proximal sesamoids, known as the 'sesamoids' are situated at the back of the fetlock joint while the distal sesamoid or navicular bone is found inside the hoof at the back of the coffin joint. Their role is to act as pulleys enabling the tendons that run over them to exert their pull on the phalanges.

# The hindlimb (Fig. 1.12)

The hindlimb has a bony attachment to the spine allowing the propulsive forces to be transmitted to and along the spine to generate movement. The hindlimb consists of:

- the pelvis
- the femur
- the tibia and fibula
- the tarsus or hock
- three metacarpals (cannon and splint bones)
- three phalanges (long and short pastern bones and the pedal bone)
- three sesamoid bones (the 'sesamoids' and the navicular bone).

## The pelvic girdle

The pelvic girdle consists of the pelvic bones, the sacrum and the first three coccygeal vertebrae.

## The pelvis (Fig. 1.13)

Each half of the pelvis is made up of three flat bones, the ilium, ischium and the pubis, which are fused into one. The upper portion of the pelvis, which is attached to the sacrum is called the ilium. The front of the pelvic floor is the pubis and the rear portion is the ischium. All three bones meet at the acetabulum which articulates with the head of the femur to make the hip joint. The ilium is the largest bone and its outermost angle is seen as the tuber coxae – the point of the hip. Where the ilium attaches to the sacrum is the sacro-iliac joint which is characterised by strong muscle attachments. At the highest point of the hindquarters the two sides of the tuber sacrale form the croup. The point of the buttocks are the thickened ends of the ischium known as the tuber ischii.

## The hip joint

The hip joint is deep in the hindquarter of the horse and is most easily seen when the hind leg is flexed. It is the joint between the pelvis and the femur and is capable of a wide range of movement. It acts to protect the internal organs, as a site for muscle attachment and to allow the efficient transfer of force to the spine.

## The femur

This very strong bone is designed to act as the medium between the hip joint and the stifle joint and is adapted for the attachment of the muscles of the hindquarter.

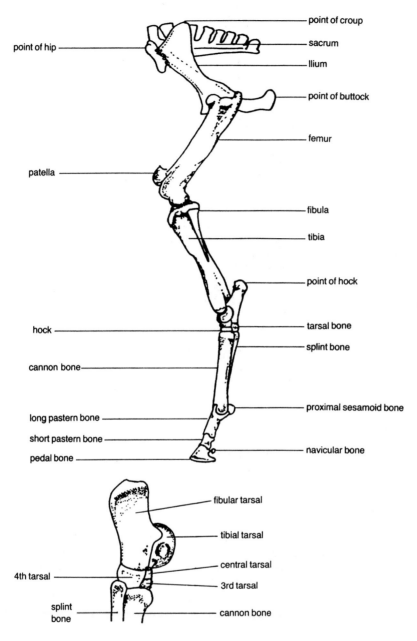

point of croup

point of hip

sacrum

Ilium

point of buttock

femur

patella

fibula

tibia

point of hock

hock

tarsal bone

splint bone

cannon bone

proximal sesamoid bone

long pastern bone

short pastern bone

navicular bone

pedal bone

fibular tarsal

tibial tarsal

central tarsal

4th tarsal

3rd tarsal

splint
bone

cannon bone

**Fig. 1.12**  Hindlimb and hock.

## The patella

The patella is a sesamoid bone and the equivalent of the human kneecap. It is associated with the stifle – the joint between the femur and the tibia.

## The tibia and fibula

The tibia is a long bone running down and back between the stifle and the hock joints.

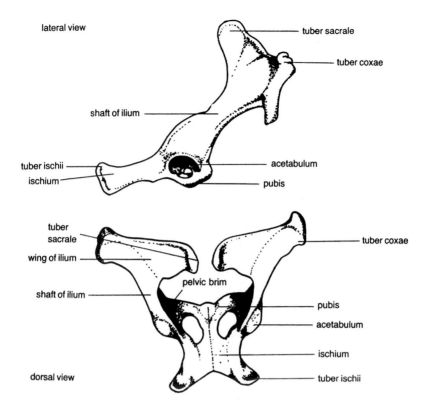

**Fig. 1.13** Pelvis.

The upper end provides attachment for the muscles acting on the hock and lower limb. The horse's fibula is so reduced in size as to be practically vestigial.

## The tarsus (hock)

The hock consists of six or seven short, flat tarsal bones arranged in three rows. In the upper row are the talus and the calcaneus; in the middle row is the central tarsus and below that the fused first and second tarsal and the third tarsal. The fourth tarsal occupies both the middle and lower row. A long bony process, the tuber calcis of the calcaneus, gives rise to the point of hock and guides the Achilles tendon of the gastrocnemius muscle over the hock, allowing tremendous leverage.

## The lower limb

Below the hock the arrangement is the same as in the forelimb.

## Diseases of the bone

Bones are deeply seated within other tissues and are not richly supplied with blood, which means that bone disease is often overlooked. Diseases of bone fall into five main categories:

- periostitis
- ostitis
- disorders of the growth plate (epiphysitis)
- infection
- fracture.

## Periostitis

Periostitis is inflammation of the surface of the bone and the periosteum. It is usually caused by sprain, blow or infection and the signs are pain, heat and swelling over the affected area. The periosteum becomes inflamed and the resulting haemorrhage lifts it away from the bone and this stimulates the osteoblasts to make new bone. A tender bony swelling then develops, often accompanied by inflammation of the surrounding soft tissue. As the inflammation subsides the bony lump remodels, becoming smaller and painless. Examples of conditions caused by periostitis are splints, ringbone and sore shins.

### Sore shins (Fig. 1.14)

Sore or bucked shins often occur in two-and three-year-old races in training. The immature bone is subjected to stress which causes microfractures and haemorrhage under the periosteum at the front of the cannon bone. The front of the cannon-bone has a convex outline and the horse may become lame. With correct treatment the horse will recover but the cannon-bone may retain a convex outline.

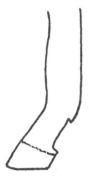

**Fig. 1.14**   Sore shins. The front of the cannon bone has a convex outline.

### Splints (Fig. 1.15)

The splint bones are attached to the cannon-bone by the interosseus ligament. In young horses this ligament is susceptible to strains and tears which result in bleeding and inflammation of the periosteum. New bone is produced which is seen as a bony enlargement or splint usually on the inside of the forelimb. Developing splints often cause lameness but as the splint settles down the swelling becomes smaller and harder and the horse returns to soundness.

## Ostitis

Ostitis involves inflammation of the bone itself as, for example, in pedal ostitis.

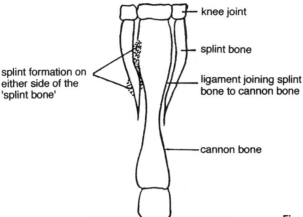

knee joint

splint bone

splint formation on either side of the 'splint bone'

ligament joining splint bone to cannon bone

cannon bone

**Fig. 1.15**  Splint formation.

### Epiphysitis

Epiphysitis occurs when the growth plate becomes inflamed and is termed a developmental orthopaedic disease.

### Infection

Infection of bone can be very serious and may require surgical intervention.

### Fractures

Fractures can be classified according to the age of the animal and the type and site of the break. Fractures of small bones may not be serious while breaking a large weight-bearing bone may result in the horse having to be destroyed.

## Joints

Joints in the skeleton arise where bones meet, giving the skeleton flexibility and allowing movement. Joints are the result of a complex process of development where several different tissues of the body interact. However, the basic structure of all joints is similar (Fig. 1.16). The joint capsule is composed of two layers:

- an outer fibrous layer which is attached to the periosteum of the bone;
- an inner synovial membrane which secretes joint oil or synovial fluid which supplies nutrition to the articular cartilage. The fluid also acts as a lubricant to the joint. The synovial membrane of a joint occasionally produces abnormal amounts of synovial fluid in response to low-grade trauma, resulting in conditions such as bog spavin and articular windgalls;
- joint or articular cartilage covering the ends of the bone to give protection. This cartilage does not have a blood or nerve supply, thus damage to the cartilage does not result in pain. Any pain experienced by the horse is caused by inflammation of the synovial membrane and the joint capsule. Articular cartilage has limited ability to repair itself, thus damage to the cartilage is not completely repaired.

The joint capsule and its ligaments provide the joint with stability. Both are attached to the periosteum, the fine membrane covering the bone, and stretching of the

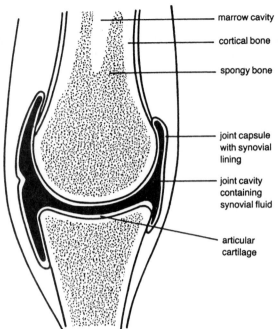

marrow cavity

cortical bone

spongy bone

joint capsule
with synovial
lining

joint cavity
containing
synovial fluid

articular
cartilage

**Fig. 1.16**   Structure of a joint.

ligaments can result in tearing of the periosteum leading to pain and new bone formation.

The joints of the limbs below the knee and hock are essentially hinge joints which allow movement in only one direction. The capsular ligaments which support the joint are very strong strap-like ligaments which have very little stretch. A ligament which is forced to be stretched by, for example, by holding a joint open beyond normal limits, will become sprained, showing inflammation, pain and swelling.

## Joint problems

Several bony and joint ailments result from the development of a faulty cartilage structure, sometimes seen in rapidly growing young stock, while others result from wear and tear, especially in competition horses. The most serious problems in the older horse involve changes to the articular cartilage.

### Osteochondrosis (OCD)

Osteochondrosis (OCD) is abnormal development of cartilage and bone, found most commonly in young, rapidly growing horses. There may be a genetic predisposition to the disease in foals bred to grow quickly and so the high planes of nutrition often fed to these foals may increase the risk of the condition occurring. The disease is most often found in the stifle, hock and shoulder joints. As bone grows and develops cartilage is turned into bone, but if this conversion is delayed by a poor blood supply, then the cartilage on the joint surface will be abnormally thick, and the lower layers of cartilage may die. This means that the cartilage is only loosely attached to the underlying bone and may detach, causing inflammation and pain.

**Articular windgalls** (Fig. 1.17)

Articular windgalls are distensions of the fetlock joint capsule often found in horses in hard work or heavier types with upright forelimbs. They are seen as swellings on either side of the fetlock between the back of the cannon bone and the suspensory ligament. They rarely cause lameness.

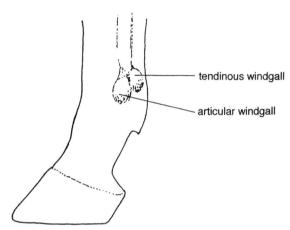

tendinous windgall

articular windgall

**Fig. 1.17**  Windgalls.

**Bog spavin** (Fig. 1.18)

Bog spavin is distension of the joint capsule of the hock, but the horse is not usually lame. It tends to occur in horses with poor hock formation or in young horses that have just gone into work. Often the fluid is reabsorbed over a period of time and no treatment is necessary.

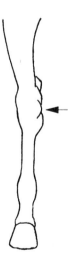

**Fig. 1.18**  Bog spavin.

**Joint sprain**

A sudden twist can result in tearing of the fibres of the joint capsule or the supporting ligaments. The severity will depend on the amount of damage, damage to the ligaments being serious as it leads to a loss of stability of the joint. The signs are heat and swelling with increased lameness when the joint is flexed. Treatment is likely to include cold therapy for the first 48 hours, support bandaging if possible, anti-inflammatory drugs and rest. Ultrasound, laser or magnetic field therapy may be useful.

## Degenerative joint disease

Degenerative or secondary joint disease is sometimes called osteoarthritis. It occurs when the articular cartilage becomes inflamed and begins to break down, leading to more inflammation until eventually there are bony changes. Examples include ringbone (pastern joint) and bone spavin (hock joint).

**Bone spavin** (Fig. 1.19)

Bone spavin is degenerative joint disease of the hock and a common cause of hind leg lameness. Poor conformation and hard work, especially involving jumping or sharp turns predispose to bone spavin. The signs include a gradual onset of lameness which is made worse by flexion; the horse may be reluctant to hold up the leg to be shod. The horse's action will change; it may drag the toe or show wear on the outside of the shoes. A swelling may be visible on the inner aspect of the hock. The treatment involves controlled exercise, relieving the pain and corrective shoeing but once bony changes have occurred the horse is unlikely to return to demanding work.

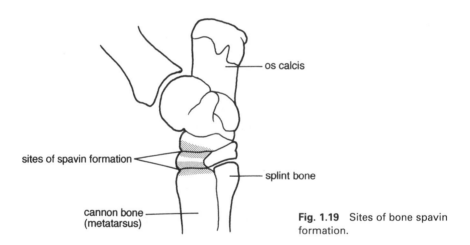

**Fig. 1.19**  Sites of bone spavin formation.

**Ringbone** (Fig. 1.20)

High ringbone is degenerative joint disease of the pastern joint and low ringbone is degenerate joint disease of the coffin joint. False ringbone, both high and low, occurs when new bone is formed on the long pastern, short pastern or pedal bone but does not involve the joint. Ringbone is seen as a hard swelling in the pastern region and the horse is lame especially on turns or circles and shows pain when the joint is flexed or twisted. As with bone spavin the prognosis for articular ringbone is guarded. Horses with non-articular or false ringbone often become sound once the inflammation has settled.

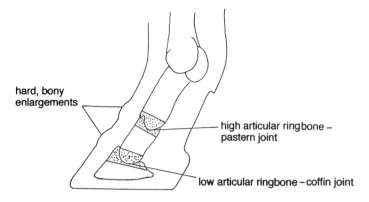

hard, bony
enlargements

high articular ringbone –
pastern joint

low articular ringbone – coffin joint

**Fig. 1.20**  Sites of articular ringbone. Non-articular ringbone does not affect the joint surface.

# Developmental orthopaedic disease (DOD)

The amount and composition of the feed in a young, growing horse's diet is vital in determining correct growth and development; the horse must grow so that athletic ability is not affected. Common growth-related disorders include epiphysitis and contracted tendons. The wobbler syndrome is also seen in young rapidly growing horses, although it can also affect older horses, and the exact cause is not known. Wobbler syndrome is covered in Chapter 6 under disorders of the nervous system.

## Epiphysitis

This refers to pain associated with abnormal activity in a growth plate, usually the lower growth plate of the radius, just above the knee or in the fetlock area, at the end of the cannon bone. It occurs in young, rapidly growing horses, most commonly yearlings but foals can be affected. There is usually swelling and heat just above the knee, the horse may or may not be lame but there is often pain if pressure is applied to the area. Where the condition is slight it may resolve itself but if severe the advice of a veterinary surgeon should be sought. The diet may be restricted to good quality hay and a micronutrient supplement with the youngster confined to the stable until the swellings go down. Foals may have their milk intake limited and be drenched with a nutrient-rich supplement. This restriction in diet will slow the growth rate so that the joints can 'catch up' and mature without excess strain. Once the bumps have subsided there should be light exercise daily and a gradual increase in diet back to normal. Epiphysitis can develop in less than a week and immediate treatment is important to aid successful recovery. Prevention is even better and energy and protein intake must be controlled and a correct mineral and trace element balance maintained.

## Contracted tendons (flexor tendon deformities)

Contracted tendons can be present at birth (congenital) or develop after birth (acquired). Rapidly growing foals between six weeks and six months are most commonly affected by acquired flexor tendon deformities, the condition appearing in one or both front limbs. The foal may stand high on its toes at birth, in which case it should be exercised regularly and allowed to grow slowly, or it may be seen to 'go up on its toes' and the limb becomes more upright and the foot becomes boxy. As soon as the condition is spotted, and it may occur very suddenly, the foal's growth rate must be slowed by cutting out any supplementary feed and restricting the mare's feed for three or four weeks. If this is carefully monitored and the micronutrient content of the diet maintained, there should not be an effect on the foal's mature size. The feet must be trimmed to lower the heels as much as possible and it may be necessary to have the foal shod until the condition resolves.

# Chapter 2
# Muscles

## The cell – building block of life

A highly complex animal like the horse is composed of billions of cells aggregated into tissues. These tissues in turn are formed into groups which work together and are called organs. Organs in turn are aggregated to form systems and the various systems are integrated to form the horse's body. The body is like a tower block housing a complex organisation and in order to function efficiently it requires a great deal of cooperation, specialisation and mutual interdependence.

All living things are made up of microscopic building blocks or cells (Fig. 2.1). In the horse the total functioning of the body involves the interaction of an estimated 400 trillion cells – the functional units of life. Internally the cell is divided into compartments called cell organelles. Organelles are well defined and clearly identifiable structures within the cell which have a specific structure and function. The interaction of these organelles within the cell contributes to what we call life. Life is an *organic* means of converting one form of energy to another, in the process a number of acts are

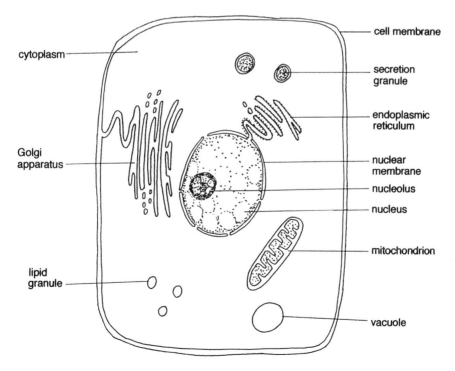

**Fig. 2.1** A typical mammalian cell.

performed which are called the vital phenomena, or the attributes of life. All life must fulfil four vital phenomena:

- growth
- reproduction
- irritability – the ability to receive and respond to external stimuli
- metabolism – the sum total of the chemical and physical changes constantly taking place in living matter.

As life forms become more complex other criteria such as conductivity become important. Others include the transmission of stimuli to other cells and organisation, the grouping of cells into tissues, the building of organs and their integration into a coherent whole.

## The cell membrane

The cell membrane forms the outermost limits of the cell and separates it from other cells. It encloses the cytoplasm which is a mass suspending the cell organelles. The cell membrane is made up of protein, lipid and water. Specific substances can cross the cell membrane and it is described as semipermeable. Water, oxygen and urea, for example, can cross with minimal trouble.

## The nucleus

The largest cell organelle is the nucleus, lying centrally and surrounded by cytoplasm. The nucleus is the 'brain' of the cell; it contains the genetic material or genes which are responsible for the transmission of hereditary characteristics from cell to cell and from parent to offspring. Genes are made up of giant molecules of DNA (deoxyribonucleic acid). The nucleus is contained by the nuclear membrane.

## The endoplasmic reticulum

Together with the ribosomes the endoplasmic reticulum is involved with the synthesis of protein within the cell. The type of protein produced is dictated by the nucleus and the types and amounts of protein manufactured will depend on the cell's function within the body. For example a cell in the skin will differ in composition to a cell in the kidney.

## The Golgi apparatus

The Golgi apparatus consists of stacks of plate-like tubules where proteins are adapted and altered for different functions. It is also involved in the secretion of protein from the cell, for example, the release of digestive enzymes into the gut.

## The mitochondria

These cylindrical organelles are responsible for the production of energy within the cell and they are known as the powerhouses of the cell. The number of mitochondria present indicates the activity of the cell. Muscle cells, for example, contain large numbers of mitochondria.

## Lysosomes

Although similar in shape to mitochondria their function is quite different. They are the digestive apparatus of the cell and break down larger molecules by enzyme action, reducing their size and composition to units small enough for the mitochondria to use. The enzymes in the lysosome can dissolve the cell if the protective membrane around the lysosomes is broken.

## Centrosomes

Also known as centrioles, the centrosomes are clearly visible during cell division when they become the centre of the spindle apparatus that separates the chromosomes of the resulting cells.

## Cell function

The individual cells of the horse's body act, interact and react with each other, they are not independent. In order to function normally there must be a continuous exchange of information which is normally chemically or electrochemically controlled. These chemical compounds may be hormones or enzymes found in the fluid surrounding the cells (interstitial fluid) or directly transferred between adjacent cells.

The transfer or transport of substances takes place via filtration, diffusion, osmosis, Donnan equilibrium and dialysis. Thus:

- *Filtration* is the passage of a liquid through a membrane due to a difference in hydrostatic pressure.
- *Diffusion* is the homogeneous mixing of two or more liquids due to the natural movement of molecules (Brownian movement).
- *Osmosis* is the passage of a solvent through a membrane from an area of low to an area of high concentration.
- *Donnan equilibrium* involves the passage of ions through a semipermeable membrane to achieve ionic balance on both sides.
- *Dialysis* is the passage of small molecules through a semipermeable membrane to achieve a molecular balance on each side.

Each of these reactions is designed to achieve harmony between the cell and its environment, in other words the cell is at ease. A cell which is not in harmony is 'diseased'.

Order and organisation are of great importance in ensuring harmony yet living things are also subject to the biological clock or temporal rhythms. There is a system of cycles that orders the lives of most living things. Seasons of the year affect the horse's sexual activity, the length of his coat and a host of other functions. Understanding and utilising biological rhythms is of prime importance in managing domestic animals in the unnatural and stressful environment in which we keep them.

Specialised cells are grouped together to form several types of tissue including:

- muscle tissue
- nervous tissue
- connective tissue
- epithelial tissue.

## Muscle tissue

The skeleton is incapable of movement on its own; all movements from a simple flick of the tail, to the most difficult dressage manoeuvre, are brought about by a complicated system of skeletal muscles. Depending on how much subcutaneous fat a horse has, it is often possible to picture many of these muscles and to feel the faint grooves that represent the divisions between them. All horses, regardless of breed, fitness and age, have the same arrangement of skeletal muscles, but some muscles may be better developed in particular horses due to their specialist training. There are, however, three types of muscle found in the body, each of which has its own characteristics and functions:

- cardiac muscle
- smooth muscle, and
- skeletal muscle.

### Cardiac muscle (Fig. 2.2)

Cardiac muscle is highly specialised and is found only in the heart. Under the microscope it appears striped and has branching fibres that interconnect and allow the heart to act as a unit. Cardiac muscle contractions are rapid and powerful and the fibres do not tire. Cardiac muscle:

- is only found in the heart;
- is striped with branching fibres;
- enables the heart to work as a unit;
- has rapid powerful contractions and does not tire;
- is not under conscious control.

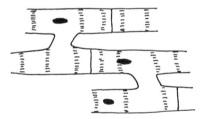

**Fig. 2.2** Cardiac muscle – banded, with central nucleus and branching fibres.

### Smooth muscle (Fig. 2.3)

Under the microscope smooth muscle does not appear striped and the cells are spindle-shaped with a central nucleus. Smooth muscle is not under conscious control and has a slower contraction time than skeletal muscle. The stimuli for contraction vary and include both nervous stimuli and chemical stimuli such as hormones. Smooth muscle is spread throughout the body organs, especially those of the gut. Smooth muscle can sustain rhythmic contractions for quite long periods which allows for movement such as the peristaltic waves of the gut which propel the digesta along its length. Smooth muscle:

- is non-striated;
- consists of spindle-shaped cells with a central nucleus;
- is not under conscious control;
- lines body cavities and blood vessels.

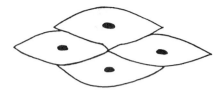

**Fig. 2.3**  Smooth muscle – spindle-shaped cells with central nucleus.

## Skeletal muscle (Fig. 2.4)

As horsemen we are most interested in skeletal muscle as we can see these muscles under the skin and can influence them through work. Under the microscope skeletal muscle, also known as striated or voluntary muscle, appears striped and it is under conscious control. Skeletal muscle:

- is striated;
- is under conscious control.

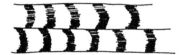

**Fig. 2.4**  Skeletal muscle – characteristic banding with the nucleus situated on the periphery of the muscle bundles.

## Muscle contraction

When muscles contract they do so by shortening their length; when they relax there is an increase in length. Total relaxation, however, never occurs, a slight contraction in one muscle being counter-balanced by slight contraction in another, leading to tension known as muscle tone. Muscle tone means that muscles are always ready for action – important in an animal such as the horse, whose main means of survival is through flight.

Each muscle is made up of many millions of specialised elongated cells called muscle fibres. Each muscle fibre itself is composed of thread-like myofibrils, which are the contractile elements of the muscle. The muscle fibres lie parallel to each other, bound together by connective tissue. The fibres combine to make up a muscle bundle and the bundles are gathered together to make up the muscle (Fig. 2.5). There is a nerve supply to each fibre to stimulate contraction.

Each myofibril is composed of sarcomeres which are crossed by regular bands which give rise to the striations seen under the microscope. The lighter coloured areas are the 'I' bands which alternate with darker 'A' bands. The bands are made up of proteins called actin (A band) and myosin (I band). Electrical impulses from the nerves supplying the muscle cause the thin filaments of actin to slide over the thick filaments of myosin to shorten the whole muscle (Fig. 2.6). Thus muscle contraction is brought about by the myofibrils sliding over one another so that the muscle shortens. This contraction requires energy in the form of adenosine triphosphate (ATP). The energy supply is maintained by the mitochondria, the 'powerhouses' of the cell, and fuel for these powerhouses is obtained from the breakdown of glucose. Muscle cells contain stores of glucose in the form of glycogen and the cells also contain a red pigment called myoglobin which, like haemoglobin in the blood, acts as an oxygen store. Energy can also be obtained from the breakdown of free fatty acids which are present in the blood or stored in the muscle.

It is essential for muscles to have a good blood supply to supply the oxygen and the

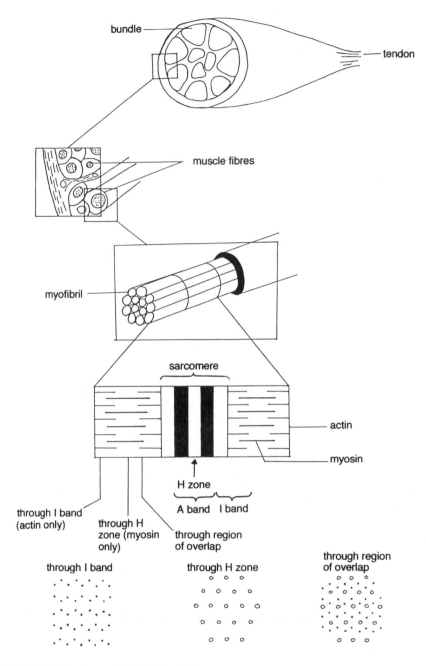

**Fig. 2.5** Structure of skeletal muscle.

other nutrients necessary for producing the energy needed for contraction, and to take away carbon dioxide and other waste products. During strenuous activity the blood supply to the muscle can be increased sixty-fold. Much of this blood is diverted from the gut and consequently digestive processes are minimal during exercise. The huge increase in blood supply indicates how important it is that the muscles receive large supplies of nutrients.

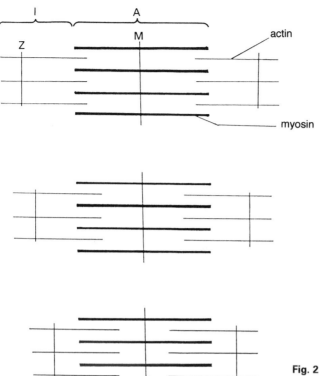

**Fig. 2.6** Contraction of a sarcomere by actin filaments sliding over myosin filaments.

## Muscle anatomy

The skeletal muscles enable the horse to adjust to the surrounding environment and make necessary movements such as grazing and running. They are attached to, and hence move, various parts of the skeleton and body. There are approximately 700 separate skeletal muscles in the horse's body, making up about one-third of its total weight (Figs. 2.7 and 2.8).

Muscles create movement by acting across joints. There are two sets of muscles, flexors (Fig. 2.9) which are placed behind the bone and pull it backwards, i.e. bending the joint, while extensors are placed in front of the bone and pull it forwards, i.e. straightening out the joint from its bent position. Remember that muscles not only produce movement: they also control and limit normal movement and prevent undesirable movements.

Each end of the muscle tapers from a larger muscle belly into a tendon – fibrous tissue which is continuous with the connective tissue of the muscle at one end and blends with the thin membrane covering the bone (periosteum) at the other. When a muscle contracts the fibres within it shorten and exert, via the tendon, a pull on the skeleton. Muscles are often large and bulky so tendons help concentrate their pull onto a small area of the bone. The horse has no muscle below the knee and hock; in order to move the hoof the muscles have to act from a distance and their power is transmitted by cord-like tendons which allow the limbs to remain streamlined and lightweight. The movement of the knee (carpal joint), fetlock and pastern joints are produced by the muscles of the forearm. Muscles which move the limb away from the

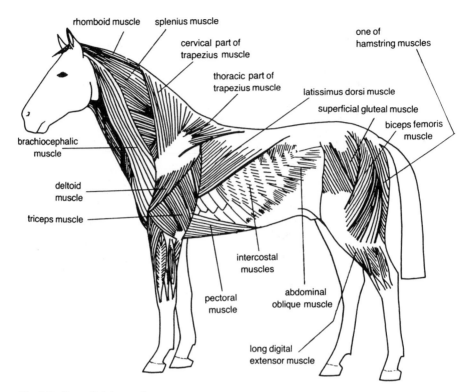

**Fig. 2.7**  Superficial muscles.

body are called abductors while those that carry the limb towards the body are adductors.

Muscle bellies vary in size and shape; some are large, flat sheets such as the latissimus dorsi muscle, others are long and strap-like, for example the brachiocephalic muscle. In both of these cases the fibres that make up the muscle belly run parallel to the long axis of the muscle. In other muscles, for example the common digital extensor muscle of the forearm, the individual fibres run obliquely to the long axis, with the muscle belly attached to either side of the tendon. These are called pennate muscles because they resemble a feather with the barbs radiating out from the quill. The length of the muscle fibres within the muscle belly determine the range of movement possible, while the power of contraction is due to the number of fibres present. Thus the long thin muscles allow substantial extension and retraction but cannot exert much force. The shorter pennate muscles do not allow as great a range of movement but because there are a large number of fibres these muscles have greater strength.

In order for muscles to produce movement they must be attached at both their ends. These ends are sometimes classified as the 'origin' and the 'insertion', the origin being the least movable of the two ends so that when the muscle contracts the insertion end is brought closer to the origin. However, in the brachiocephalic muscle either end can be the origin or the insertion; if the forearm is kept still and the head dipped, the insertion is at the back of the head and the origin at the base of the neck. If the head is kept still and the forearm moved then the attachment at the head becomes the origin and that at the forearm becomes the insertion.

Muscles are always arranged in opposing groups which perform opposite actions;

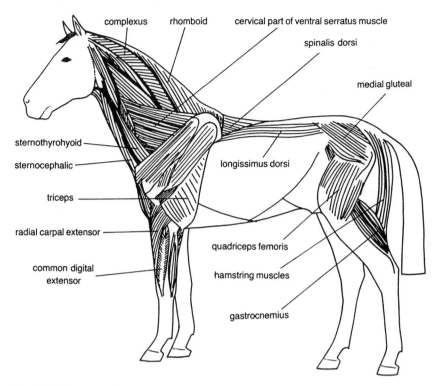

**Fig. 2.8** Deep muscle.

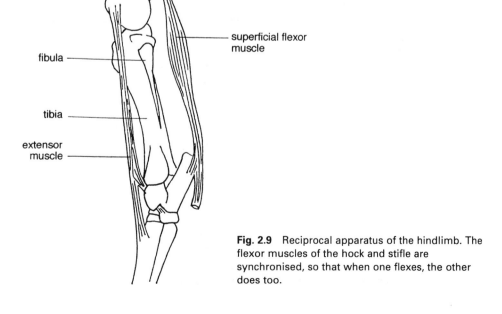

**Fig. 2.9** Reciprocal apparatus of the hindlimb. The flexor muscles of the hock and stifle are synchronised, so that when one flexes, the other does too.

this results in smooth and even movements. Muscles use energy to contract but do not have a way of stretching themselves again, instead the contraction of the opposing muscle is used to relax the tensed muscle. Thus as one group contracts the other relaxes to a corresponding degree; if the splenius at the top of the neck contracts, the head is lifted but the sternocephalic on the underside of the neck acts in opposition so that the degree of head-lifting is controlled.

The name may tells us what the main action of the muscle is; for example, the digital extensor extends the toe. Some muscles are named after their places of attachment; the brachiocephalic, for example, extends from the arm (brachium) to the head (cephalic).

## Muscles of the neck (Table 2.1)

### The brachiocephalic muscle

Behind the lower jaw or mandible lies the parotid gland, the largest of the salivary glands. Below and behind the ear the parotid gland meets the brachiocephalic muscle. The brachiocephalic muscle is a long, flattened muscle arising from the mastoid process of the temporal bone behind the ear, the wing of the atlas and the transverse processes of the second, third and fourth cervical vertebrae. The muscle runs down the length of the neck and inserts onto the humerus, forming the upper boundary of the jugular groove. When the muscle contracts it pulls the forearm forwards and the position of the horse's head will affect its efficiency. Horses move more freely in front when the head and neck are extended, unlike the position demanded of the dressage horse. It is a powerful muscle with a two-way action; when the head is extended and the neck held firmly by its own muscles, contraction of the brachiocephalic carries the arm and knee forward. When the horse is standing still contraction helps turn the head.

- Origin – wing of atlas.
- Insertion – humerus.
- Acts on the cervical vertebrae, extends the shoulder joint and produces sideways movement of the head and neck.

### The sternocephalic muscle

The sternocephalic muscle or sternomandibularis, is a long, narrow muscle which extends from the sternum to the jaw, forming the lower boundary of the jugular groove. Underneath the neck the trachea can be felt through the thin sternothyohyoid muscles. The oesophagus lies on the left side along the upper surface of the trachea and can be seen dilating when the horse swallows food or water.

- Origin – sternum.
- Insertion – back of jaw.
- Flexes the head and neck forward and down.

### The splenius muscle

- Origin – thoracic vertebrae.
- Insertion – wing of atlas and cervical vertebrae.
- Flexes the cervical vertebrae to lift the head and to turn the head and neck from side to side.

## Muscles of the shoulder (Table 2.2)

In the absence of a bony attachment, the muscles of the shoulder help to tie the limb to the body. Bearing in mind that two-thirds of the horse's body weight is taken on the forehand, these muscles act as weight supporters and shock absorbers.

### The trapezius muscle

The trapezius is a flattened triangular sheet of superficial muscle, the base of which arises in the area of the neck, withers and thorax from the funicular part of the ligamentum nuchae and the supraspinous ligament back to the tenth thoracic vertebra. The point of the muscle inserts into the spine of the scapula.

Trapezius muscle – cervical part

- Origin – cervical vertebrae.
- Insertion – scapular.
- Draws the scapula up and back to lift the shoulder

Trapezius muscle – thoracic part

- Origin – thoracic vertebrae.
- Insertion – scapula.
- Draws the scapula up and back to lift the shoulder.

### The rhomboideus

Underneath the trapezius is the rhomboideus which ties the scapula into the sides of the spinous processes of the thoracic vertebrae and the ligamentum nuchae. Like the trapezius it has cervical and thoracic parts.

- Origin – occiput.
- Insertion – top of scapula.
- Lifts the shoulder up and forward.

### The deltoideus

The deltoideus arises from the scapular spine; it can be felt on the outside of the shoulder joint as it runs down to meet the brachiocephalic muscle before inserting on the humerus.

- Origin – scapula.
- Insertion – humerus.
- Flexes the shoulder joint to abduct the forelimb.

### The triceps

The triceps is made up of three muscles running from the scapula to the point of the elbow. They make up a rounded muscle mass lying alongside the ribs just above the elbow joint – it is the bottom of the triceps that is generally used as a guide when clipping the front legs in a hunter clip. The long head of the triceps originates on the scapula and flexes the shoulder as well as extending the elbow joint. The lateral and medial heads are shorter and originate on the humerus and extend the elbow joint.

- Origin – scapula/humerus.
- Insertion – olecranon process (point of elbow).
- Extends the elbow joint.

**Table 2.1**  Muscles of the neck

| | Trapezius | Splenius | Sternocephalic |
|---|---|---|---|
| Location | | | |
| Body Joint action | Draws scapula upwards and backwards<br>Lifts shoulder | Lateral flexor of cervical vertebrae<br>Elevates head and turns head and neck to one side | Flexor of cervical vertebrae and inclines to one side<br>Flexes head and neck forwards and downwards |
| Origin | Dorsal midline and supraspinous ligament above 3rd cervical to 10th thoracic vertebrae | Spines of 4th to 6th thoracic vertebrae | Manubrium of the sternum and cariniform cartilage |
| Insertion | Cervical part inserts along whole scapular spine, thoracic part only along proximal part of the spine | Nuchal crest, transverse vertebral processes of 3rd to 5th cervical mastoid process and wing atlas | Mandible to caudal border of ramus |
| Nerve supply | Spinal accessory nerve, dorsal branch | Last six cervical nerves, dorsal branches | Spinal accessory nerve, 11th cranial nerve, ventral branch |
| Blood supply | Dorsal artery, deep cervical artery | Deep cervical artery, dorsal artery | Carotid artery |
| Development problems | Underdeveloped: dip in neck, little lifting of shoulder or forehand, lack of coordination and forward movement | Stiff neck in lateral flexion; tight neck | Overdeveloped: horse takes a pull; no control of athletic performance |

| | Rhomboideus | Brachiocephalicus | Multifidus cervicus | Longissimus capitis |
|---|---|---|---|---|
| | | | | |
| Joint action | Draws scapula upwards and forwards | Cervical vertebrae; flexor laterally extends shoulder joint | Rotates head to opposite side of flexion | Rotate atlas |
| Body action | Elevates shoulder | Sidewards movement of head and neck, when acts singly (see 'forearm') | Extends neck and flexes to side of contraction | Extend head and neck, flex head and neck laterally if acting singly |
| Origin | Occiput — dorsal midline of neck thoracic spine 2–7 | Wing of atlas and mastoid process, temporal bone, nuchal crest | Last five cervical vertebrae articular processes | Transverse processes of 1st two thoracic vertebrae |
| Insertion | Scapular cartilage — medial surface on dorsal border | Humerus — deltoid tuberosity and fascia shoulder and arm | Cervical vertebra — spinous and articular processes | Mastoid process wing of atlas, tendon in common with splenius and brachiocephalicus |
| Nerve supply | 6th and 7th cervical nerves, ventral branches | Spinal accessory nerve, cervical nerve, axillary nerve | Last six cervical nerves, dorsal branches | Last six cervical nerves, dorsal branches |
| Blood supply | Dorsal artery, deep cervical artery | Inferior cervical artery, carotid artery, vertebral artery | Vertebral artery | Vertebral artery and deep cervical artery |
| Development problems | Loss of activity in shoulders/forehand. Affects coordination; stiff/tight muscles cannot stretch | Gait not level in front: worse on turns and circles; not going forwards, choppy strides | Resistance in neck action, feels tight, poor contact with bit | Head unlevel; neck tight and stiff. One side difficult to flex and does not take contact. Head shaking, unsteady. Cannot extend head |

**Table 2.2**   Muscles of the shoulder

| | Brachiocephalicus | Supraspinatus | Infraspinatus | Subscapularis |
|---|---|---|---|---|
| Location | | | | |
| Joint action | Extensor | Extensor and support — acts as lateral ligament | Supports and stabilises acts as lateral ligament | Support; adducts humerus |
| Body action | Protracts fore limb, raises shoulder and pulls it forward | Advances the fore limb | Abducts forearm and rotates outwards | Adductor of fore limb; prevents limb moving outwards |
| Origin | Wing of atlas and mastoid process, nuchal crest | Scapula — cartilage and spine; supraspinous fossa | Scapula — infraspinous fossa and cartilage | Subscapular fossa, medial side |
| Insertion | Humerus — above deltoid tuberosity and distal crest, elongated line attachment | Humerus — lateral tuberosity | Humerus — caudal part of lateral tuberosity | Humerus — medial tuberosity |
| Nerve supply | Spinal accessory nerve and dorsal and ventral branches; axillary nerve, cervical nerve | Suprascapular nerve | Subscapular nerve | Subscapular nerve |
| Blood supply | Inferior cervical artery, carotid artery, vertebral artery | Suprascapular artery | Circumflex scapular artery | Subscapular artery |
| Development problems | Cause shoulder tightness or joint instability | | | |

| | Superficial pectoral | Deep pectoral | Coracobrachialis | Deltoideus |
|---|---|---|---|---|
| Location | | | | |
| Joint action | Supporter | Pulls humerus back | Flexes shoulder joint; holds joint in apposition | Flexes shoulder joint |
| Body action | Adductors of fore limb | Retractor and adductor; helps raise thorax relative to the limb | Adducts arm; supports fore limb | Abducts fore limb |
| Origin | Sternum — xiphoid and costal cartilage | Sternum — xiphoid cartilage, cartilages ribs 1–4 | Scapula — cranial border of coracoid process | Scapula — lateral caudal edge |
| Insertion | Humerus — humeral crest and antebrachial fascia | Humerus — medial tuberosity | Humerus — Craniomedial part of shaft proximal end | Humerus — deltoid tuberosity |
| Nerve supply | Pectoral nerve | Pectoral nerve | Musculocutaneous nerve | Axillary nerve |
| Blood supply | Cranial circumflex humeral artery | Intercostal artery, internal and external thoracic, inferior cervical, anterior circumflex | Anterior circumflex artery | Subscapular artery |
| Development problems | Short stride and an inability to spread over a fence. Sore on girthing up | | | |

### The latissimus dorsi

The latissimus dorsi lies behind the shoulder covering the side of the chest and extending up onto the back. It has a broad origin at the midline in the thoracic and lumbar regions which inserts on the humerus.

- Origin – thoracic/lumbar vertebrae.
- Insertion – humerus.
- Flexes the shoulder joint and draws the scapula down and back, retracting the forelimb.

### The pectorals

The pectoral muscles pass down and out from the sternum to insert on the numerus to form a triangular sheet with the base on the sternum and the apex on the humerus. The superficial pectorals are easily seen on the front of the chest.

- Origin – sternum.
- Insertion – humerus.
- Supports and pulls the humerus back so that the forelimb is adducted.

## Muscles of the forearm

### Digital extensor muscles

The muscle mass at the front of the forearm originates on the humerus and radius and their role is to carry the limb and foot forward. The extensor carpi radialis acts on the knee and the common digital extensor acts on the knee and digit (foot).

- Origin – upper ends of radius and ulna.
- Insertion – via digital extensor tendons to long pastern, short pastern and pedal bones.

### Digital flexor muscles

The muscle mass at the back of the forearm originates on the humerus and point of the elbow. It includes the muscles that flex the knee, fetlock and foot. The tendons of the flexor muscles run down the lower limb to influence the bones of the limb and effect movement.

- Origin – upper ends of radius and ulna.
- Insertion – via superficial and deep digital flexor tendons to short pastern bone and pedal bone.

## Muscles of the trunk (Table 2.3)

The trunk consists of the back and loins, the chest and the barrel or abdomen.

### Abdominal muscles

The four layers of the abdominal muscles are strong, extensive muscles which form most of the abdominal wall. They support the digestive and reproductive organs. By compressing the abdomen they aid in defaecation, urination, expiration, coughing and parturition. They also arch the back and can flex the trunk laterally.

### Intercostal muscles

The intercostal muscles and other deeper muscles are responsible for the movements involved with breathing in and out. The external intercostals extend downward and backward from each rib to the next rib back. Their action increases the size of the thorax by rotating the ribs up and back. The internal intercostals lie beneath the external intercostal muscle and extend from each rib down and forward to the next rib in front. They rotate the ribs backwards, decreasing the size of the rib cage and thorax.

- Origin – thoracic vertebrae.
- Insertion – ribs.

### The longissimus dorsi

The longissimus dorsi is the largest and longest muscle in the body. Along with other muscles it forms the contours of the horse's back. These muscles lie above the spine, and between the processes of the vertebrae, extending longitudinally from the croup towards the withers.

- Origin – pelvis/sacrum.
- Insertion – thoracic vertebrae.
- This is the muscle on which the saddle, and hence the rider, sits. Its role is to transmit to the forehand the propulsion generated by the hind limbs.

## Muscles of the hind limb (Table 2.4)

The hindquarters extend out and back from the point of the croup and consist of a mass of muscle clothing the pelvis and femur and running down the thigh to the hock and lower leg.

### The gluteal muscles

The gluteal muscles make up the bulk of the muscle mass that gives the quarters their rounded appearance. The gluteals arise from the shaft of the ilium and insert onto the femur.

- Origin – pelvis.
- Insertion – femur.
- Strong hip extensors involved in rearing, kicking and galloping.

### The biceps femoris

The hind part of the quarters is made up of a muscle mass called the biceps femoris extending from the sacral and coccygeal vertebrae to attach to the femur and stifle joint.

- Origin – sacral vertebrae.
- Insertion – femur.
- Extends and abducts the hindlimb, in other words it is involved with propulsion, rearing, and kicking.

### The semitendinosus muscle

The semitendinosus muscle is a long muscle extending along the rear of the biceps femoris down the back of the thigh. The division between these two muscles is known as the poverty line and is clearly seen in thin or fit horses.

- Origin – pelvis.
- Insertion – tibia.
- Extends the hip and hock and flexes the stifle so that the limb is rotated inwards and provides propulsion. These muscles make up the hamstring group and are important in locomotion.

**Table 2.3**  Muscles of the trunk

| | Latissimus dorsi | Seratus ventralis |
|---|---|---|
| **Location** | | |
| **Joint action** | Draws scapula down and back | Cervical and thoracic part acts as 'sling' for trunk |
| **Body action** | Retracts fore limb | Lifts body in relation to the scapula; suspends trunk between scapulae |
| **Origin** | An aponeurosis continuous with the thoracolumbar fascia | Ribs — lateral surfaces of 1st–9th |
| **Insertion** | Humerus — teres tuberosity | Scapula — serrated face on medial surface |
| **Nerve supply** | Thoracodorsal nerve | Cervical nerves — 5th–8th |
| **Blood supply** | Subscapular artery | Dorsal artery, vertebral artery intercostal artery |
| **Development problems** | | Stiff in forehand; shows in turns and circles as stiffness. |

**Table 2.3** contd.

| | Latissimus dorsi | Levatores costarum | Longissimus costarum |
|---|---|---|---|
| Location | | | |
| Joint action | Draws humerus up and back; supports dorsal part of thorax flexes shoulder joint | Rotation and lateral flexion of spine | Extends spine; depresses and retracts ribs; expiration |
| Body action | Retracts fore limb and draws trunk forwards when limb fixed | Draws ribs forwards for inspiration | Lateral flexion of trunk |
| Origin | Thoracic spines, withers and an aponeurosis continuous with the thoracolumbar fascia over caudal thorax | Transverse processes of thoracic vertebrae | Lumbar transverse processes last 15 ribs — anterior lateral surfaces lumbodorsal fascia |
| Insertion | Humerus — teres tubercle | Lateral surfaces and anterior borders of upper ends of ribs | Posterior borders of ribs; transverse process of the last cervical vertebrae |
| Nerve supply | Thoracodorsal nerve | Intercostal nerve | Thoracic nerve |
| Blood supply | Subscapular artery, intercostal artery, lumbar artery | Intercostal artery | Intercostal artery |
| Development problems | | Cause sore, tight backs and a stiff wooden feel to the rider | |

**Table 2.4**  Muscles of the hind limb

| | Biceps femoris | Semitendinosus | Semimembranosus | Gluteus medius |
|---|---|---|---|---|
| **Location** | | | | |
| **Joint action** | Extends hip joint; flexes stifle joint; main belly flexes hock; anterior part extends stifle | Extends hip and hock and flexes stifle | Extends hip joint | Extends hip joint |
| **Body action** | Extends and abducts the hind limb and propulsion; rearing; kicking | Propulsion of trunk; rotates limb inwards; rearing | Adducts hind limb | Abducts limb strong hip extensor rearing, kicking, propulsion |
| **Origin** | Ischiatic spine, and tuber ischium and sacral vertebrae; sacroiliac ligaments | Tuber ischium — mid ventral area, and ilium — mid shaft | Tuber ischium — medial ventral border and sacrosciatic ligament | Ilium — gluteal surface and crest and aponeurosis of longissimus lumorum |
| **Insertion** | Femur — 3rd trochanter, patella and lateral ligament tibial crest, crural fascia to hock | Tibial crest and fascia part joins tarsal tendon of biceps femoris which attaches to tuber calcis | Femur — medial epicondyle; stifle — medial side | Femur — trochanter major |
| **Nerve supply** | Posterior gluteal nerve, sciatic nerve, and branches tibial and caudal, gluteal, peroneal nerves | Great sciatic nerve | Great sciatic nerve | Cranial and gluteal nerve |
| **Blood supply** | Gluteal artery and obturator branch; deep femoral artery; posterior femoral artery | Posterior gluteal artery; obturator artery; deep femoral artery; posterior femoral artery | Posterior gluteal artery; obturator artery; femoral artery | Gluteal, iliolumbar artery; lumbar artery; iliacofemoral artery |
| **Development problems** | Shortening of forward stride, resist lateral movements, discomfort in hind joints | | | |

**The digital extensor muscle**

Below the stifle the digital extensor and hock flexor muscles make up the gaskin or second thigh. Digital extensor muscle

- Origin – femur.
- Insertion – lower limb.
- One of the muscles of the second thigh that attaches to the tendons of the lower leg, transmitting movement to the toe.

**The gastrocnemius**

The gastrocnemius runs down the back of the limb ending in a powerful tendon. It is associated with the tendon of the deeper lying superficial flexor muscle and the combined tendon is palpable above the hock as the Achilles' tendon. The tendon of the gastrocnemius attaches to the hock while the superficial flexor tendon runs over the hock and down the back of the limb to the foot.

- Origin – femur.
- Insertion – hock.
- Attached to the Achilles tendon (one of the largest tendons in the body) and moves the hock.

# The importance of muscle in equine performance

## Muscle fibre types

There are several different types of fibre within each muscle. This is the same for horses and humans and has been studied using a technique called muscle biopsy, a safe and painless way of taking tiny samples of living muscle tissue for study under the microscope.

Initially muscle fibre types are identified by colour; red muscle is associated with long-term or endurance work (chickens, for example, have dark leg meat and they use their legs for standing on all day). This dark red colour reflects the high myoglobin content and consequently the muscle's ability to store and use large amounts of oxygen; it is known as high oxidative muscle. The breast meat of chickens, on the other hand, is white. This muscle is used for power, for example getting a chicken off the ground and flying. This muscle has a lesser ability to use oxygen and is known as low oxidative muscle.

More scientifically, muscle can be divided into two major groups depending on its contractile behaviour:

(1) Slow twitch muscle has a slower contraction time and a greater ability to use oxygen, which means that it can work steadily for long periods of time.
(2) Fast twitch muscle has fast, powerful contractions. Further work has shown that fast twitch fibres differ in their ability to use oxygen.
　(a) Fast twitch, high oxidative fibres can generate power but also have a good ability to use oxygen and can therefore continue working for long periods of time. This makes these fibres very important to horses that need to sustain speed over long distances.
　(b) Fast twitch, low oxidative fibres are designed to produce explosive power rapidly. They do not use large amounts of oxygen and tend to fatigue quickly. These fibres are used for galloping and jumping.

## Muscle fibre recruitment

Most muscles consist of a mixture of these three fibre types. During muscle contraction it is unlikely that all the muscles need to exert maximum strength; in other words, not all the fibres in one muscle are stimulated at once. There is an orderly selection of muscle fibres depending on the amount of exertion; for walking and standing only slow twitch fibres are used but as the speed increases fast twitch, high oxidative fibres are recruited and when the horse is accelerating, galloping and jumping the fast twitch, low oxidative fibres are brought into play. The fact that muscles contain a mixture of fibre types means that they have a wide range of responses and can respond to the varying demands that the horse makes.

## Distribution of muscle fibres

Studies of human athletes have shown that the best marathon runners have a very high proportion of slow twitch fibres while sprinters have more fast twitch fibres. This difference appears to be genetically determined, in other words, some people are born with a proportion of slow twitch to fast twitch fibres that makes them more likely to be better marathon runners than sprinters.

A similar trend can be seen in different breeds and types of horses; even an unfit Quarter horse, which is a sprinting specialist, has a greater proportion of fast twitch fibres than the Arab (Table 2.5).

**Table 2.5**   Slow twitch fibres in different breeds of horse

| Type of horse | % slow twitch fibres |
| --- | --- |
| Quarter-horse | 7 |
| Thoroughbred | 13 |
| Arab | 14 |
| Standardbred | 18 |
| Shetland | 21 |
| Pony | 23 |
| Donkey | 28 |
| Endurance horse | 28 |
| Heavy horse | 31 |

The physique of these two types of horses is also different; fast twitch fibres have a great diameter in order to generate power. In those horses better suited to endurance-type work the muscle fibres are thinner, allowing blood carrying oxygen and other nutrients to reach the fibres easily. Thus the Quarter horse has a bulky, muscular physique, much like the powerful human sprinter, while the long distance horse, the eventer and the 'chaser are rangy and lean.

## Fatigue

The aim of getting a horse fit is to be able to work it for longer before it gets tired, in other words to delay the onset of fatigue. A horse is said to be fatigued when it can no longer continue the exercise at that level – a horse cannot gallop for ever! If the horse is not allowed to slow down exhaustion will set in eventually, exhaustion being the complete inability to continue work.

There are four major factors which contribute to fatigue:

- glycogen depletion
- lactic acid build-up
- dehydration and heat stress
- lameness.

## Glycogen depletion

A horse involved in long, slow work will be using a majority of slow twitch, high oxygen-using fibres. Oxygen is brought to the muscle fast enough to supply the energy demands because the horse is not working hard and fast. The oxygen is used to 'burn up' glycogen to produce ATP, which is then used for muscle contraction.

Eventually all the glycogen stores in the muscles and the liver will be used up, there will be no energy source, the muscles will not be able to contract and the horse is tired and no longer able to work. Once all the glycogen is used up it takes between 46 and 72 hours to replace it all.

## Lactic acid build-up

As the speed increases so does the energy demand from the muscle and the blood is no longer able to supply oxygen quickly enough to satisfy these demands. At the same time the fast twitch, low oxidative fibres are recruited, and these use the energy produced from glycogen in the absence of oxygen, a process called anaerobic respiration. This results in the by-product of anaerobic respiration being produced in the muscles. At fast speeds there is so much lactic acid being produced that it builds up in the muscles. This acid condition stops the muscle functioning correctly and eventually the horse has to slow down. Once the horse has slowed down sufficiently to return to aerobic work the blood can carry away the excess lactic acid and the muscle will start to work properly again. The horse will feel more comfortable and the rider will notice that the horse has picked up and is ready to gallop again. This means that any successful training programme must aim to reduce the amount of lactic acid produced in the muscles.

# Chapter 3
# The Lower Leg

As the horse evolved into a fleet-footed herbivore, the proportions of the limbs changed so that the modern horse stands on the equivalent of the tip of the human finger (Fig. 3.1). To achieve greater speed the lower limb was kept as light as possible so that the horse has no muscle below the knee The pull of the muscles is transmitted to the bones of the lower leg and foot via long tendons which can be easily felt running down the back of the horse's leg. The length of these tendons plus the fact that they lie close to the skin mean that they are susceptible to damage.

It is important to be able to identify the structures of the lower limb in the healthy horse so that the first signs of over-use or lameness can be located and acted upon before permanent damage is done. The cannon and two splint bones can be easily felt under the skin. Each splint bone ends in an obvious small lump about three-quarters of the way down the cannon bone.

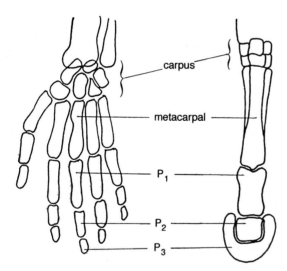

carpus

metacarpal

$P_1$

$P_2$

$P_3$

**Fig. 3.1** Comparison between the human hand and the equine limb.

## The tendons and ligaments of the lower leg (Fig. 3.2)

### Tendon structure

Tendons attach muscle to bone and are relatively inelastic as their job is to exert pull on the skeleton, initiated by muscle contraction. A tendon is not a separate entity, it is a strong extension of a muscle which attaches to a bone. The muscle is elastic but the tendon is almost rigid compared to muscle. The tendon and the muscle act together to allow movement, bear weight and to accommodate stretch.

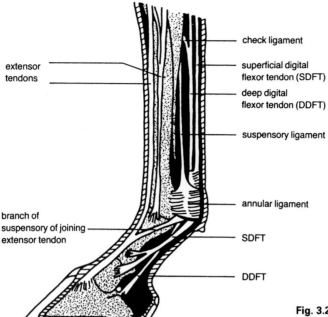

extensor tendons

check ligament

superficial digital flexor tendon (SDFT)

deep digital flexor tendon (DDFT)

suspensory ligament

annular ligament

branch of suspensory of joining extensor tendon

SDFT

DDFT

**Fig. 3.2** Ligaments and tendons of the lower limb.

## Tendon sheaths

Tendons run from the forearm muscles in grooves of the bone across the knee and fetlock. They are held in position because the grooves are converted into canals by connective tissue called annular ligaments. Annular ligaments encircle tendons at the top and bottom to keep the tendons in the proper track. As the tendons move in these canals they are subject to friction from all sides. To prevent damage the tendons are surrounded by tendon sheaths. These have an outer layer attached to the lining of the canal and an inner layer (epitenon) attached to the surface of the tendon (Fig. 3.3). Oil-like synovial fluid is secreted between the two layers to allow the surfaces to run over each other smoothly. The two layers form the mesotenon which carries blood vessels to the tendon.

Inside this the tendon consists of groups of fibres called fascicles, which run longitudinally, i.e. in the same direction as the forces acting on the tendon. These fibres consist of closely packed bundles of collagen fibres arranged parallel to one

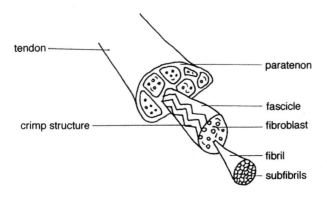

tendon

paratenon

fascicle

fibroblast

crimp structure

fibril

subfibrils

**Fig. 3.3** Tendon structure.

another and following helical spiral along the length of the tendon. The fibres also show 'crimp'; rather than being straight they bend in a regular zig-zag pattern. This gives the tendon a degree of elasticity, or rather an ability to lengthen. When the muscle contracts and puts pressure on the tendon, the crimp straightens before exerting its pull on the bone to which it is attached. Providing that the tendon is not overstretched it returns to the crimp formation when the load is removed. Tendons have high tensile strength but restricted elasticity. At 3% extension the crimp disappears and at around 8% extension fibres rupture.

Collagen is a type of protein which is produced by tendon fibroblasts, special cells arranged parallel to the fibril. All collagen is replaced every six months. There are several types of collagen which are found in different parts of the body. Normal tendon is composed of Type 1 collagen which is relatively elastic. However, if the tendon is damaged, the repair tissue is made of Type 3 collagen which is not as resilient, resulting in weakness so that the tendon is more susceptible to re-injury. In addition the new collagen bundles are laid down randomly, not in parallel, which further weakens the tendon. Controlled exercise has a significant role in re-aligning the new collagen.

## Extensor tendons

The common digital extensor tendon runs down the front of the cannon from the knee attaching to the pedal bone within the hoof. The lateral digital extensor tendon runs from the side of the knee, outside the common digital flexor tendon, to insert onto the long pastern bone. Both the superficial and deep digital flexor tendons begin above the knee, the superficial tendon is joined by a strong fibrous band, the radial or superior check ligament, which fuses with it at the back of the knee.

## Flexor tendons

The deep and superficial digital flexor tendons pass down through the carpal canal in a synovial sheath to the cannon region. At the lower end of the cannon the superficial flexor tendon flattens and widens to form a ring which surrounds the deep flexor tendon. The deep flexor tendon runs through this ring behind the fetlock, surrounded by a synovial sheath. Below the fetlock the superficial flexor tendon divides into two parts, attaching to either side of the long and short pastern bones. The deep flexor tendon runs down through this fork, within the digital synovial sheath, to attach to the bottom of the pedal bone at the semilunar crest, crossing the underneath of the navicular bone (distal sesamoid). The navicular bursa lies between the deep flexor tendon and the navicular bone.

## Ligaments and the suspensory apparatus

A ligament originates from, and is attached to, bone. Ligaments are even less elastic than tendons. Thus a ligament has no muscular attachment, it connects bone to bone.

### The check ligament

In the upper part of the cannon the deep flexor tendon lies underneath the superficial flexor tendon and is attached to the back of the knee by the fibrous carpal check ligament. The check ligament can be palpated just below the knee if the horse's foot is picked up so that the tendons are relaxed.

### The suspensory ligament

The suspensory ligament differs from other ligaments in that it is a modified muscle and contains some muscle tissue which gives it considerable elasticity compared to other ligaments. It lies between the deep flexor tendon and the cannon bone and is sometimes mistaken for the splint bone as it feels very rigid when the horse's leg is bearing weight. The suspensory ligament is a flat band originating from the back of the knee and passing down the back of the leg in a channel between the cannon bone and the two splint bones. At the level of the sesamoid bones it divides into two branches which pass forwards to join the extensor tendon on the front of the pastern. The rest of the suspensory ligament is attached to the sesamoid bones.

The suspensory ligament is part of the stay apparatus which is discussed in Chapter 17. Its job is to suspend the fetlock, support the leg and to prevent over-extension of the fetlock joint. Its support of the joint is helped by the superficial and deep flexor tendons and along with the proximal sesamoid bones it carries much of the horse's weight during movement.

## Blood supply to the lower leg (Fig. 3.4)

The median artery passes down behind the knees through the carpal canal with the deep digital flexor tendon and continues as the common artery on the inner side of the flexor tendons. It then passes between the back tendons and the suspensory ligament and divides above the fetlock into the lateral and medial digital flexor arteries passing across the fetlock to follow the borders of the deep digital flexor tendon into the foot.

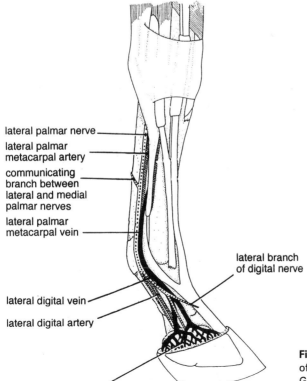

lateral palmar nerve

lateral palmar metacarpal artery

communicating branch between lateral and medial palmar nerves

lateral palmar metacarpal vein

lateral branch of digital nerve

lateral digital vein

lateral digital artery

coronary venous plexus

**Fig. 3.4** Blood vessels and nerves of the forelimb. (Adapted from Goody, P.C. (1983) *Horse Anatomy*, J.A. Allen.)

Within the foot the two digital arteries enter the underside of the pedal bone to form a terminal arch. Branches from this arch pass through the bone to nourish the sensitive structures within the hoof. Veins run alongside the arteries, draining from a coronary venous plexus which circles the upper part of the foot. On the outer side of the limb the lateral digital vein merges into the lateral palmar metacarpal vein while on the inner aspect the medial digital vein joins the common digital vein before merging with the cephalic vein which continues above the knee.

## The nerves of the lower leg

Nerves accompany the arteries; the lateral palmar nerve runs alongside the lateral palmar metacarpal artery on the outer aspect of the leg. On the inner aspect the medial palmar digital nerve runs parallel to the common digital artery. The two nerves are connected by a communicating branch which can be felt running diagonally across the superficial flexor tendon in thin-skinned horses. Both palmar nerves branch dorsally into the front of the pastern, the remainder of the nerves penetrating the foot and supplying the sensitive tissues within the hoof. The nerves can be 'blocked', i.e. injected with local anaesthetic, either below or above the fetlock during the location of the seat of lameness. Chronic lameness can be treated by severing the nerves to remove sensation from the area, a process called denerving.

## Tendon and ligament injury and healing

### Bursal enlargements

Bursae are sacs containing synovial fluid which run over bony areas to help tendons or muscles slide over the underlying bone. These can become inflamed and swollen.

### False bursae

Capped hock and elbow are enlargements of the point of hock or elbow known as false bursae due to repeated irritation or trauma causing fluid accumulation.

### Tendon sheaths

Tendon sheaths are long sacs containing synovial fluid which enclose all or part of a tendon and lubricate its movement. The digital flexor tendon sheath above the fetlock and between the suspensory and flexor tendons may become enlarged, a condition called tendinous windgalls. A thoroughpin is an enlargement of the deep flexor tendon above the hock. It is situated higher up and further back than a bog spavin and the swelling can be moved back and forwards.

### Tendon injury

The athletic horse is prone to lower limb tendon and ligament strain. Early recognition and prompt and correct treatment are essential if the horse is to regain full athletic potential.

### Causes

- Constriction by an overtight bandage may cause localised inflammation in and around the superficial flexor tendon, causing swelling and 'bowing' of the tendon.

However, the injury does not normally affect the fibrils and recovery should be good.
- A direct blow to the back of the leg results in localised injury and, usually, fibril damage. There is bruising and bleeding into the tendon and the resulting damage is healed by Type 3 collagen so that there is a potential for re-damage if the injury is not treated properly.
- Tendon strain results in partial or total rupture of the fibrils with extensive bleeding into the tendon and substantial inflammation. Even minor strains should be treated as serious injuries. The causes of tendon strain include:
  - poor conformation e.g. back at the knee;
  - poor or infrequent shoeing leading to long pasterns and low heels;
  - fatigue leading to lack of co-ordination when galloping and jumping;
  - sudden changes in the ground e.g. going from firm to soft ground at speed;– uneven ground;
  - re-occurring slight injury. Do not ignore the early signs.

## Signs

- Swelling, heat and pain which may be slight in early stages.
- The horse may not be lame, unless the injury is severe.

Even minor fluctuations in the amount of heat and swelling in the lower leg should not be ignored. Unless the tendons are given time to recover from these minor injuries the damage will accumulate and may result in severe tendon strain. The extent and position of the damage within the tendon can be assessed using ultrasound scanning. Scanning at regular intervals during recovery can also give a picture of the healing process.

## Treatment

The first priority is to relieve the swelling in order to:

- restore normal alignment of fibrils
- minimise inflammation
- reduce pain.

This can be done using a combination of cold treatment, such as icepacks at frequent intervals and anti-inflammatory drugs. In most cases the horse will be on box rest until the heat has gone from the leg and will wear support bandages on both the injured and sound leg. Generally speaking the quicker the swelling goes down the better the healing will be.

# Tendon repair

Fibroblasts migrate to damage area to make more collagen. However, the fibrils are laid down in a haphazard way and the resulting scar tissue tends to be weak. Controlled exercise will help encourage longitudinal arrangement of the fibrils and will also prevent adhesions from forming. In-hand walking is usually recommended once the horse is sound in walk and the heat has gone from the leg. These exercises can be gradually built up so that by eight weeks after the injury the horse is doing 60 minutes walking work under saddle and 30 minutes trotting by three to four months. After this the horse is ideally turned away until nine months after injury. It must always be remembered that the horse will be sound *before* full healing has occurred and that it takes a minimum of 15 months for maximum healing to take place after a serious injury.

Alternative treatments for tendon injury include, firing (a controversial treatment which is not encouraged by the veterinary profession), tendon splitting and carbon fibre implants.

## The hoof

The foot or digit of the horse is equivalent to the human middle finger, consisting of three bones known as:

- first, second and third phalanges, or
- proximal, middle and distal phalanges; or
- long pastern, short pastern and pedal bone.

These bones give rise to the fetlock, pastern and coffin joints. The joint between the cannon bone and the long pastern bone is the fetlock joint, between the long and short pastern bones is the pastern joint and between the short pastern bone and the pedal bone is the coffin joint.

The hoof surrounds the pedal bone and the navicular bone and part of the short pastern bone (Fig. 3.5).

The horse's hoof is a very specialised structure, designed to:

- resist wear
- support the horse's body weight, and
- absorb concussion.

The hoof is a continuation of modified skin, similar to horns and claws in other animals, and consists of two distinct parts:

- the external hoof which is the equivalent of the epidermis, and
- the internal or sensitive foot, which is equivalent to the corium.

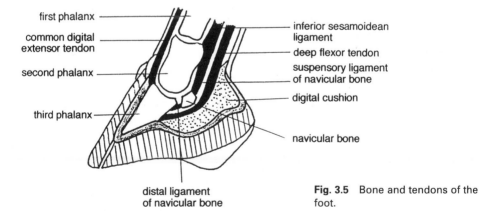

first phalanx

common digital extensor tendon

second phalanx

third phalanx

distal ligament of navicular bone

inferior sesamoidean ligament

deep flexor tendon

suspensory ligament of navicular bone

digital cushion

navicular bone

**Fig. 3.5**   Bone and tendons of the foot.

### The external hoof (Fig. 3.6)

The external hoof is insensitive and non-vascular, i.e. it does not have a blood supply. It consists of three parts:

- the wall
- the sole
- the frog.

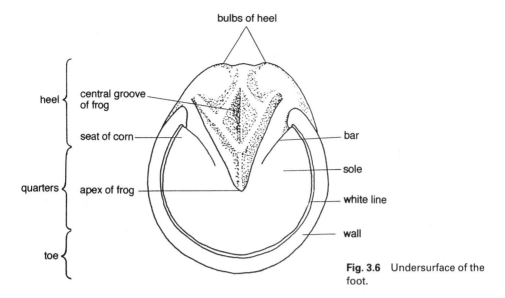

**Fig. 3.6** Undersurface of the foot.

## The wall

The wall is produced by and grows down from the coronary band and is the part that can be seen when the foot is on the ground. it consists of dense horn and is divided into the toe, quarters and heels. At the heels it is reflected back, inwards and forwards, to form the bars of the hoof. The bars

- give strength at the heels and allow the hoof to withstand the weight of the horse. It is difficult to balance a piece of paper on its edge but if each end of the paper is folded over, like the bars, it will stand quite easily;
- allow for expansion when the horse's weight lands on the hoof. Except at the walk, when the foot lands virtually level, the hoof is placed heel first, then the frog, and finally the toe. Each time this happens the frog is designed to take the weight, force the angle of the bars open and prevent the heels from caving in and contracting.

The bars must be allowed to grow. If they are pared away by the farrier the horse's heels will start to contract.

The area of sole between the walls and the bars is known as the seat of corn. In poorly shod horses, or ones with overgrown feet, the shoe will press on this area and give rise to bruised areas called corns.

Two sets of lines can be seen on the smooth glossy outer wall; vertical lines run in the direction of hoof growth and indicate the direction of the tubules which grow down from the papillae of the coronary band. Rings consisting of alternating ridges and depressions run parallel to the coronary band and indicate the growth rate of the hoof, in much the same as the rings within a tree trunk indicate its age. The rings will deviate if the growth rate of the hoof has been abnormal – for example, if the horse has had laminitis.

The colour of the hoof wall depends on the colour of the horse's skin at the coronet. White feet are said to be more brittle than black feet.

The wall is covered by a thin layer of epidermis called the periople which originates from a rim of soft grey horn at the coronary band, the perioplic cushion. This rim is thickest at the top of the hoof and at the heels forms a wide cap to blend with the frog. It is best seen when the hoof is wet. The periople is carried down the hoof by the growth of the wall, dries out and forms the cuticle which tends to flake off and does not extend much below half way down the hoof. It is argued that the periople controls the movement of moisture in and out of the foot and that when the horse is shod the periople should not be rasped away. As the periople extends only a short way down the hoof it is acceptable to rasp the toes but it is important not to rasp the upper hoof.

The internal surface of the wall carries the insensitive laminae which consist of 500–600 horny leaves each of which has 100–200 secondary laminae. These dovetail with the sensitive laminae of the sensitive foot to create a very strong bond between the two (Fig. 3.7). The junction between the insensitive and sensitive laminae is shown on the underside of the foot by the white line. This indicates the thickness of the wall and enables the farrier to assess where to fit the nails. The wall consists of about 25% water and is thicker at the toe than at the heel, enabling the farrier to nail higher up the wall at the toe than at the heel. It grows about one inch (2.5 cm) in three months, so that it takes the toe nine to twelve months to grow from coronary band to ground and the heel about six months. As the horn grows down from the coronary band it becomes keratinised and compressed and thus stronger and harder. The toe is harder than the heel, allowing the heel to expand as described. Some hoof preparations act as a mild blister to the coronet, increasing blood supply and thus hoof growth.

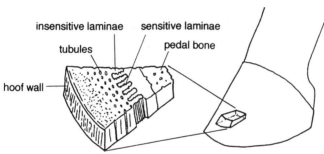

insensitive laminae    sensitive laminae

tubules    pedal bone

hoof wall

**Fig. 3.7**   Hoof structure.

## The sole

The sole is the ground surface of the hoof. It is crescent-shaped and concave so that it arches over the ground, protecting the sensitive structures within the foot. It contains more water (33%) than the wall and is thus less dense and resistant than the wall. It supports the weight of the body rather than bearing it. Soles are of variable thickness and a horse with relatively flat soles which can be compressed will be more prone to bruising and sore feet.

## The frog

The frog is a wedge of soft elastic horn containing about 45% moisture and situated between the bars and separated from them by the paracuneal groove. At the rear it becomes the bulbs of the heels while at the front the dorsal tip of the frog is called the apex. The frog has a central groove dividing the frog into two crura. The frog and the paracuneal grooves are the site of thrush, a foul-smelling condition caused by *Shaerophus necrophorus* and involving disintegration of the frog, which occurs when the horse stands in wet bedding without proper foot care. Thrush may eventually penetrate the sole affecting the sensitive laminae leading to lameness and contracted heels.

There is some controversy about the frog's true function and whether it should make contact with the ground. Its functions are to

- absorb concussion
- assist circulation
- aid grip.

In theory the frog should come below the level of the sole and come into contact with the ground when the horse moves. When the frog hits the ground it is compressed and expands, putting pressure on the digital cushion, which in turn squeezes the lateral cartilages and wall of the foot and the wall expands. If the horse is shod so that the frog does not come into contact with the ground this cushioning effect is lost and the frog shrinks and the heel contracts.

## The horn

The horn which makes up the external hoof consists of epithelial cells in the form of horny tubules, which have become impregnated with a protein called keratin, a process known as keratinisation. These tubules contain fluid obtained from the coronary corium and the surface of the hoof. This fluid is lost by evaporation from the surface; too much loss results in brittle feet, while too little makes the hoof soft. applying oil or grease to the surface of the hoof inhibits natural water evaporation from the hoof and is not recommended for healthy feet. Horn is dissolved by alkali, thus wet bedding containing ammonia from urine will damage the feet. Fortunately horn is a bad conductor of heat, allowing the farrier to hot shoe the horse.

## The internal foot

The corium or sensitive tissue of the foot is a specialised vascular continuation of the dermis of the skin and provides nutrition to the foot and attachment for the insensitive foot. There are five layers of corium:

- perioplic corium
- coronary corium
- laminar corium
- sole corium
- frog corium.

A very thin layer of epidermis covers each corium which gives rise to the growth of epidermal cells which are keratinised to form the horny components of the hoof.

- The perioplic corium is situated above the coronary corium and separated from it by a small groove, it broadens at the heel to become continuous with the frog corium. The perioplic corium supplies the periople with nutrients.
- The coronary corium is an enlarged band above the sensitive laminae which produces the wall much as skin produces hair and nourishes the wall of the hoof. The coronary corium is pigmented in dark hoof and bears papillae which produce the wall of the hoof.
- The laminar corium consists of the sensitive laminae which attach to the periosteum of the pedal bone and suspend this bone within the hoof by interlocking with the insensitive laminae. The primary laminae have lateral secondary laminae giving a total surface area of eight square feet which supports the weight of the horse.
- The sole corium or sensitive sole attaches the sole of the pedal bone to the horny sole and supplies nutrition to the sole.

- The epidermis of the frog corium or sensitive frog produces horny tubules which are flexible and only partly keratinised, hence the soft nature of the frog. It is attached to the digital cushion in the heel of the foot and nourishes the digital cushion.

## The digital or plantar cushion (Fig. 3.8)

The digital cushion is a wedge-shaped fibro-elastic pad situated in the back part of the foot, filling the heels and lying above the frog and below the deep flexor tendon. The bulbs of the cushion are soft and fatty while the rest is more fibrous. It is not well supplied with nerves and a pricked digital cushion may not give the horse any pain and a serious infection may develop. Its role is to help absorb concussion. The lateral cartilages lie on either side of the digital cushion.

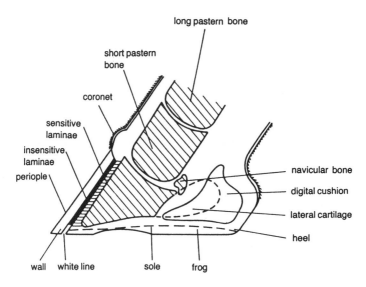

**Fig. 3.8** Structure of the foot, showing the digital cushion and lateral cartilage.

## The lateral cartilages (Fig. 3.8)

The lateral cartilages are two plates of gristle which attach to the wings of the pedal bone and curve back inside the wall, reaching just above the coronary band. In young horses the soft cartilage is very flexible, but as the horse ages the cartilage becomes tougher and is less able to withstand distortions of the limb which may occur during exercise. Injury may cause ossification of the lateral cartilages, resulting in sidebone. The palmar venous plexus lies between the cartilage and the digital cushion.

## The pedal and navicular bones

These two bones are highly vascular and fit closely together. The deep flexor tendon fans out to run over the navicular bone and attach to the undersurface of the pedal bone. The navicular acts as a pulley as the tendon exerts pull on the pedal bone during locomotion.

### The blood supply to the foot

The common digital artery, along with the nerve supply runs down the lower leg next to the flexor tendons. Just above the fetlock it divides to supply the pastern bones and the pedal bone. The veins form dense networks called plexi which penetrate the sensitive foot and supply the hoof. When the foot takes the horse's weight it expands which raises the blood pressure and empties the veins. When the foot is raised, the blood pressure is reduced and the veins fill.

## The functions of the foot

There are three main functions of the foot:

(1) to reduce concussion
(2) to prevent slipping
(3) to aid circulation.

### Reducing concussion

The hoof is adapted to accommodate concussion when it hits the ground with the wall bearing the majority of the impact. In the unshod horse, the frog strikes the ground first, then the heels, bars, quarters and finally the toe. As the frog comes under pressure the heels and bars expand, this expansion is limited by the toe which is immovable. Thus shoes are not nailed at the heel. Concussion is transmitted through the wall to the laminae and to the periosteum of the pedal bone and the rest of the bones of the limb. There is slight yielding of the pedal bone which is cushioned by the lateral cartilages. There is also some movement in the joint between the pedal bone and the short pastern. Concussion is also reduced by the cushioning effect of the frog and the digital cushion, but this is only applicable if the frog is in contact with the ground. The angulation of the scapula, humerus and fetlock joint and the support of the suspensory apparatus also reduce the concussive effects.

### Anti-slip

When the ground is soft the toe cuts in to prevent slipping but this is not effective on hard or greasy going. When the foot sinks into the ground, the dome shape of the sole has a suction effect which gives firm grip. This is so effective that the horse will have to work very hard in soft ground. The contact of a properly formed frog with the ground is an important anti-slip device, especially on firm ground. However, shoes tend to raise the frog clear of the ground, depriving the horse of its anti-slip mechanism. This is counteracted by using modifications to the shoe such as calkins or studs.

### Circulation

As there is no muscle below the horse's knee it cannot rely on muscle massage of veins to promote venous return of blood to the heart. As the foot comes under pressure the blood in the three venous plexi (coronary, dorsal and palmar venous plexus) is squeezed into the digital veins. As the weight comes off the foot arterial blood enters the foot, venous blood is prevented from flowing back into the foot by valves. Frog pressure is needed for this to work and the theory is probably an oversimplification as horses that have had the frog pared away do not seem to suffer from bad circulation or concussion. It may be that the spreading of the heels and role of the lateral cartilages is more important. Indeed, one theory poses that as the heels spread when the horse lands blood is drawn into the foot, and as the heels contract blood is squeezed out of the foot.

# Hoof care

## Hoof oils and creams

Many horses develop multiple splits around the bottom of the hoof wall, especially in the summer, and it has been suggested that damage to the periople can lead to drying of the hoof wall, making it prone to cracking. Add to this long toes and loose shoes and the cracking will become worse. Once the horse develops poor quality hoof horn, the underlying tissues are not adequately protected and can be bruised, resulting in blood leaking into the horn, further weakening it. Apart from those products purely designed to improve the appearance of the hoof, hoof oils and creams claim to condition the hoof wall.

Some external hoof care dressings aim to waterproof the hoof wall to protect against the damp in much the same way that we apply barrier creams to our hands. They are also said to counter brittleness and contracted feet. Modern opinion is that they are mainly cosmetic and may actually upset the normal movement of moisture in and out of the hoof.

'Moisturising' creams and oils aim to regulate the moisture balance of the hoof. Horses' hooves can lose moisture to dry ground, bedding and when there is heat in the feet. The idea is that these protect the hoof from the extremes of outside influences while allowing the hoof to 'breathe' naturally. The hoof also needs protection from the effects of standing in dung-and urine-soaked bedding; ammonia and urea given off by excreta is a major cause of soft hoof walls and soles.

Some hoof preparations recognise that the horse evolved in arid conditions where the hooves would have been hard and dry and aim to harden and condition soft and brittle horn. 'Natural' dry horn may break up when subjected to shoeing, however; in the British climate horses are just as likely to have waterlogged soft horn as dry and brittle horn.

## Feeding for better feet

In recent years more attention has been given to the effect of the horse's diet on the quality of hoof growth. The hoof wall consists of body cells which have been strengthened by a protein called keratin; the cells grown down from the coronary band at the rate of about one cm per month. The growth of the horny hoof wall requires certain nutrients including biotin, methionine, cysteine, zinc and sulphur. The stabled horse's diet is liable to be deficient in one or more of these nutrients, particularly if the hay is not of good quality and the horse's access to grazing is limited.

### Sulphur

Each nutrient has a different role to play. Sulphur, for example, is essential in all body cells and is concentrated in hair, skin and hoof. The laminae of the hoof are held together by disulphide bonds (S-S) and the coronary band needs sulphur, a lack of which results in reduced keratinisation and hence poor hoof growth and quality. Unfortunately sulphur is lost during the drying and processing of hay and concentrates and may well be lacking in the diet. Adding a bio-available source of sulphur, such as MSM, to the diet has been shown to increase both hoof growth and horn quality. Some sources of sulphur also appear to attract water and hence moisturise the hoof resulting in improvement in both hoof quality and growth rate.

## Biotin

Biotin is one of the B vitamins. Horses with hoof horn that tends to crumble at the lower edges of the wall have responded to biotin supplementation over a period of nine to twelve months. Biotin is also effective within the hoof, strengthening the white line and the lower part of the hoof wall. Biotin is present in many feeds including oats and barley but is not easily available to the horse, and the high levels required for hoof repair must be added to the feed in the form of a supplement.

## Methionine and cysteine

These are sulphur-containing amino acids and are the building blocks of the protein keratin found in the hoof. Methionine is an essential amino acid, which means it must be supplied in the diet.

## Zinc

Zinc is required in hooves for growth and ensuring healthy tissue and is often included in hoof supplements. Horses with weak or brittle hooves are usually lacking several nutrients, so a horse that does not respond to specific supplementation may require a broader spectrum supplement containing a range of micronutrients.

Some horses even when fed a hoof-improving supplement show no sign of improvement in cracking or brittle feet, although the growth rate of the hoof may have increased. American research suggests that this may be due to an infection called white line disease which is treated topically. Maintaining good hoof condition in horses depends on a combination of regular skilled attention from the farrier and feeding a good quality, well-balanced diet which provides the necessary minerals, vitamins and amino acids.

# The balanced foot

There is probably no such thing as the 'perfect foot' and when the horse is being shod it is more important that the farrier should match the foot with the leg, so that the shape and proportions of the foot are the most suitable for that limb, than it is to make the food 'ideal'.

## Assessment of balance

Before trimming the foot and nailing on the shoe the foot balance should be assessed when the horse is stationary (static) and when it is moving (dynamic).

### Static hoof balance

The foot should be looked at from the front (anterior view), underside (solar view) and side (lateral view).

#### *The front (anterior view)*

A vertical axis drawn through the centre of the cannon bone should bisect the hoof into two equal halves (Fig. 3.9). A line running across the top of the coronary band should be horizontal, i.e. the same distance from the ground on both sides of the hoof, showing that the hoof wall is at the same angle on both sides (Fig. 3.10). The wall should not flare out or run under.

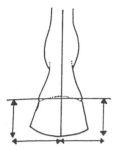
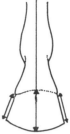
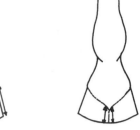

**Fig. 3.9** Correct foot shape: a vertical axis through the centre of the cannon bisects the foot. A line running across the top of the coronary band is horizontal.

**Fig. 3.10** The distance from the coronary band to the floor is the same on both sides of the foot.

### The underside (solar view)

The frog is the best guide to the foot's symmetry. A trimmed frog is shaped like a wedge that starts between the heels and ends in a point (the apex) just in front of the hoof centre. The frog should exactly bisect the foot and the hoof should be equal in shape and proportion on either side of the frog (Fig. 3.11). If the hoof wall is not evenly proportioned the foot should be reshaped and the shoe set symmetrically around the frog, so that it too is bisected equally by the centre of the limb.

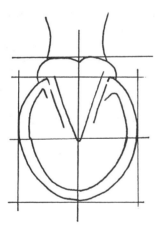

**Fig. 3.11** Foot balance – solar view. The foot should be symmetrical about a horizontal and vertical axis.

### The side (lateral view)

It is essential that the hoof-pastern axis (HPA) is in alignment. Ideally, the hoof wall and angle at the heel should also align (Fig. 3.12). If the HPA is broken back great strain is thrown upon the stay apparatus and dorsal wall laminae. If the horse has long toes and low heels the chances of tendon injury are increased and the toe should be dressed back and the horse shod with upright heels and a rolled toe. Long toes delay and prolong the breakover of the leg over the foot with the heel remaining on the ground longer. This compresses the front of the joints and the navicular bone, contributing to poor stride length, stumbling and forging. A broken forward HPA is not as serious as a broken back HPA but can lead to stumbling and excessive landing on the heels. Poor HPA conformation is usually induced by shoes being left on too long and/or short

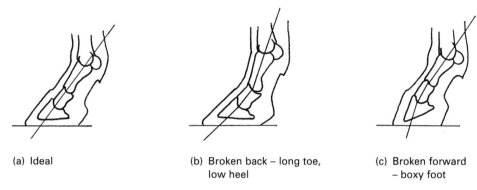

(a) Ideal  (b) Broken back – long toe, low heel  (c) Broken forward – boxy foot

**Fig. 3.12** Hoof pastern angles.

shoeing. The ideal hoof angle is said to be 45–50° in front and 50–55° for the hind feet. The angle depends on the individual horse's conformation, and in practice tends to be more upright than the 'ideal'.

## Dynamic hoof balance

The horse's movement and soundness are the greatest tests of hoof balance. The farrier cannot influence the flight of the horse's foot through the air but he can influence the way the foot lands and takes off.

The hoof has good side-to-side balance if it lands level. This can be judged by standing directly in front of the horse as it is walked towards you. An out of balance foot may 'toe out'; as the foot lands, the outside toe (which is usually flared) lands first, as the bodyweight passes over the foot the inside heel is snapped down. The weight of the horse is rolled over the inside toe as the foot breaks over and lifts off. This type of movement is liable to cause the inside heel to shunt up higher than the outside heel. At first glance the inside heel appears higher and is often trimmed down to 'level it' with the outside heel, exacerbating the problem. Instead the shoe should be set wider to support the limb more evenly (Figs. 3.13 and 3.14).

From the side the well balanced foot should land level or slightly heel first. Horses that land toe first are usually showing signs of pain in the rear area of the foot and are prone to stumbling.

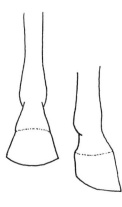

**Fig. 3.13** A horse with toe-out conformation places the lateral toe first, then slams down the medial side.

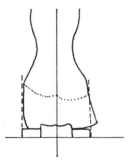

**Fig. 3.14**   Unbalanced foot trimmed to remove the flare and shod to support the under-run side.

# Infection in the foot

The horse's foot may become infected for many reasons. Corns, bruising, 'pricked' foot and puncture wounds are common causes of lameness.

Corns are bruised areas caused by the shoe putting pressure on the seat of the corn where the wall reflects back to form the bars. Commonly this is due to the shoes being left on too long or the horse being shod too close at the heel. The sole may be bruised with a single blow such as treading on a stone. Neglected or severe bruises may become infected. Infection can also enter the foot if a nail is driven into the sensitive tissue during shoeing or if the horse treads on a sharp object.

Infection leads to inflammation which gives rise to intense pain as the swelling is restricted by the hoof wall. The horse will be reluctant to put weight on the foot, there will be a strong digital pulse and heat in the foot, and the leg may also fill. Hoof testers can be used to pinpoint the site of injury although the horse may respond to finger pressure. Unless treated, the pus resulting from the infection will track along the line of least resistance, migrating under the sole and up between the laminae to emerge at the coronet. The vet will check the horse's tetanus status and remove the shoe and open up the abscess to drain it and eliminate the infection. Hot poultices left on for 24 hours for two to three days, followed by tubbing the foot in warm salt water are usually successful if the drainage is adequate. The position of the wound is significant as the pedal bone or navicular bone may be involved if the puncture is deep.

## Navicular syndrome

Navicular syndrome is a poorly understood condition where multiple causes of pain lead to similar signs of lameness. The navicular bone acts as a stabiliser and keeps the DDFT attachment to the pedal bone at a constant angle during the weight bearing phase of the stride and when the foot is in flight. It prevents the tendon being flexed and twisted at every step which would eventually tear it loose. The navicular bone also supports the joint between the short pastern and pedal bone by increasing the bearing surface of the short pastern and, along with ligaments, limits the amount of flexion and rotation of the joint.

### Causes

It is possible that blood clotting in the tiny arteries that serve the bone leads to pain and bony changes. Also repeated pressure and vibration of the navicular bone against the deep flexor tendon could lead to degeneration and bursitis.

**Signs**

Navicular syndrome occurs in the front feet of horses, rarely ponies, and usually affects both feet leading to a shortening of stride, unlevelness on turns and a reluctance to work on hard ground. The horse is often described as 'footy' or 'pottery' with intermittent lameness, especially in circles. The horse may point its toe at rest. Horses with all shapes of foot may develop navicular. Commonly horses with long toes and low heels are affected; conversely those with narrow upright feet may also develop the condition.

**Diagnosis**

The horse tends to place the toe first, especially on hard ground and the stride is shorter than expected. Flexion of the fetlock and lower joints may make the horse more lame and it will also be worse when lunged on the hard with the lame foot to the inside. Nerve blocks will indicate that the lameness is in the foot and X-rays reveal characteristic changes in the navicular bone. There is however a large 'normal' variation in the bone which makes interpretation of the X-rays difficult.

**Treatment**

There is no single 'cure' for navicular syndrome. Treatment relies on a combination of the following methods:

- Shoeing and trimming – the foot must be balanced with plenty of heel support, e.g. an egg bar shoe.
- Exercise – the horse should be exercised regularly and turned out daily to maintain the blood supply to the foot.
- Warfarin prolongs blood clotting time and must be used with care.
- Isoxsuprine dilates the peripheral blood vessels and may be very successful if treatment is early enough.
- Desmotomy – cutting the suspensory ligament of the navicular bone to relieve pressure – has shown encouraging results.

## Pre-navicular syndrome

Horses may show pre-navicular syndrome, which if treated can prevent irreversible change in the navicular bone.

**Signs**

- Subtle decline in performance, e.g. poor attitude to work, stumbling, choppy gait until warmed up, reluctance to jump.
- Minor discomfort, e.g. stiff on leaving stable, uncomfortable but not lame.
- Clues that the heels are sore, e.g. pointing a toe, landing on toe first, wearing toe of shoe quicker than heels.

**Prevention**

While there is no recipe for the successful prevention of navicular syndrome, the following points should prolong the horse's active life:

- Turnout – horses are not designed to stand for 23 hours a day in a stable, and regular turnout so that the horse can exercise itself is a more healthy option.

- Exercise – the horse should be exercised regularly and at a level to suit its degree of fitness.
- Correct bodyweight – obesity puts extra strain on all the limbs.
- Fitness – horses should be fit enough for the work demanded of them.
- Shoeing – the horse should be regularly and correctly shod.

# Chapter 4
# The Respiratory System

## Function

The horse requires a constant supply of oxygen to stay alive. At all times, in all living cells, energy liberation continues without interruption. This energy results from the oxidation of complex carbon-containing substances. In simple terms, glucose is broken down in the presence of oxygen to release carbon dioxide and energy. The waste product, carbon dioxide is toxic and must be eliminated from the body. Respiration is the process by which the horse takes oxygen into its body and also rids its body of carbon dioxide.

Essentially respiration is the exchange of gases between the horse and its environment. The horse has a system of respiratory organs which are designed to bring oxygen into the cells of the body and to expel carbon dioxide and water. Two types of respiration are involved: external respiration involving the exchange of gases between the respiratory organs and the bloodstream and internal or tissue respiration, involving the exchange of gases between the bloodstream and the body cells.

## Anatomy

The respiratory system consists of the airways of the head and neck and the lungs. It is in essence a series of tubes, starting at the nostrils and ending as a multitude of tiny, thin-walled sacs called alveoli which are in intimate contact with a dense network of blood capillaries. The structures involved are the nasal cavity, pharynx, larynx, trachea, bronchi, lungs, pleurae and thoracic cavity.

### Within the head and neck

The airways of the head and neck are shown in Fig. 4.1. The nostrils are the entrance to the respiratory system. The horse draws in air only through the nostrils and not through the mouth, and they can expand in order to take in more air. The nostrils lead to the nasal cavity which is divided into two by the nasal septum. Each side contains three delicate bones called turbinates which are covered by a thick, soft mucus membrane which is a yellow brown colour. The upper (dorsal) and lower (ventral) turbinates are long, rolled up like a scroll and perforated by many holes. Together with the nasal hairs and membrane covering the turbinates this contributes to the accuracy and sensitivity of the horse's sense of smell by providing a large surface area for warming and filtering the air that enters through the nostrils.

The third turbinate bone (the ethmoid turbinate) is a group of plate-like projections in the back part of the nasal cavity. The surface of the mucus membrane that covers this bone is involved with the sense of smell.

Each side of the nasal chamber is connected to four air sinuses. These are pockets in the bone which lie immediately beneath most of the surface bones of the forehead and

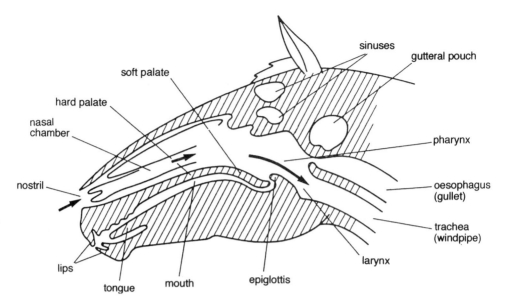

**Fig. 4.1**   Airways of the head.

occupy some space under the facial bones beneath the eyes. Lining the inside of each sinus is a thin layer of epithelial tissue which may become inflamed, resulting in sinusitis. Sinuses appear to have no specific purpose other than rounding out the facial areas and making the skull lighter in weight.

Once warmed and filtered, air passes the pharynx and larynx to go down the trachea (windpipe). The pharynx is situated at the back of the throat and is a funnel-shaped organ involved in both the digestive and respiratory systems as it opens into the mouth and the nasal cavity (Fig. 4.2). At the bottom of the pharynx is the soft palate which is overlapped by the epiglottis. Most of the time this overlapping shuts off the mouth and allows the free passage of air into the next part of the system – the larynx. When the horse swallows, however, the epiglottis flips over the opening of the larynx, the soft palate moves up and food is admitted from the mouth into the pharynx and is then swallowed. This mechanism is effective in separating the processes of breathing and eating but makes mouth-breathing under stress very difficult for the horse.

The larynx is a movable framework of cartilage and muscle that connects the pharynx and trachea; it supports the epiglottis and is also known as the voice box because it contains the vocal cords.

The trachea runs from the larynx to the lungs and consists of a heavily walled tube kept permanently open by closely spaced C-shaped rings of cartilage set in its wall. The trachea passes down and back along the ventral surface of the neck and enters the thoracic cavity at the thoracic inlet.

## Within the chest

The lungs occupy most of the thoracic cavity. The right lung is bigger than the left and has an intermediate lobe (Fig. 4.3). The structure of the lungs is shown in Fig. 4.4. At the region of the heart the trachea divides into two primary bronchi, each bronchus entering one lung at the hilus. Within the lung the bronchi divide and subdivide to terminate in the alveoli. The scheme within the lungs is as follows

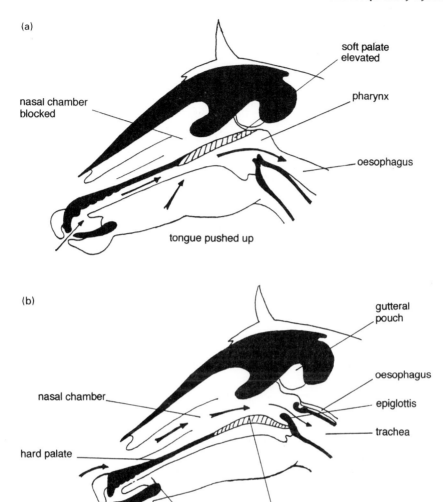

**Fig. 4.2**  Function of the pharynx in (a) swallowing and (b) breathing.

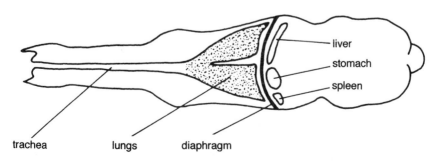

**Fig. 4.3**  Relationship between the stomach, diaphragm and lungs.

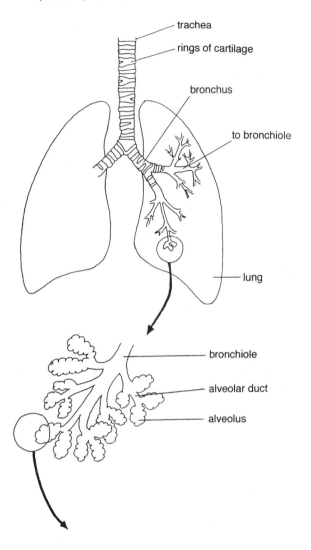

trachea

rings of cartilage

bronchus

to bronchiole

lung

bronchiole

alveolar duct

alveolus

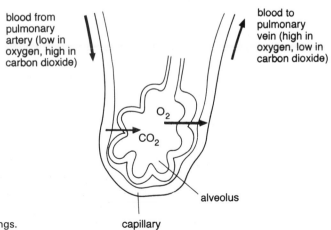

blood from pulmonary artery (low in oxygen, high in carbon dioxide)

blood to pulmonary vein (high in oxygen, low in carbon dioxide)

$O_2$

$CO_2$

alveolus

capillary

**Fig. 4.4**  Structure of the lungs.

- trachea
- primary bronchi
- secondary bronchi
- bronchioles – lobular and intralobular
- terminal bronchioles
- respiratory bronchioles
- alveolar sacs
- alveolar ducts
- alveoli.

The C-shaped rings of cartilage become plates in the primary bronchi and disappear completely in the secondary bronchi when these become less than 1 mm in diameter. The secondary bronchioles become bronchioles that continue to branch and reduce in diameter until they become respiratory bronchioles. Respiratory bronchioles have very thin walls and terminate in alveoli. The alveolar sacs are in the middle of a cluster of alveoli that are connected to the sac by delicate alveolar ducts. The lungs have a huge surface area due to the vast number of alveoli, estimated at 3000 million, which give a total surface area the size of an Olympic swimming pool.

The alveoli are the true respiratory structures. Here the exchange of gases between the inspired air and the bloodstream takes place. Each alveolus is wrapped around by a dense network of tiny blood-vessels called capillaries (Fig. 4.4); the alveolar-capillary wall consists of a continuous, extremely thin, alveolar membrane, a basement membrane and an equally thin capillary endothelium. The air contained within the sacs is in such close contact with the blood that oxygen is able to move from the air in the alveoli into the blood and carbon dioxide from the blood diffuses into the air in the alveoli and is removed when the horse exhales.

Air movement in and out of the lungs has little effect on alveolar size; inspiration and exhalation are achieved by the action of smooth muscle dilating and lengthening, and compressing and contracting the bronchial tree. This includes all structures up to the alveoli with the main breathing activity being in the terminal bronchioles. Ventilation of the alveoli is accomplished by air currents caused by the expansion and contraction of the bronchioles rather than the bellows-like movement of the alveolar walls.

The inner surfaces of the alveoli and terminal bronchioles are coated with a surfactant fluid which reduces the surface tension of the fluids within the lung and helps prevent collapse of the alveoli. The surfactant has low surface tension in small areas and high surface tension in large areas. Without surfactant, therefore, the small alveoli would collapse into larger ones and fail to reinflate, leading to laboured breathing and poor gaseous exchange.

The respiratory tract is lined and protected by special cells, many of which have frond-like cilia which give the airways a surface of resembling a deep-pile carpet. These cilia can move creating currents which convey tiny bits of debris, carried in mucus, up the tubes to the pharynx, where the horse coughs up or swallows the phlegm. Larger particles are coughed or sneezed out of the system.

## Blood supply

The pulmonary blood system begins with the pulmonary artery which leaves the right ventricle of the heart and carries deoxygenated blood. The pulmonary artery divides to give the right and left pulmonary arteries and these eventually subdivide to form the capillaries which surround the alveoli. Here gaseous exchange takes place and oxygenated blood is carried back to the heart via the pulmonary vein.

The tissue of the lung itself is nourished by blood carried in the bronchial circulation; the right and left bronchial arteries invade the lung, the blood returns via the bronchial veins to the anterior vena cava.

### The pleurae

The pleurae are membranes which cover the inner wall of the thorax and the organs found within the thorax. They are lubricated to slide over one another as the horse breathes in and out.

### The diaphragm

The diaphragm separates the thorax and lungs from the abdomen which contains the digestive organs. It is a strong, dome-shaped sheet of membranous muscle attached to the ribs and involved in breathing.

## The physiology of respiration

The process of respiration can be broadly divided into two parts:

(1) External respiration – breathing and transportation.
(2) Internal respiration – the production of energy within the cell.

### External respiration

Breathing is the obvious and well-known process of bringing air and blood into intimate contact in the lungs and consists of two phases, inhalation and exhalation. Transportation is the carrying of oxygen and carbon dioxide between the alveoli and the bloodstream.

The horse draws air in through its nostrils; air passes through the larynx, down the trachea and into the lungs. Here, oxygen passes from the air into the bloodstream and carbon dioxide passes from the blood into the lungs, a process called gaseous exchange. The alveoli fill with air due to changes in the size and shape of the lungs; as the lungs are held within the thoracic cavity, the lungs change in shape as the thoracic cavity moves. The pleurae hold the lungs so that they conform with the inner walls of the chest. There is no pushing or pulling by the chest wall or diaphragm on the lungs as they inflate and deflate. The lungs are filled by the action of the dome-shaped diaphragm and ribs. When the ribs are pulled forward and outwards, the chest expands; simultaneously the diaphragm contracts, flattening the dome and thus enlarging the 'box' in which the lungs are contained and drawing in air to fill the available space. As the diaphragm contracts, the abdominal muscles relax allowing the abdominal organs to move down and back. This process is called inhalation or inspiration.

Breathing out or exhalation is accomplished by the thorax decreasing in size, causing the air to flow out as the elastic lungs contract. There are three groups of muscles that affect exhalation; abdominal muscles, muscles of the chest and smooth muscle around the bronchioles. As the abdominal muscles contract, pressure is put on the organs in the abdomen which in turn press on the diaphragm and push it forwards to its resting position. The chest muscles rotate the ribs inward and back. The smooth muscle around the bronchioles contracts and forces air out of the lungs.

The external intercostal muscles and the levatores costarum move the ribs outward, upward and forward, thus increasing the size of the chest cavity. The internal intercostals rotate the ribs back to their resting position and the transverse thoracic muscles complete exhalation by compressing the thorax. In quiet breathing the muscles of inhalation do not contract fully and the muscles of exhalation are not used at all; the recoil of the chest wall and the collapse of stretched lung tissue accomplish the movement.

The respiration rate varies between species. The average resting respiration rate for the horse is 8 to 16 breaths per minute, the rate being higher for young stock. After strenuous exercise the rate can be up to 120 breaths per minute. Table 4.1 shows the resting respiration rates for various domestic animals and man.

**Table 4.1** Respiratory rates per minute of eight domestic animals

| Horse | 8–16 |
| --- | --- |
| Cow | |
| Dairy | 18–28 |
| Beef | 12–20 |
| Sheep | 12–24 |
| Goat | 12–20 |
| Pig | 15–24 |
| Dog | 19–30 |
| Cat | 24–42 |
| Man | 12–30 |

(Adapted from Dukes Physiology of Domestic Animals.)

## Lung air volumes (Fig. 4.5)

A number of air volumes apply to the breathing process:

- Total lung capacity – all the air the lungs can hold, about $42\,000\,cm^3$ in the horse.
- Vital capacity – the total functional capacity, the deepest inhalation followed by the deepest exhalation, about $30\,000\,cm^3$.

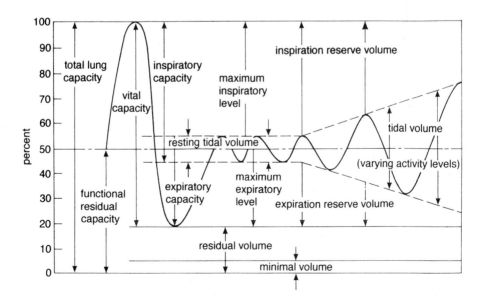

**Fig. 4.5** Lung air volumes.

- Normal capacity, the amount of air remaining in the lungs after a normal quiet exhalation, about $24\,000\,cm^3$.
- Tidal air – the volume of inhaled or exhaled in a normal quiet breath, about $6000\,cm^3$.
- Complemental air – the volume of air that can be taken in by the deepest possible inhalation after a normal quiet inhalation, about $12\,000\,cm^3$.
- Supplemental air – the air that can be forced out after a normal exhalation, about $12\,000\,cm^3$.
- Residual air – the air which remains in the lungs even after deep exhalation as the lungs never collapse completely, about $12\,000\,cm^3$.

## Dead space

The anatomical term 'dead space' is used to describe the air passages between the nostrils and the alveoli. It is called dead space as there is no gaseous exchange in this area. The anatomical dead space amounts to about $2000\,cm^3$ in the horse. The air contained in these passages mixes with the new air taken in at each breath and warms and humidifies it. This helps protect the delicate alveoli from sudden alterations in the temperature and composition of incoming air.

Alveolar dead space exists in those alveoli that are not being used. In resting horses this can be a large percentage of the lungs but decreases to nearly zero in horses that are working hard and breathing heavily.

## Regulation of breathing

Breathing is regulated by the coordinated action of the muscles of the chest, diaphragm and thorax. These are controlled by the respiratory centre of the brain which is located in the medulla oblongata of the brain. This centre is influenced both by sensory nerves and chemical changes in the blood, and controls the rate and depth of breathing. Motor nerve fibres leave the centre and pass down the spinal cord to emerge as peripheral nerves which pass to the respiratory muscles. The diaphragm is activated by the right and left phrenic nerves which emerge at the level of the seventh cervical vertebrae. Other motor fibres emerge from the spinal cord at the thoracic and abdominal level to go to the muscles that control breathing in and out. Pain of any origin can cause the rate and depth of respiration to increase because the respiratory centre has a potential connection to nearly all parts of the body.

The responses of the respiratory centre can be modified by chemicals carried in the blood stream. An increase in the amount of carbon dioxide in the blood results in acidity in the brain, the centre is stimulated to give stronger and more frequent stimulation of the motor nerves so that the carbon dioxide can be removed from the blood. An exercising horse has elevated levels of carbon dioxide and lactic acid in the blood due to increased muscle metabolism. The responses of the respiratory centre in the brain can be modified by chemicals carried in the blood stream. An exercising horse has elevated levels of carbon dioxide and lactic acid in the blood due to increased muscle metabolism. This results in the respiratory centre becoming more acidic and it is stimulated to give stronger and more frequent stimulation to the motor nerves so that the horse breathes more rapidly and deeply, and the carbon dioxide and lactic acid can thus be removed from the bloodstream.

Breathing can be controlled voluntarily but only within limits. Horses may hold their breath or speed up breathing, but only for a limited time. Vocalisation is a modification of breathing, air being channelled over the vocal cords to result in sound. Breathing can also be controlled to produce abdominal strain; if an animal breathes out with the glottis closed, the tightening of the abdominal muscles causes a rise in pressure inside the abdomen. This pressure is transferred to the abdominal organs and helps staling, giving birth and defaecation.

The respiratory rate is linked to the horse's gait. At gallop the stride rate equals the respiration rate and is described as locomotory-respiratory coupling and means that the muscles of breathing and movement do not work against each other. As the galloping horse lifts the limbs, the head is raised, the gut moves back and the horse breathes in. As the horse lands, the head drops, the gut moves forward and the horse breathes out (Fig. 4.6).

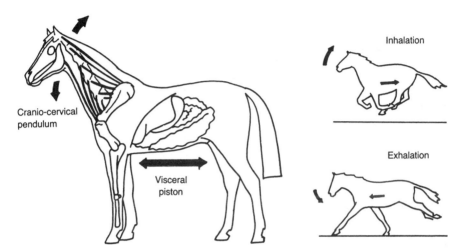

**Fig. 4.6** Synchronisation of stride and breathing. As the head moves up and the gut back the horse breathes in; the head moves down as the horse lands, the gut moves forwards and the horse breathes out.

## Clearing air passages

The airways of the bronchioles are kept clear by the cilia of the epithelial cells that line them. These fibrils beat in rhythmic waves to push fluid, mucus or foreign matter up the tubes and this matter may then be sneezed or coughed out of the horse.

Coughing is a forcible exhalation made with the glottis closed which raises pressure within the chest. The glottis then opens, reducing the pressure in the trachea and bronchi while high pressure remains in the deeper air spaces. The sudden drop of pressure in the trachea causes it to collapse inwards; air forced out of the depths of the lung passes through the narrowed trachea at considerable speed, expelling foreign matter. The horse has a poorly developed cough reflex; a horse coughing regularly, if infrequently, is showing signs of respiratory distress. An equine sneeze is an upper respiratory cough, air being expelled through the nostrils with considerable force.

## Air, gaseous exchange and blood transport

Normal atmospheric air has an approximate composition of 79% nitrogen and 20% oxygen with 1% composed of variable proportions of carbon dioxide and water vapour. Air breathed out of the lungs contains 79% nitrogen, 16% oxygen and 4% carbon dioxide saturated with water vapour. 4% of oxygen has been exchanged for carbon dioxide during the process. The venous blood coming to the lungs is relatively high in carbon dioxide and low in oxygen. Gaseous exchange takes place across the alveolar membrane and oxygen is taken into the red blood cells while carbon dioxide is released from them. Oxygen is carried in the red blood cells by haemoglobin, or respiratory pigment, which contains iron attached to a polypeptide called globin. Normal haemoglobin levels vary between species but the level in the horse is about 11 g per 100 ml of blood. Haemoglobin can combine loosely with oxygen and carbon dioxide. It is part of the blood buffer system which maintains body pH at about 7.4. Haemoglobin can readily combine with carbon monoxide and become incapable of carrying oxygen.

## The oxygen dissociation curve (Fig. 4.7)

This S-shaped curve shows the relationship between oxygen tension and haemoglobin saturation and indicates that blood can become almost fully saturated at relatively low oxygen levels. In other words haemoglobin has a high affinity for oxygen. The steep part of the curve corresponds to the range of oxygen levels found in the tissues; over this part of the curve, a small drop in oxygen level will bring about a relatively large fall in the percentage saturation of the blood. So, if the oxygen level falls as a result of tissues utilising oxygen at a faster rate, haemoglobin will respond by giving up more of its oxygen.

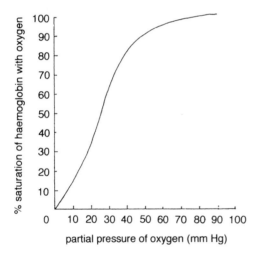

**Fig. 4.7**   Oxygen dissociation curve.

## The Bohr effect (Fig. 4.8)

The concentration of carbon dioxide affects the affinity of haemoglobin for oxygen. With increasing carbon dioxide level the haemoglobin must be exposed to higher oxygen levels in order to become fully saturated but it will also release oxygen at higher oxygen levels. In other words, at high carbon dioxide levels haemoglobin is less efficient at taking up oxygen but better at releasing it. Release of oxygen is therefore favoured in the tissues where carbon dioxide concentrations are naturally high due to its release during energy production. In the lungs carbon dioxide tension is lower and this favours oxygen uptake.

Once gaseous exchange has occurred the oxygenated blood passes back to the heart and then to the rest of the body. At the tissues, where oxygenated blood

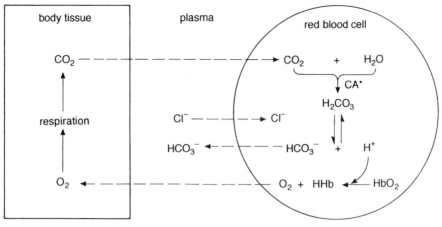

*carbonic anyhydrase

**Fig. 4.8**  Summary of red cell chemistry related to the carriage of respiratory gases.

encounters areas of low oxygen and high carbon dioxide levels, oxygen passes into the tissues while carbon dioxide diffuses into the blood. The deoxygenated blood returns to the heart and then the lungs.

## Internal respiration

Three phases are involved in internal respiration:

- transport of oxygen and carbon dioxide to and from the body cells;
- the exchange of oxygen and waste products between the blood and the body cells;
- the creation of energy within the cell.

Every living cell undergoes respiration but the rate of respiration can vary widely. For example, nervous tissue can exist for more than four minutes without oxygen while bone cells require little oxygen and can survive for hours without it. Oxygen is brought in the bloodstream and so hard-working tissues (brain, liver, kidneys, cardiac and skeletal muscle) have a plentiful capillary supply while relatively inactive tissues such as bone, cartilage, tendons and the cornea, have a limited blood supply.

### Energy for life

In order for a cell to stay alive and functioning it has to be able to extract and use the chemical energy locked inside the end-product of soluble carbohydrate digestion, glucose. When a molecule of glucose is broken down, carbon dioxide, water and energy are released; in the cell some of this energy is released as heat which can be used to perform work, as in a steam engine. However, in the cell some of this energy is captured by transferring the energy lost from the glucose directly to another chemical compound called an *energy carrier molecule*. This reaction takes place in the power house of the cell, the mitochondria. The reaction is complex and imperfectly understood but all life processes utilise energy in the form of a common basic unit. In all living cells from bacteria to man the major energy carrier molecule is adenosine triphosphate (ATP). This molecule consists of an adenosine body with three phosphate attachments. When one of the phosphates is lost to form adenosine diphosphate (ADP) energy is released (Fig. 4.9). This energy can be used by the cell to perform work such as muscle contraction.

Energy is stored in the horse's body in the form of glucose, glycogen, fat and protein. When needed this energy is transferred to ATP and then used to fulfil the cell's energy requirements.

adenosine $\text{P}$ $\text{P}$ $\text{P}$ $\longrightarrow$ adenosine $\text{P}$ $\text{P}$ + $\text{P}$ + energy

**Fig. 4.9**  Energy for life – ATP. (Courtesy of *Horse Talk* magazine.)

The horse requires energy to carry out the processes necessary for life such as breathing, reproducing and eating. He also needs energy to do the work we demand. Energy exists in several forms including light, heat, electrical, chemical and mechanical energy. All living things survive because they have the ability to convert one form to another, for example the chemical energy derived from the digestion of food is transferred to the mechanical energy required by the galloping horse to evade a predator.

Energy originates from the sun as radiant solar energy. While animals cannot utilise this for growth or work, plants can harness it in the process of photosynthesis (Fig. 4.10). Photosynthesis involves the creation of carbohydrate from carbon dioxide by plants, utilising solar energy. Thus chemical energy in the form of carbohydrate is now available for the horse which eats the plant. A by-product of photosynthesis is oxygen which animals need to breathe to stay alive; this is one of the reasons why the destruction of rain forests poses a serious threat to the environment.

The free energy of solar radiation is thus trapped by plants as chemical energy which can be used by the horse. The two major sources of chemical energy for the horse are carbohydrates and fats. Except during starvation proteins are of little importance as energy sources. When sufficient oxygen is present both carbohydrates and fats are completely broken down and the energy released completely.

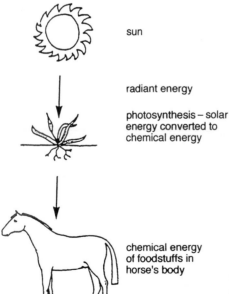

sun

radiant energy

photosynthesis – solar energy converted to chemical energy

chemical energy of foodstuffs in horse's body

**Fig. 4.10**  The energy chain. Transformation of solar energy to chemical energy. (Courtesy of *Horse Talk* magazine.)

## Energy storage

The horse is able to store energy within its body for future use. One way it can do this is in the form of glycogen which consists of many glucose molecules joined together. Glycogen is stored in the liver and in the muscle cells. The glycogen in the liver supplies glucose for all tissues of the body including nerves and blood cells. The glycogen stored in the muscles is only used by the muscle for contraction.

When there is too much energy or carbohydrate in the horse's diet the excess is converted to fat and stored in the various fat depots of the body. There is more than 30 times the amount of energy stored within the horse's fat reserves than in all the glycogen in the body. However, there is no point in fattening up horses to provide a built-in energy store for hard work. The rate at which muscles can use this energy source is limited and the built-in store can only be used during long, slow work. Additionally, with the exception of liver glycogen, glycogen storage is specialised for specific purposes and the glucose derived from it is not available for general use. Additionally, one gram of fat contains 2.25 times the energy of a gram of glycogen. Fat is a concentrated energy store. Proteins can be synthesised into fatty acids and triglycerides when there is excess protein in the diet.

The reactions that convert glycogen to glucose and then break down glucose to carbon dioxide, water and energy are known as glycolysis and Krebs cycle.

## Glycolysis (Fig. 4.11)

Glycogen consists of many molecules of glucose polymerised to form a complex carbohydrate. In glycolysis, successive molecules of glucose in the polymer chain are split off the main body by a process called phosphorylation. The hormones glucagon and adrenalin both activate the enzyme, phosphorylase, which allows the process to take place.

The resulting glucose molecules are phosphorylated, in other words they each have a phosphate group attached to them. The phosphorylated glucose can continue down the glycolytic pathway or, if the phosphate group is removed, the glucose can pass out of the cell and be transported in the blood to other cells which need energy. Muscle cells do not contain the enzyme (phosphatase) needed to remove the phosphate and so the glucose is trapped in the muscle cell to be broken down within the cell. Most liver glycogen is converted to glucose and sent off in the blood to fuel the body.

During the glycolysis of glucose to pyruvic acid only two ATP molecules are produced – however, quite a lot of energy is lost as heat making this reaction only 25% effective. In order for the pyruvic acid to be converted to carbon dioxide and water, respiratory oxygen is necessary. Glycolysis is known as anaerobic respiration as it does not require the presence of oxygen to take place, but it is relatively inefficient, producing small amounts of energy and large amounts of heat. Anaerobic respiration also has the disadvantage that, in the absence of oxygen, the pyruvic acid is converted to lactic acid which can accumulate in the muscle cells, contributing to fatigue.

## The Krebs cycle or the tricarboxylic (TCA) cycle (Fig. 4.12)

The conversion of pyruvic acid to carbon dioxide and water liberates hydrogen atoms which are oxidised through the oxidative phosphorylation process to produce ATP (Fig. 4.13). The complete oxidation of one molecule of glucose to carbon dioxide and water gives rise to a total of 38 units of ATP. The breakdown of glucose in the presence of oxygen (aerobic respiration) is much more efficient than anaerobic

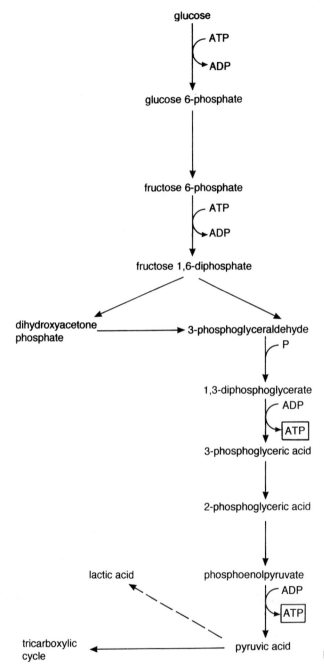

**Fig. 4.11**   Glycolytic pathway.

respiration, but there is still considerable heat loss. This heat is utilised by the horse's body to keep warm.

## Fat metabolism (Fig. 4.14)

Fats or lipids occur in three main forms: triglycerides, phospholipids and cholesterol. All triglycerides and phospholipids contain fatty acids of one type or another,

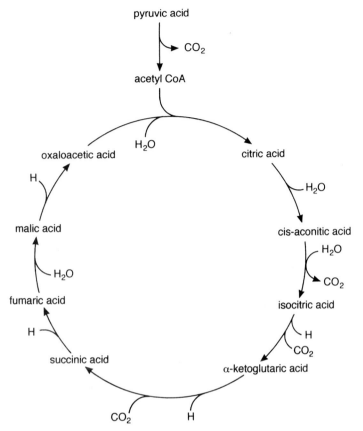

Liberated hydrogen is used to synthesise ATP by oxidative phosphorylation

**Fig. 4.12** Tricarboxylic (Kreb's) cycle.

characterised by a long chain of carbon atoms joined to hydrogen atoms. The less hydrogen in the chain the less saturated and more fluid the fatty acid will be. Thus highly unsaturated fats are oils while highly saturated fats are waxes.

During digestion in the stomach and small intestine fats are split into glycerol, monoglycerides and fatty acids which pass across the intestinal wall. Once across this barrier the fats are resynthesised into triglycerides and pass into the lacteals. The tiny droplets of fat are transported away from the intestine and into the blood stream via the lymphatic system.

Most of the absorbed fat is hydrolysed into fatty acids and glycerol in the blood. Unutilised fats are stored as energy reserves in fat depots or adipose tissue. Fat cells are specialised connective tissue cells which are capable of storing triglycerides. Depending on the species and the type of fat in the diet the fat within the cells may be more or less liquid. In sheep and cattle the fat is notably firm while in horses, dogs and cats it is more liquid. When carbohydrate intake is low the utilisation of body fat increases and the fat depots are reduced.

**Triglyceride metabolism** (Fig. 4.15)

The liver plays a major role in breaking down fat to provide energy. The liver can also resynthesise triglycerides to form specialised fats or fatty acids needed by the body.

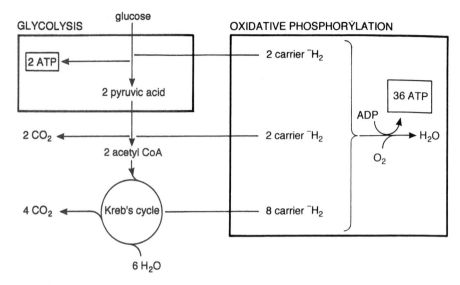

**Fig. 4.13**  Summary of the formation of ATP during the aerobic breakdown of glucose to carbon dioxide and water.

triglyceride $\rightleftharpoons$ glycerol + 3 fatty acids

**Fig. 4.14**  Fat metabolism.

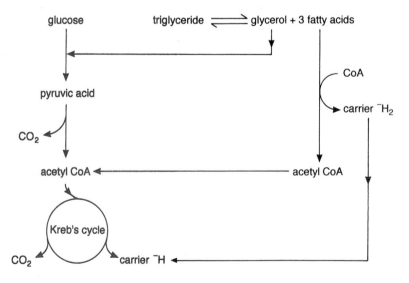

**Fig. 4.15**  Energy release from fat.

During times of stress, starvation or reduced carbohydrate intake the liver acts as a reception and conversion centre where the triglycerides from fat depots are broken down to provide energy.

The first stage is the conversion of triglycerides to fatty acids and glycerol. The glycerol passes through the phosphogluconate pathway to release energy. The fatty acids are converted into acetyl-CoA which then enters the Krebs cycle and is processed in the same way as glucose. The breakdown of one molecule of fatty acid produces more ATP than one molecule of glucose – fat is very energy-dense.

## Protein metabolism

Proteins are often called the building blocks of the body. They are the most complex molecules that occur in nature and are made up of chains of amino acids. During digestion proteins are broken down to amino acids and transported across the intestinal wall into the blood capillaries by which they are taken to the liver via the portal circulation. In the liver the amino acids may be processed or transferred directly to the bloodstream. The processing reactions include the synthesis of amino acids into body protein, the creation of hormones and enzymes, the conversion of toxic ammonia into urea and the use of amino acids as fuel. The process of converting protein to carbohydrate is called gluconeogenesis. Under normal conditions it is a low level activity but during disease or starvation it can become the major source of body energy, hence the wasting away of muscle that is seen.

# Respiratory disease

Respiratory disease is a serious problem for the equine athlete; even a mildly affected horse will perform below par. All respiratory problems will affect the efficient function of the lungs, especially at peak performance, when the horse uses five times more lung capacity than at rest. Viral infection, dusty, poorly ventilated stables, mouldy hay and a badly planned exercise programme all contribute to the development of respiratory disease.

## Types of respiratory disease

Respiratory disease has two main causes: infective agents such as viruses, and non-infective agents like fungal spores. However, in practice it is often difficult to separate the two as respiratory problems are often progressive.

### Viral infections

- Influenza: the horse suffers from a dry, frequent cough at rest; after an incubation period of about three days there is a short fever during which the horse will be depressed, off its feed and lethargic. The lymph glands beneath the jaw may be enlarged.
- Equine herpes virus 1 (EHV-1): Two strains of the virus exist – sub-type 1 causes abortion in mares, mild respiratory symptoms and occasionally, paralysis while sub-type 2 (rhinopneumonitis) affects only the respiratory tract and inflames the lining of the nose and eyes for one to three weeks. The horse may have a fever and a thick nasal discharge. The virus can lie dormant in the horse after infection for several years, waiting for the horse to be stressed, and then it flares up again.

- Adenovirus, rhinovirus, picornavirus: these all produce mild respiratory problems, but are generally much less significant.

## Bacterial infections

Bacterial infections commonly follow viral infections; taking advantage of the vulnerability of the horse's body tissues. *Streptococcus zooepidemicus*, *Streptococcus pneumoniae* and *Streptococcus equisimilis* are commonly involved.

### Strangles

Strangles is caused by *Streptococcus equi*. The disease leads to loss of appetite, fever, depression and a highly infectious, purulent nasal discharge. The lymph glands of the throat become very enlarged and may develop into abscesses. Abscesses may also form in the gut with serious consequences.

### Pneumonia

Pneumonia is caused by *Rhodococcus equi*. Bacteria rely heavily on dust in the air to spread them to other animals and this bacterium causes pneumonia in foals, especially in dry and dusty environments.

The first time a horse is infected by respiratory disease it will be more severely affected than during subsequent infections. This is because the horse develops a degree of immunity. The length and degree of protection will depend on the type of infective agent and how long ago the horse was last infected; immunity wanes with time. If infection occurs when the horse has a high immunity then, providing that the horse is not stressed, there may not be any outward signs of disease. However, if the horse is stressed by travel or work then clinical signs will develop or the horse's performance slumps.

## Non-infective agents

Non-infective agents such as fungal spores initially appear as 'the poor performance syndrome'. Typically the horse performs well in the early part of a race and rapidly fades in the later stages, recovery from work is slow and there may be an occasional cough at the beginning of work. A galloping horse with reduced lung capacity will not be able to get oxygen into his bloodstream quickly enough and his performance will suffer. If this loss of performance is not noticed and acted upon then the horse can develop small airway disease where the lower airways of the lungs become inflamed. If the horse is still not treated, or if he is over-stressed, the cells lining these airways may become hypersensitive or allergic, a condition called chronic obstructive pulmonary disease.

### Small airway disease

The cells of the lower airways are inflamed and become susceptible to further damage, leading to poor performance.

### Exercise induced pulmonary haemorrhage (EIPH)

Bleeding from the nose after exercise, also known as epistaxis, occurs in many horses; it is believed that such bleeding originates from the lung tissue itself and may be a sequel to an allergic state in the lower respiratory tract. EIPH occurs in varying degrees; a horse may not show any external signs other than blowing more than would be expected. Or it may have a thin, blood-stained nasal discharge. In extreme cases the horse will have to pull up, bleeding heavily. The galloping horse has a great oxygen demand and in an attempt to satisfy this the blood supply to the lungs is increased. The resultant increase in blood pressure causes some of the thin-walled blood-vessels in the lung tissue to burst, blood escapes into the alveoli, preventing oxygen exchange and putting more stress on the remaining lung tissue. The debris that accumulates as a product of inflammation will have a similar effect – not allowing oxygen to pass into the bloodstream. Any damage to the alveoli is reflected by weakness in the adjacent capillary wall, predisposing it to rupture and bleeding in to the lung. EIPH tends to occur at the top of the lung, near the diaphragm, where the normal blood supply is least; the lung inflates more slowly due to the thickness of the damaged walls and the inflammatory debris, the tissue tears and bleeds. The partial blockage causes the negative pressure in the alveoli to increase and their blood-vessels rupture and bleed into the lungs.

### Chronic obstructive pulmonary disease (COPD)

Once the mucus lining of the small airways of the lungs have been damaged they may become 'sensitised' to environmental influences, to which they develop an allergy. These allergens may be:

- *Non-specific* – for example, cold air or dust which causes irritation of the tissues, or
- *Specific* – for example, the fungal spores found in hay, which cause COPD. The horse may be allergic to pollens, causing a hay-fever type condition.

Frequently it would appear that respiratory disease is progressive. Horses rarely develop COPD overnight; there is a build-up of stress on the respiratory system with infection, poor environment and exercise all contributing to inflammation and damage until the lung becomes hypersensitive and COPD results.

## Development of respiratory disease

The respiratory tract can be damaged by: infection, inflammation and allergy.

## Infection

Many horses these days travel widely to competitions and mix with many other horses. They are therefore particularly vulnerable to viral infection. Viruses contaminate the air that an infected horse breathes out and infect water droplets that are coughed into the atmosphere. Viruses cannot live for long outside the horse but they are highly infectious to surrounding horses that may inhale infected water droplets or touch a discharge from eyes or nose. A horse will recover from a simple, uncomplicated viral infection in about a week, but the virus will have damaged the cells lining the airways so that they are much more susceptible to a secondary bacterial infection. This infection leads to a thick purulent nasal discharge.

## Inflammation

Small airway disease is associated with local inflammation (Fig. 4.16) which may follow infection, irritation or allergy. Inflammation leads to swelling of the lining of the airways so that the internal diameter is reduced, making breathing less efficient.

## Allergy

Blood cells attracted by the inflammation may then meet allergens such as fungal spores (*Aspergillus fumigatus* and *Micropolysporum faeni*). This causes the muscle of the airways to go into spasm, thus reducing the diameter even further. Debris (dead cells and mucus) from the inflammatory reaction accumulates, physically blocking the air flow. At the same time the cilia lining the tubes becomes broken or tangled so that

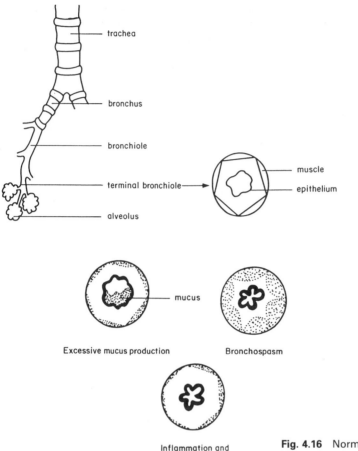

Fig. 4.16   Normal and obstructed small air passages of the lung.

the mucus produced is not moved out of the airways and infection makes this mucus more tacky and difficult to get rid of. Effectively the airways are narrowed and then blocked by mucus making respiration an effort and less effective.

## Signs of respiratory disease

(1) *Increased respiration rate:* the healthy horse has a resting respiration rate of 8–12 breaths per minute and an increase over this indicates stress of some sort, for example, fever or respiratory problems.

(2) *Amount of effort needed:* the normal lung has plenty of spare capacity so, at rest, there should be little or no visible movement of the chest as the horse breathes. If the horse is clearly making an effort to breathe there is likely to be a respiratory abnormality. The effort made breathing out or on expiration becomes more noticeable, and in severe cases the horse will develop a 'heaves line', the muscles of the abdomen involved with breathing out become enlarged and the horse can be seen making an extra exhalatory effort.

(3) *Nasal discharge:* there may be an abnormal discharge from the nose and/or eyes; in the early stages of a viral infection this will be watery, but later becomes thick and purulent, indicating a secondary bacterial infection.

(4) *Fever:* the early stages of a viral infection usually causes a sharp rise in body temperature (normally 38°C or 100.5°F), but this is often very shortlived and is easily missed. Where performance is important temperatures should be routinely taken morning and evening.

(5) *Loss of appetite:* the horse may go off its feed for a few days, this usually coinciding with the fever.

(6) *Coughing:* a cough will develop. This may be an occasional cough in the stable which becomes more severe during and after exercise.

(7) *Reduced work tolerance:* All of these things will combine to stop the horse working as efficiently. Indeed, the first thing the rider or trainer notices may be the fact that the horse is 'not himself'.

(8) *Exercise induced pulmonary haemorrhage:* bleeding from the lungs as previously discussed indicates respiratory disease.

## Diagnosis of respiratory disease

### Auscultation

Auscultation is listening to the lungs with a stethoscope. Although it is useful to listen to the horse's lungs and to gain information by percussion of the chest, especially after exercise, it is difficult to ascertain the amount of damage. The use of X-rays to examine the internal situation is not generally practical in an animal as large as the horse.

### Endoscopy

Probably the most important development in diagnosis of respiratory disease came with the introduction of the fibre optic endoscope. This is a flexible tube which is introduced into the airways via the nose of the standing horse. This allows the vet to see into the airways at least as far as the entrance to the chest; remote control moves the tip so that the whole area can be visualised in detail. Looking at the upper airways can pinpoint any physical obstruction which may need surgical correction. The vet can ascertain if there is mucus and pus in the airways and where this is originating the endoscope will also allow these fluids to be collected and examined in more detail. Chronic pulmonary disease is characterised by excess mucus at the lowest point in the trachea which forms thick plugs that can only be removed by coughing. Traces of blood in the fluids will indicate EIPH.

### Ultrasound

Ultrasonic examination of the chest will show the position of gross abnormalities in severe lung disease.

### Swabbing

Bacteria and viruses can be identified by taking swabs from the nose and pharynx. However, viruses can only be retrieved in the early stages of the infection and consequently are often missed.

### Blood testing

The signs of viral respiratory disease are often vague and diagnosis relies heavily on changes in the blood picture. Remember that each horse has a different 'normal' picture and it is important to know what is normal for a horse before you try to diagnose the abnormality. The test should be done as soon as infection is suspected and a further test taken two weeks later to monitor progress. The vet will be looking for changes in levels of white blood cells and serum proteins; horses may also become anaemic subsequent to a viral infection.

### Lung function

All horses with respiratory disease have low levels of oxygen in their blood after exercise and blood gas analysis can be a useful diagnostic tool. The effort made in breathing can be measured using a ventigraph, which is a diaphragm sensitive to pressure changes. It is inserted into the oesophagus until it lies just within the chest. The greater pressure required in breathing using a diseased lung can be quantified and recorded. Lung function can be assessed during exercise – the gases passing in and out of the horse's lungs as it works on a treadmill can be analysed and compared with expected normals. This method can identify very low grade problems that manifest themselves only as a slight fall in performance.

### Hay sampling

The degree of fungal spore contamination of hay and straw should be checked. Even the cleanest-looking forage will be contaminated to some extent.

## Control of respiratory disease

The most satisfactory method of control is prevention and this falls into two main categories: vaccination and environmental control.

### Vaccination

The most widely used vaccine is against equine influenza. Equine 'flu consists of a group of viruses of which only the three most common strains are included in the vaccine. Regular and frequent vaccination effectively protects the horse in the vast majority of cases, but the vaccine occasionally 'breaks down'. Susceptible horses should be vaccinated more frequently. It is frustrating that vaccination still leaves the horse vulnerable to other respiratory viruses that produce similar, if milder signs.

Horses can also be vaccinated against EHV-1. One such vaccine (Pneumabort-K) controls abortion in mares, but its efficacy against the respiratory form of the virus is untested. The other vaccine currently available (Rhinomune) is designed to prevent respiratory damage. Neither vaccine has been shown to protect the horse against the paralysis that may accompany EHV-1 infection. The immunity conferred by vaccination is short-lived and boosters are needed every three months.

Horses can be vaccinated against the strangles, but the vaccine is not available in the UK because it is not considered to be adequately effective.

### Environmental control

Respiratory disease must not be allowed to progress into COPD, the environment should be as dust and fungal spore-free as possible.

- *Hay:* in severe cases change to a fungal spore-free alternative such as haylage, good silage, barn-dried hay, alfalfa, grass nuts, hydroponic grass or high-fibre cubes. If this is not a viable alternative the hay will have to be soaked; the idea is that the fungal spores swell and are swallowed, not inhaled. In order to accomplish this, hay must be thoroughly soaked. Opinions vary as to how long hay should be soaked and the amount of nutrition lost by soaking. In practice many yards put the evening's hay in soak that morning and the next morning's hay in soak the evening before. Each batch of hay should be soaked in clean water as the discoloured water can soon become foul-smelling, especially in hot weather. It is wise to have a fungal spore count carried out as hay can look and smell clean and yet be heavily contaminated with fungal spores.

- *Dust-free bedding:* wood shavings although often dusty contain few spores; let the dust settle after putting in new shavings before returning the horse to its box. Bedding should be kept scrupulously clean.
- *Drainage:* bad drainage means a damp bed; paper and peat are very prone to dampness. A damp bed produces ammonia, which irritates the lungs and paralyses the hair-like cilia which waft the mucus away from the alveoli and up the bronchial tree.
- *Stable ventilation:* fresh air is essential. The stable should be draught-free with air vents in the roof apex which are large enough to carry away stale air. The air inlets – half door and window – should be in adjacent, not the same, walls so that air movement outside will always get into the stable. Air movement around the stable should be free – buildings, hedges and trees will obstruct air flow.
- *Clean stable:* the dust from floor to ceiling should be vacuumed or washed away; dust, cobwebs, ledges and cracks all harbour spores.
- *Soak hay for horses in rest of yard:* spores can be blown on the wind; the position of the muck heap and where hay and straw are stored must all be away from the stabling.
- *Fresh air:* the horse should be turned out as much as possible, especially in acute cases of COPD, regardless of the weather and time of year.

## Treatment of respiratory disease

There is no one 'cure' for respiratory disease, in many cases the condition is far advanced before the signs are noticed and treatment requested. Even when the horse's performance is below par it is not obvious that it is the fault of the respiratory system. Consequently, the veterinary surgeon uses a series of principles which are applied in all cases of respiratory disease, whatever the cause, and adds any specific treatment that may be indicated in each individual case.

### Rest

In the acute stages it is important to allow the horse complete rest. Whether this is in or out depends on the weather and what the horse is used to. Fresh air is necessary but draughts, cold winds and rain should be avoided. If the disease is suspected to be infectious the horse should be isolated and its companions watched for any signs of disease for the next two to three weeks. Regular temperature taking may indicate a problem before the horse shows any clinical signs. When lung damage has become so bad that bleeding occurs when the horse is worked hard, several weeks of rest are essential to allow the blood vessels to heal. The horse's return to work must be gradual, fast work will stress the newly healed vessels.

### Viral infection

No specific treatment can be given as antiviral drugs are so expensive as to make their use for horses unrealistic.

### Secondary bacterial infection

The bacterial infection that moves into the cells damaged by the viral infection can be readily and effectively treated with antibiotics.

### Bacterial infection

On the relatively few occasions that bacteria are the sole cause of respiratory disease, e.g. strangles, it may be better to delay antibacterial treatment until the abscesses have formed and good drainage has been achieved. If antibacterials suppress the infection rather than clear it up it may flare up again later.

### Getting rid of the mucus

In respiratory disease the cilia that waft away the mucus are reduced in number, and more mucus is produced which is more viscous than usual. If a cough suppressant is used the horse stops coughing and large particles of debris will be left in the airways to cause damage. In the early stages it is better to give the horse a mucolytic agent which helps move the mucus by making it more liquid. Consequently coughing is reduced because the horse can clear the mucus far more easily. Sputolosin (dembrexine) used over a 10-day period will dramatically reduce coughing and increase the clearance of mucus.

### Stopping the coughing

The only situation in which cough suppressants may be of value is when coughing is so frequent that the resulting irritation stimulates more coughing. A short course of anti-inflammatory corticosteroids is a good approach.

### Relieving the bronchospasm

Horses in severe respiratory distress will suffer bronchospasm; the small airways contain smooth muscle which, in response to antigens or irritant substances present in the airway, contract causing narrowing of the passages. This can cause quite severe distress in the horse which will have real difficulty in taking in enough air to breathe and is equivalent to an asthma attack in humans. Ventipulmin (clenbuterol) is a spasmolytic which acts by causing the smooth muscle to relax, opening the airways and allowing more air to pass into the lungs. Ventipulmin has the added advantage of acting on the cilia, stimulating their activity and hence the movement of mucus out of the airways.

### Preventing the attack

If exposure to the allergens responsible for a horse's 'asthma attack' is unavoidable a spasmolytic (sodium chromoglycate) can be given as a liquid that can be inhaled using a mask and a nebuliser. Treatment by inhalation on three or four successive days will protect a horse for up to three weeks and can be given in anticipation of exposure to fungal spores if, for example, stabled away from home.

When we train horses for supreme athletic performance we can see them muscle up, we can carry out blood tests to ensure that all is well, but all performance depends on getting maximum oxygen to the tissues, using one system that cannot be seen – the respiratory system. Many horses, due to poor environment and unobserved signs of respiratory disease, will have small amounts of airway obstruction; even the smallest obstruction will limit the amount of oxygen getting into the lungs and hence the tissues. Oxygen is essential for efficient energy production and thus muscle contraction; a lack of oxygen will limit performance and is seen as the 'poor performance syndrome'.

# Chapter 5
# The Circulatory System

All large animals need a transport system to supply all their cells with food, oxygen and other materials. The main transport system of the mammal is the circulatory system, sometimes known as the vascular system.

The circulatory system consists of a four-chambered pump known as the heart and a system of tubes or blood-vessels which circulate the transport medium, the blood (Fig. 5.1). As a general rule, the vessels which carry blood away from the heart are known as arteries whereas the vessels which carry blood back to the heart are known as veins. In addition there is a system of vessels which carry lymph or tissue fluid to the large veins and these are known as lymph vessels.

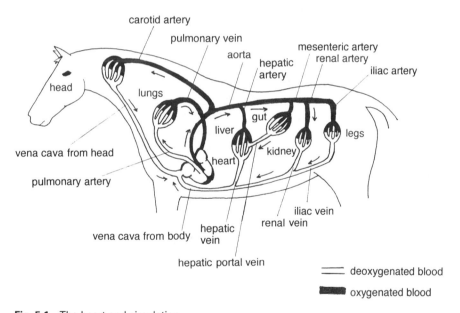

**Fig. 5.1** The heart and circulation.

## The heart

This is central to the circulatory system and is basically a large muscular pump which has the ability to contract and send blood through the network of vessels which supply the tissues of the horse's body. The heart of a 16 hh horse would weigh approximately 4 kg (9 lb). As the horse gets fitter, the heart size may increase up to about 5.5 kg (12 lb). A large heart has been associated with great racehorses such as Eclipse and Pharlap.

The heart is surrounded by a sac known as the pericardium or pericardial sac which is a completely closed sac containing a small amount of fluid for lubrication (Fig. 5.2). The heart wall consists of three layers, the epicardium, the endocardium and the important muscular layer –the myocardium. The myocardium consists of cardiac muscle which is also known as involuntary striated muscle.

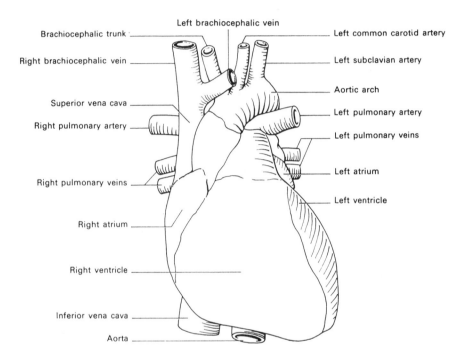

Fig. 5.2   External appearance of the heart.

The heart is divided into four hollow chambers (Fig. 5.3). The right-hand side is separate from the left-hand side, so that blood does not mix between the two. The right-hand side of the heart is responsible for moving deoxygenated or venous blood, i.e. blood that has had most of its oxygen removed as it travelled around the horse's body. Veins carry this deoxygenated blood via the body's largest vein, the vena cava, to the right auricle or atrium of the heart. Once full the right auricle contracts, pushing blood into the more muscular right ventricle (RV). The tricuspid valve snaps shut to prevent any back flow of blood. This is the first noise of the heart sounds which can be heard using a stethoscope, the 'lub' part of the characteristic 'lub-dup'. The right ventricle then contracts, pushing blood into the pulmonary artery which takes blood to the lungs (Fig. 5.4).

It is important to note that the pulmonary artery and vein are the exception to the general rule that arteries carry oxygenated blood and veins carry deoxygenated blood. The pulmonary artery carries deoxygenated blood to the lungs and the pulmonary vein carries oxygenated blood from the lungs to the heart.

Once in the lungs the blood comes into close contact with the alveoli and the carbon dioxide it is carrying is exchanged for oxygen by a process known as gaseous exchange. The now oxygenated or arterial blood then returns back to the heart via

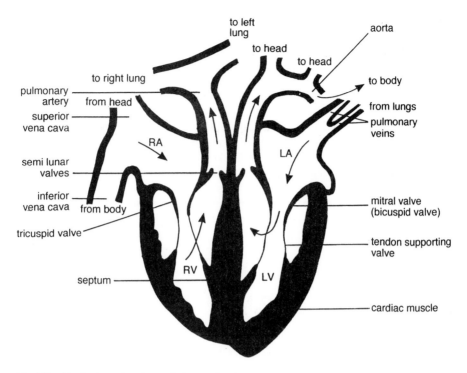

**Fig. 5.3**   Vertical section through the equine heart.

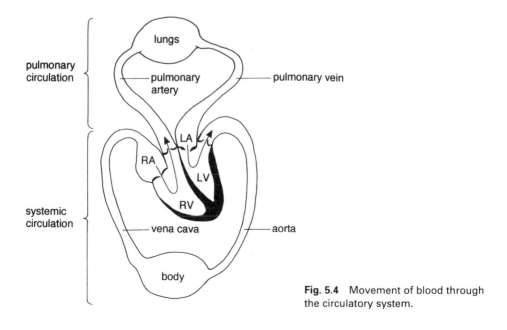

**Fig. 5.4**   Movement of blood through the circulatory system.

the pulmonary vein to the left auricle. Once it is full, blood is forced into the left ventricle (LV) and again the bicuspid valves shut to prevent any back flow of blood.

The left ventricle has the thickest muscular wall of any of the four heart chambers because blood from the left ventricle is forced out at great pressure into the aorta, which is the largest artery in the body. Blood from the left ventricle has to travel a greater distance to all parts of the horse's body and not just to the lungs, hence the thicker muscular wall (Fig. 5.1).

Valves at the entrance of the aorta known as semi-lunar valves prevent back-flow and lead to the second sound of the heart beat the 'dup' part of lub-dup.

The heartbeat therefore has four phases involving the filling and contraction of each of its four chambers, but because the auricles and ventricles empty almost simultaneously, often only two phases can be heard through an ordinary stethoscope. All four may be heard when the resting heart rate is low. These four sounds are:

$S_4$ – LU systolic
$S_1$ – LUB systolic
$S_2$ – DUP diastolic
$S_3$ – DUP diastolic

## Regulation of the heart beat

The heart is essentially a self-contained organ which can carry on working without the direct intervention of the voluntary or involuntary nervous system. This explains why isolated hearts can continue to beat for a long time if kept in the correct environment. The heart has its own in-built nervous system in the form of a pacemaker otherwise known as the sino-atrial (S-A) node or SAN (Fig. 5.5). The SAN is situated in the right atrium (RA). An impulse originates at the SAN and spreads in all directions at a rapid rate, causing contraction of the atria. The muscle fibres of the atria are not continuous with those of the ventricles and so this impulse stops at the atrial-ventricular border.

The mass of ventricular tissue is much larger than that of the atrial tissue and so a special conducting system is required. This system is situated at the base of the septum or wall between the left and right atria. A small area of tissue similar to the SAN, but known as the atrio-ventricular (AV) node conducts the impulse at a much slower rate, ensuring a pause between the contraction of the atria and the ventricles. From the AV node, the impulse travels through a series of modified cardiac fibres (Purkinje fibres)

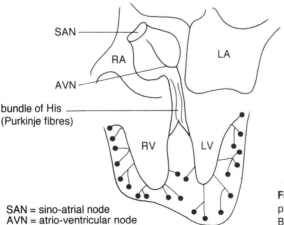

SAN = sino-atrial node
AVN = atrio-ventricular node

**Fig. 5.5**  Position of the natural pacemaker of the heart (SAN) and the Bundle of His.

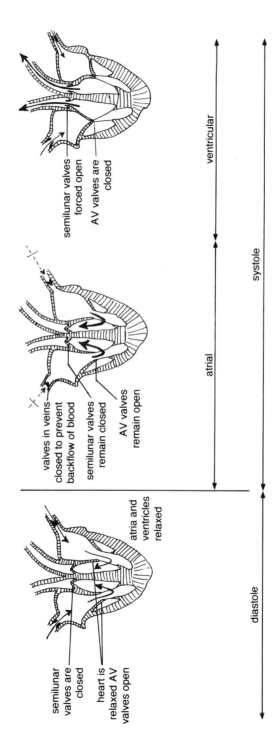

semilunar
valves are
closed

heart is
relaxed AV
valves open

atria and
ventricles
relaxed

valves in veins
closed to prevent
backflow of blood

semilunar valves
remain closed

AV valves
remain open

semilunar valves
forced open

AV valves are
closed

diastole

atrial

systole

ventricular

**Fig. 5.6**  Diagrammatic representation of the cardiac cycle.

which are arranged into a special bundle known as the Bundle of His. These structures cause the contraction of the ventricles.

The heart does have a nervous supply, but it is not responsible for starting the heart beat. Its role is to modify the rate and force of contraction of the heart according to the needs of the horse at the time.

The heart is therefore either filling with blood or contracting to pump it round the body. The period of the ventricles relaxing and filling is known as *diastole* and the period of active contraction is known as *systole* (Fig. 5.6).

# Blood vessels (Fig. 5.7)

## Arteries

Blood is carried from the heart to the tissues of the body in vessels known as arteries. If an artery is cut, bright red blood will spurt from the wound in time with the heart beat. These arteries gradually decrease in size and form branches as they become further away from the heart. This leads to a reduction in blood pressure as blood moves into the tissues.

The walls of the arteries contain several tissues including elastic, collagen and nerve fibres and smooth muscle. The proportion of elastic to muscle tissue changes from the large vessels to the smaller arteries at the outer limits. This results in two types, elastic and muscular arteries. The elastic arteries are those found closer to the heart and these act as a reservoir of blood.

The larger vessels give rise to smaller ones which have smooth muscle in their walls. These are known as arterioles, because they are able to contract and can regulate blood flow to various organs. The arterioles then supply the capillaries with blood. These are very thin-walled vessels whose walls are one cell thick. Here the blood gives up its oxygen, nutrients and hormones and collects waste products such as carbon dioxide. The capillaries then converge to form very small veins or venules and then progressively larger veins (Fig. 5.8).

## Veins

Veins have a similar structure to that of arteries, but the walls are much thinner and the proportion of muscular tissue is much less. The larger veins contain valves which prevent the back flow of blood. Muscular contractions of the horse's body helps to keep blood moving towards the heart. This is one reason why horses often develop filled legs when standing in a stable for a long time. This forced inactivity inhibits the venous return to the heart and once the horse starts walking again the swelling will often disappear.

Eventually venous blood will enter the great veins or vena cavae and be returned to the right auricle of the heart. If a vein is cut, dark red blood will trickle from the wound.

The horse's normal resting heart beat is 36–42 beats per minute. This can be taken by using a stethoscope or feeling for the pulse where an artery passes over bone, for example under the jaw.

When the horse is exercised, the demand for oxygen increases so that he can produce the energy required to contract muscles and move. In order to get this increased oxygen to the cells that require it, the heart has to beat faster to pump the blood to the tissues. The heart of the galloping horse can reach rates of up to 240 beats per minute, so that it takes only five seconds for a red blood cell to go around the body.

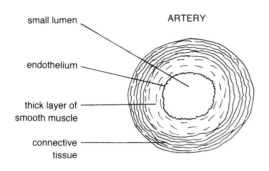

small lumen

ARTERY

endothelium

thick layer of smooth muscle

connective tissue

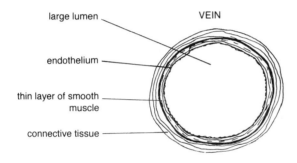

large lumen

VEIN

endothelium

thin layer of smooth muscle

connective tissue

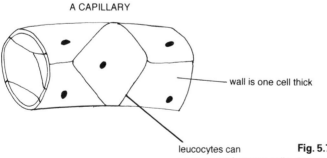

A CAPILLARY

wall is one cell thick

leucocytes can squeeze out between cells

**Fig. 5.7** Sections through the three types of blood vessels.

This can be compared to a human, whose resting heart rate is about 60 beats per minute, rising to a maximum of only 180.

## Heart abnormalities in the horse

Horses seldom die from heart disease, unlike humans. However, certain abnormalities of the equine heart tend to be quite common. It has been suggested that approximately

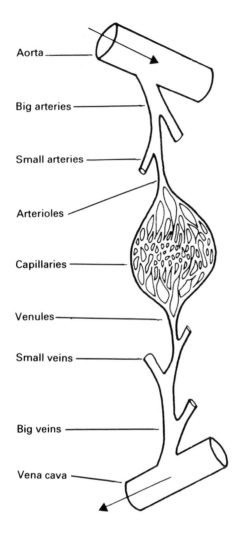

Aorta

Big arteries

Small arteries

Arterioles

Capillaries

Venules

Small veins

Big veins

Vena cava

**Fig. 5.8** Capillary network and the direction of blood through it.

50% of all horses have a heart which makes some odd noise or beats rather unevenly, but most of these horses seem to perform quite well.

Heart abnormalities in horses tend to be placed into one of two groups:

(1) Arrhythmias (unevenness of beat)
(2) Murmurs (extra noises).

## Arrhythmias

These tend to be more likely to upset the horse's athletic performance than heart murmurs. Arrhythmias may be found with a stethoscope, but more likely an electrocardiogram which records the electrical activity of heart muscle cells will reveal an arrhythmia.

Perhaps the most common arrhythmia is the dropped beat, i.e. just a 'lub' is heard instead of the normal 'lub-dup'. This is a fairly common phenomenon in fit horses at rest and when these horses work, the normal heart rhythm kicks into play. This is probably why most veterinary surgeons attach little significance to this condition. Atrial fibrillation is a more serious arrhythmia. The atria or auricles empty themselves by a series of flutters which fail to stimulate the ventricles properly. These then contract infrequently. This condition will produce a sudden drop in the horse's athletic performance. It is essential that the horse is given veterinary treatment in the form of drugs and rested until the heart beat returns to normal. This condition is also frequently seen in people who are stressed. It is possible that stress may also be involved in horses, but other known causes include infections such as strangles, influenza and herpes. These infections can produce inflammation of the heart muscle itself and this is known as myocarditis.

## Murmurs

These are without doubt the most common heart abnormalities in horses and they are often found during routine veterinary examinations, for example during the pre-purchase examination. Like arrhythmias, these murmurs can be found with the use of a stethoscope. A horse with a murmur will be heard to have one or more extra sounds during the normally quiet phase of the cardiac cycle. The interpretation of these abnormal sounds requires considerable expertise and experience. Some murmurs are benign in nature in that they have no effect on the horse's performance. Others are pathological and may severely affect the horse's health, let alone performance.

Heart murmurs are a result of turbulence within the normal flow of blood through the heart. A common cause seems to be a lesion on one or more of the heart valves. Some murmurs are fairly quiet whereas others are quite loud. A grading system has been established to describe the loudness of murmurs, ranging from 1 (faint murmur) to 6 (very loud).

When a heart murmur is detected it is important to have it investigated by the veterinary surgeon to establish whether it will affect the horse's performance.

## Heart monitors

Many trainers and owners of performance horses measure their horses' heart rates to monitor fitness. It is obviously impossible to use a stethoscope while the horse is moving. Heart meters or cardiotachometers are now available which give a readout of the cardiac cycle at a given time. They have been developed so that they can record the heart beat at fast speed for playback later. These machines are small and portable. Electrodes are placed in contact with the horse's skin and the machine is attached to the rider by a belt or is strapped to the horse's neck or saddle.

These heart monitors give a basic ECG (electrocardiograph) reading and can be very useful indeed in the training process.

In a healthy heart, the ECG will produce a standard trace on the machine known as PQRST complex (Fig. 5.10). The SAN pacemaker (see Fig. 5.5) creates an impulse which then travels over the RA and LA leading to contraction of the atria and producing the P wave on the ECG trace. The impulse is then slightly delayed at the AVN producing the gap between the P wave and the start of the QRS complex. This gap is known as the PQ interval. From the AVN, the impulse then passes along the Bundle of His to the ventricles to produce ventricular contraction creating QRS complex on the trace. The ventricles, having contracted, have to repolarise ready to accept the next contraction of the following heart beat (Fig. 5.11). This repolarisation shows as the T wave on a standard trace.

These traces from an ECG can be used to measure heart rate, rhythm and changes in conduction of impulses where heart problems are suspected.

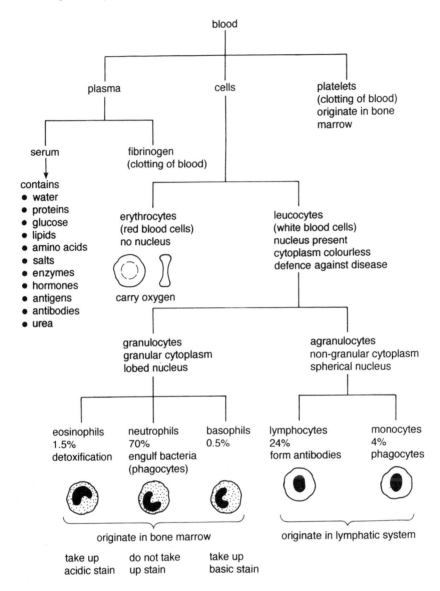

**Fig. 5.9**   Summary of the constituents of blood.

## The blood

The blood is the body's transport system and it consists of a fluid called plasma, in which are suspended red cells, white cells and platelets. It carries gases, nutrients, hormones and salts in solution and acts as a communication system reaching the whole body. A summary of blood constituents is shown in Fig. 5.9.

### Plasma

Plasma consists mainly of water (about 92%) with many substances dissolved in it, such as glucose, amino acids, hormones, salts, plasma proteins and antibodies. The plasma

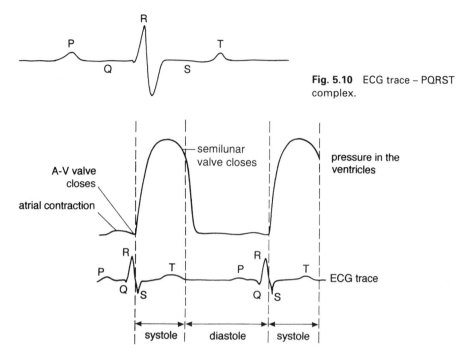

**Fig. 5.10** ECG trace – PQRST complex.

**Fig. 5.11** Relationship of pressure in the ventricles to the ECG during the cardiac cycle.

proteins consist of two major types, albumin and globulins. Albumin is the most abundant protein in the plasma and is important in binding and transporting many substances in the blood. The globulins are also made in the liver and their production is stimulated by the presence of antigens. Most of the antibodies are globulins and they are strongly associated with immunity and resistance to disease.

Plasma is often referred to as the 'internal environment' which bathes all the cells of the body. The kidneys are responsible for maintaining a constant level of water and other substances within the plasma.

The constituents of cells and plasma can easily be seen if a tube of blood, which has been prevented from clotting is left to stand. The heavier particles such as the cells and platelets settle to the bottom leaving the straw coloured plasma above. Approximately 45% of blood is made up of cells, the remaining 55% being plasma. (See Fig. 5.12 and Table 5.2.)

## Red blood cells (erythrocytes)

These are specialist cells designed to carry oxygen and some carbon dioxide. The red cells have lost their nucleus to make room for haemoglobin, an oxygen-carrying protein. The pigment part of the haemoglobin molecule requires iron.

Haemoglobin is able to form a reversible combination with oxygen and carbon dioxide:

haemoglobin + oxygen = oxyhaemoglobin
haemoglobin + carbon dioxide = carbohaemoglobin

In the lungs, the haemoglobin in the red cells combines with oxygen to form oxyhaemoglobin. As blood takes up oxygen it becomes a brighter red colour. This

**Table 5.1**   Components of blood plasma

| Substance | Source | Destination | Notes |
|---|---|---|---|
| Water | Absorbed in colon | All cells | Excess removed by kidneys |
| Plasma proteins e.g. fibrinogen and antibodies | Fibrinogen made in liver<br>Antibodies made by lymphocytes | Remain in the blood | Fibrinogen aids blood clotting.<br>Antibodies fight disease |
| Lipids, including cholesterol and fatty acids | Absorbed from the small intestine and also derived from bodies fat reserves | The liver for breakdown or the adipose tissue for storage | Breakdown of fats yields energy |
| Carbohydrates, e.g. glucose | Absorbed from the small intestine or derived from glycogen breakdown | To all cells for energy, released by the process of cellular respiration | Excess glucose is converted to glycogen and stored in liver and muscles |
| Urea and other excretory substances | Derived from amino acid breakdown in the liver (deamination) | To kidneys for excretion | |
| Mineral ions, e.g. Na, Cl | Absorbed in small intestine and colon | To all cells | Excess are excreted by kidneys |
| Hormones | Secreted into the blood by endocrine glands | To all parts of the body | Hormones only have an effect on their target organs. They are broken down in the liver and excreted by the kidneys |
| Dissolved gases, e.g. $CO_2$ | $CO_2$ is released from all cells as a waste product of respiration | To the lungs for excretion | Most $CO_2$ is carried as bicarbonate ($HCO_3^-$) in the plasma |

oxygenated blood is returned to the heart and pumped around the body to the various tissues, where some of the oxyhaemoglobin gives up its oxygen. When blood gives up its oxygen it becomes a much darker, deeper red colour. In the tissues, the red cells collect some carbon dioxide, forming carbohaemoglobin which is then returned to the lungs via the heart and the carbon dioxide is released and breathed out. However, most carbon dioxide is carried as bicarbonate ($HCO_3^-$) in the plasma (Fig. 5.13). The red cells are shaped like a biconcave disc, which increases the surface area for the exchange of oxygen.

Because the red cells have no nucleus, they have a limited life span of about three to four months. They therefore have to be constantly manufactured by the red bone marrow. A huge number of red cells disintegrate and are replaced daily. In the horse, it has been estimated that 35 million red blood cells are produced every second of the day! Old red blood cells are broken down and the iron containing part is used to make new red cells. The pigment portion is converted to the bile pigments bilirubin and biliverdin which are then excreted via the digestive tract.

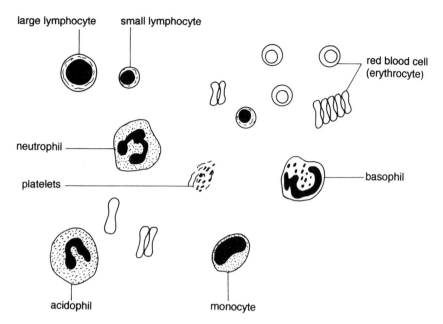

**Fig. 5.12**   Constituents of blood as seen at high magnification.

**Table 5.2**   The components of blood

| Component | Structure | Function |
|---|---|---|
| Plasma | Water containing many substances in solution | (1) Liquid medium in which cells and platelets float<br>(2) Transports $CO_2$<br>(3) Transports food substances<br>(4) Transports urea<br>(5) Transports hormones<br>(6) Transports heat<br>(7) Transports antibodies<br>(8) Transports blood clotting |
| Red cells | Biconcave discs, no nucleus, contain Hb | (1) Transport oxygen<br>(2) Transport small amount of $CO_2$ |
| White cells | Variable shape with nucleus | (1) Engulf and destroy bacteria (phagocytosis)<br>(2) Production of antibodies |
| Platelets | Small fragments with no nucleus | Aids blood clotting |

## White blood cells (leucocytes)

These cells form a major part of the body's defence mechanism. There are several types of white cell which respond to different types of challenge or infection.

White cells are made in the bone marrow and in the lymph nodes. Unlike the red blood cells, all white cells contain a nucleus and this is often quite large and lobed. White blood cells are capable of some independent movement, rather like an amoeba, and can squeeze out through the thin walls of blood capillaries into all parts of the body.

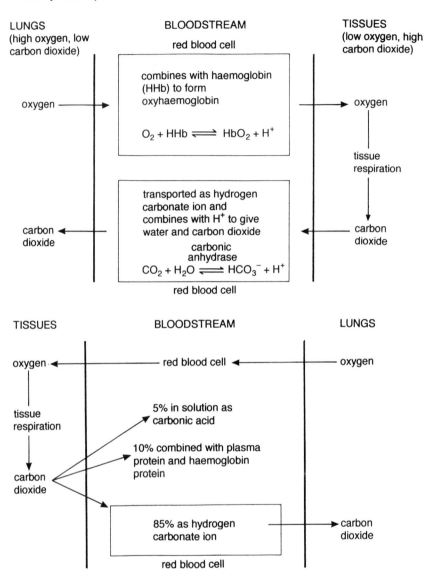

**Fig. 5.13** Summary of the transport of oxygen and carbon dioxide by the blood. The reactions shown are reversed when the blood reaches the capillary network surrounding the alveoli in the lungs.

They are then able to engulf and digest unwanted foreign substances such as invading bacteria.

They are far fewer in number than the red blood cells and they are larger. The horse has approximately 9000 per cubic millimetre of whole blood compared with seven million red cells per cubic millimetre. In general, the white cell count can vary and will rise to meet specific problems such as disease and infection. However, their number can also increase in response to normal physiological events, such as pregnancy, digestion of food and exercise.

White blood cells or leucocytes are classified as follows:

- Granulocytes – neutrophils, eosinophils, basophils
- Agranulocytes – monocytes, lymphocytes.

The life span of the white blood cells varies considerably. Granulocytes may last only a few hours whereas monocytes may last for months and lymphocytes for years. Within the blood system itself, the white blood cells tend to be non-functional and are simply being transported to sites within the horse's body where they are required.

## Granulocytes

As the name implies, these contain granules within their cytoplasm which stain with common stains used in blood staining tests. These stains contain an acid dye, eosin, which is red or a basic dye, methylene blue, which is blue. The granulocytes are named according to the colour of stain which the granules in their cytoplasm pick up. Thus the eosinophils stain red and the basophils blue. Neutrophils stain indifferently.

### Neutrophils

The commonest type of granulocyte is the neutrophil which accounts for over 70% of the white blood cells. These neutrophils are actively phagocytic, in other words they engulf bacteria and debris at the site of infection. A localised collection of pus is known as an abscess and the pus contains vast numbers of these neutrophil granulocytes. The neutrophils also degrade dead tissue in the area.

The number of neutrophils in the blood increases rapidly whenever acute infection is present, and this is one of the purposes of taking a blood sample. A blood test may show the presence of infection before the horse starts to show clinical signs. Neutrophils therefore, constitute the first line of defence against infection by migrating to any area invaded by bacteria, passing through the capillary walls to the site of infection.

### Eosinophils

Also known as acidophils, these white cells are found in much smaller quantities and account for approximately 2% of all white cells. Eosinophils are known to increase in number in certain chronic diseases such as parasite infections. They are also responsible for the detoxification of foreign proteins introduced into the body via the lungs or the gut. Their number also increases in allergic reactions.

### Basophils

These are also rare in normal blood. Since they contain the anticoagulant, heparin, it is thought that they may release this substance in areas of inflammation.

## Agranulocytes

As the name implies, these white cells show few granules in their rather sparse cytoplasm. These cells include monocytes and lymphocytes.

### Monocytes

These are the largest of the white cells and like the neutrophils they engulf foreign matter such as bacteria. However, while the neutrophils are active mainly in acute infections, the monocytes tend to be called into action for more long term, chronic infections such as tuberculosis in humans. When monocytes from the blood enter the tissues they develop into larger cells known as macrophages.

*Lymphocytes*

These are variable in appearance and size and have a relatively large nucleus surrounded by a small amount of cytoplasm. One of the major functions of the lymphocytes is their response to foreign substances or antigens. This involves the production of antibodies that circulate in the blood, or in the development of cellular immunity which is discussed in more detail in Chapter 14.

## Platelets

In addition to red and white blood cells, the blood also contains some tiny colourless corpuscles known as platelets or thrombocytes. Each platelet looks like a small rounded or oval disc and there are approximately 400 000 of them per cubic millimetre of blood. They are produced from large cells in the bone marrow called megakaryocytes. Platelets are also relatively short-lived with a life span of between nine and eleven days.

Platelets are important in the clotting of blood, particularly where blood vessels are damaged. The surface of platelets appears to be quite sticky and when blood is shed, the platelets tend to stick together in clusters. By adhering together and sticking to the surface of damaged blood vessels, they effectively form a plug or a clot thereby preventing further blood loss. Platelets are also responsible for the conversion of an element prothrombin which is present in the blood, to thrombin. Thrombin then assists in the blood clotting process (see below).

Two-thirds of all platelets in a healthy horse are in constant circulation in the blood. The remaining third are held in the spleen, ready for emergency use. If the spleen is removed, there is a persistent excess of platelets in the blood, known as thrombocytosis.

## Blood clotting

Whenever blood escapes from the body via a wound or injury, it quickly changes from a fluid to a thick jelly-like material called a clot. This process of clotting (or coagulation) is an essential process that prevents the valuable blood pouring from a wound which may otherwise result in the horse bleeding to death. Formation of a clot will also prevent the entry of bacteria into the horse's body.

The process of clotting is a highly complex one and is dependent upon a large number of factors. The times for clot formation vary between domestic animals. The horse seems to have a particularly long blood clotting time compared with other animals (Table 5.3).

The process of clotting (Fig. 5.14) depends upon the change in state of a blood protein found in the plasma called fibrinogen. Fibrinogen is normally found dissolved in the blood plasma, but when blood is shed, fibrinogen changes into a long fibrous

**Table 5.3** Average blood clotting times of some animals in minutes

| | |
|---|---|
| Horse | 11.5 |
| Cow | 6.5 |
| Dog | 2.5 |
| Sheep | 2.5 |
| Pig | 3.5 |
| Human | 5 |

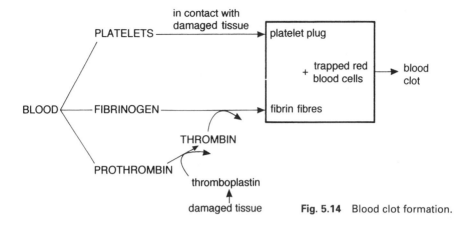

**Fig. 5.14** Blood clot formation.

network of molecules of fibrin. This network gradually contracts to form a clot and within its meshes are trapped various blood constituents such as red and white cells (Fig. 5.15). As the clot shrinks, a clear yellow fluid escapes from the wound and this is serum. It is quite simply plasma without the fibrinogen, which has been converted to fibrin. On the surface of the wound, the clot dries to form a scab and the healing process will take place underneath this mechanical protective covering.

Although clotting checks bleeding, it also helps to prevent potential leaks. For example, migrating worm larvae which may damage the lining of blood vessels, can result in the formation of clots within the blood vessel which will strengthen the damaged part. These clots, when remaining fixed are called thrombi. A thrombus can become so large that it completely blocks the blood vessel, preventing the flow of blood to further parts which may die as a result. The thrombus can also become loose and

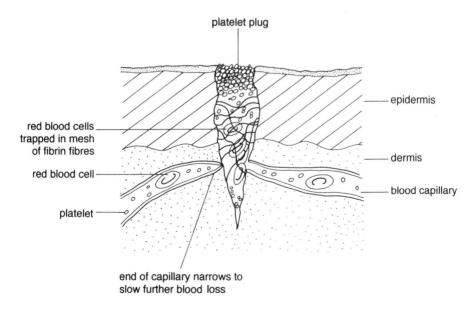

**Fig. 5.15** Vertical section through a blood clot. (Adapted from Jones, G. and Jones, M. (1987), *Biology GCSE Edition*, Cambridge University Press.)

float freely in the blood stream where it may cause a lethal blockage, called an embolus, elsewhere.

## Blood tests

There is no doubt that horses perform at their best when their blood constituents are within a normal range. Blood can change quite rapidly in response to disease, stress and electrolyte imbalances and regular blood tests will quickly identify problems often before clinical signs are shown by the horse. Changes in the blood will also occur as the horse's fitness increases. The blood parameters will also vary between individual horses.

Some horses such as racehorses and eventers are routinely blood tested to monitor their health and fitness. Each individual horse on such a yard may then have their results computerised and an overall picture of their blood patterns can be very useful when planning their training programmes and assessing their individual fitness. They should be used as an aid to diagnosis and to identify health problems. Blood tests also help a trainer to decide whether or not a horse should compete.

The blood tests generally fall into one of two categories:

(1) Haematology – the study of blood cells
(2) Biochemistry – the study of the chemistry of the substances in blood plasma.

When a blood sample is taken, the veterinary surgeon will not request that every possible test is undertaken on that sample. Some tests can be extremely expensive and will only be requested if there is suspicion of a particular problem. Other tests are fairly routine and basic.

It is wrong for horse owners to assume that when a vet takes a blood sample it will instantly reveal any problems. It depends completely upon the tests carried out on that sample. Most blood tests consist of investigating several routine blood parameters. Often the results from one of these routine analyses may suggest whether further tests should be carried out, but this is not always the case. Table 5.4 shows routine haematological and biochemical tests which are carried out on blood samples.

## Blood typing

Many breed societies now require that horses are blood typed before they are registered. This allows horses to be accurately identified. Although parents can be proven *not* to have produced individual offspring, they cannot be proven to be the parents.

The process of blood typing includes the mapping of the horse's blood group and certain proteins and enzymes within the serum which together produce a unique identification of the individual horse. Blood typing is carried out by using the genes which have control over the red blood cell antigens found on their surface. These antigens are known as blood factors and vary between groups of red blood cells, hence they can be used to identify blood groups. Also some of the serum proteins and enzymes such as albumin and transferrin are under gene control and can also be used. The blood factors and serum proteins and enzymes can be identified by biochemical and immunological assays on blood samples taken from the individual horse.

Because blood typing is genetically determined it remains the same throughout the horse's life and serves as a unique and permanent record of identification.

**Table 5.4**　Haematology and plasma biochemistry tests

| Blood test | Function | Normal range (SI units*) |
|---|---|---|
| **Haematology** | | |
| Red blood cells (erythrocytes) | Oxygen-carrying capacity | 6.5–12.3 |
| Haemoglobin | Low = anaemia | 11.2–16.2 |
| Haematocrit (packed cell volume) | Proportion of cells to plasma<br>Low = unfit or disease<br>High = electrolyte imbalance or exhaustion | 0.32–0.43 |
| Mean corpuscular volume (MCV) | Size of erthryocytes. New ones are larger than older ones<br>High = red worm damage | 36–46 |
| Mean corpuscular haemoglobin concentration (MCHC) | A guide to the oxygen-carrying capacity of blood<br>Low = severe anaemia | 29–37 |
| Total white blood cells | Vary in response to disease<br>Low = viral<br>High = bacterial infection | 5–10.5 |
| % neutrophils to total white blood cells | High shows bacterial infection | 60 |
| Neutrophilis | High = bacterial infection | Normal = 6. Range 2–7 |
| Lymphocytes | High = chronic bacterial/viral infection | Normal = 4. Range 1–6 |
| Monocytes | Seen in some viral infections | 0–0.4 |
| Eosinophils | Seen in allergic responses and parasitic infections | 0–0.3 |
| Basophils | A sign of inflammation | 0÷0.1 |
| **Plasma biochemistry** | | |
| Total protein albumins | Shows nutritional status and gut function.<br>Reflects feed quality<br>High = rhabdomyolysis<br>Low = poor liver function, poor feeding or intestinal disease | 60–80 gl<br>27–40 gl |
| Globulins (antibodies) | Increase with infection | 17–34 gl |
| Plasma viscosity (PV) or erythrocyte sedimentation rate (ESR) | Measure of blood condition<br>High = unfit or viral infection or poor performance syndrome | 1.4–1.7 centipoises |
| Plasma fibrinogen | Chronic infection, internal parasites | 0–3.0 gl |
| Calcium (Ca) | Vital for bone health and muscular function<br>Low Ca may be due to stress, laminitis or muscular problems | 2.6–3.9 mmol/l |
| Phosphorus (P) | Bone health | 0.8–1.8 mmol/l |
| Ca:P ratio | Phosphorus should be lower than calcium | 3 : 1 |
| Urea | High = kidney problems | 3.5–7.3 mmol/l |
| Bilirubin | Bile salt | 10–40 mmol/l |
| Enzymes – body function tests | | |
| Aspartate aminotransferase (AST/SGOT) | High = rhabdomyolysis, liver problems | 0–250 u/l |
| Creatine kinase (CK/CPK) | Muscle enzyme – rises with muscle breakdown, tying up | 0–100 mmol/l |

* Measured in standard SI units

## The lymphatic system

This is basically a system of fine tubes which run through the body in a similar way to blood vessels. The capillaries which carry blood allow leakage of plasma into the tissues. The white blood cells are also able to squeeze through gaps in the capillary wall, but red blood cells cannot. The result of this is that white blood cells and plasma continuously move out of the capillaries and bathe all the tissues within the body. This fluid is called tissue fluid and supplies all cells with nutrients and oxygen. Carbon dioxide and waste products then diffuse back into the capillaries.

Because each cell is bathed with tissue fluid, it provides a constant environment, i.e. a constant temperature and osmotic pressure. This consistency is vital for the health of cells and is known as homeostasis.

The main function of the lymphatic system is to help drain away the tissue fluids and eventually return them to the blood. Within the tissues, alongside the capillaries, are other small vessels called lymphatic capillaries. The tissue fluid slowly drains into these tubes and the fluid once within the lymphatic vessels is known as lymph (Fig. 5.16). The smaller lymphatic vessels link up with larger, blind ending ones which carry the lymph to the subclavian veins where it rejoins the blood in the horse's chest. The smaller tubes have a thin wall which is one cell thick, whereas the larger vessels have connective tissue in their walls.

The walls of the lymphatic vessels do not contain muscle tissue and therefore they are unable to actively propel the lymph along the vessels. The intermittent pressure of surrounding muscles helps to push lymph along the vessels and valves within the larger lymphatic vessels prevent back flow and keep the lymph moving in one direction only. Before the lymph drains back into the blood it passes through lymphatic tissue. This

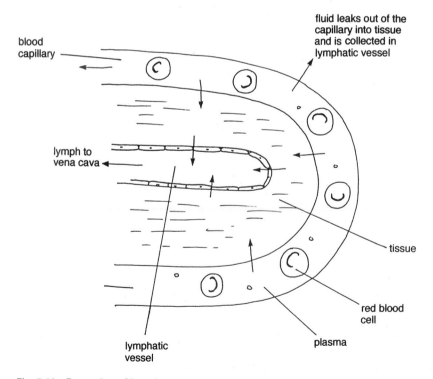

**Fig. 5.16**  Formation of lymph.

consists of lymphocytes and the cells which produce them and macrophages. The function of these is to destroy any bacteria or toxins which may have been drained away from the tissues and so help to reduce the chances of infection.

This lymphatic tissue may collect together in groups surrounded by connective tissue and these constitute the lymph nodes (Fig. 5.17). The lymph nodes are found in areas such as the neck, base of the bronchi and along the larger blood vessels in the abdominal cavity. Lymph nodes may become enlarged and tender when the horse has an infection. An example is the mandibular gland which sits between the angles of the lower jaw. This often becomes swollen in young horses as a result of bacteria passing from the lining of the airways of the head to the lymphatic vessels. Some bacteria, for example *Streptococcus equi* which causes strangles may result in the production of an abscess containing pus which eventually bursts through the skin under the jaw.

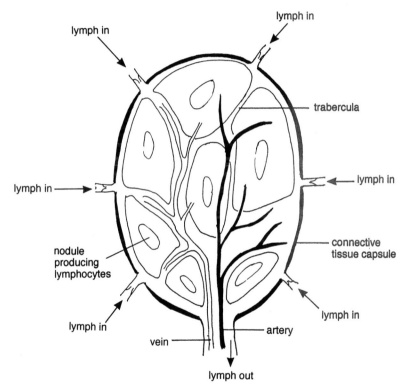

**Fig. 5.17** Diagram of a lymph node showing incoming lymph vessels.

## Filled legs

The main function of the lymphatic system is to drain away excess fluid from parts of the body. The pressure in the blood vessels of the horse is greatest in the lower leg, due to the influence of gravity. Often the water balance within the vascular system and tissue system can become unbalanced or upset due to differing concentrations of salts and proteins between the two. This may lead to excess water within the lymph system which leads to filled legs.

Too little exercise and too much feed can disturb this delicate protein and blood salt balance and the lymphatic system becomes unable to drain away all the excess water.

**Table 5.5**   The lymphatic system

---

- Lymph makes up 2–3% of the total body fluids of the horse.
- Lymph absorbs and transports fats from the intestines to the blood.
- Lymph returns fluid to the anterior vena cava and the subclavian vein.
- Horses have large groups of lymph nodes where other animals would have just one or two.
- Due to the structure of some of the larger lymphatic vessels and their entrance to the lymph nodes, it would seem that a substantial proportion of the lymph fluid is not exposed to the phagocytosis and other disease-clearing processes until deep within the node itself.

---

Lack of exercise, for example when a horse is standing in the stable, will exacerbate the problem because exercise helps to move the lymph back up the leg against the pull of gravity. The result is a filled leg, which disappears when the horse is exercise.

Other causes of filled legs include toxins which damage the walls of the blood and lymph vessels, allowing the drainage of lymph into the lymphatic system at an abnormally high rate. Allergic reaction, viral or bacterial infections can all have a similar effect. High protein diets may also cause an upset leading to filled legs.

Often bacterial infections will spread to the lymphatic vessels, causing inflammation. This happens with the condition known as lymphangitis which is more severe than filled legs and may result in a permanently swollen leg, more commonly in the hind legs as they are furthest away from the horse's heart. Also, localised infections within the lymphatic vessels may become so bad that ulcers burst through the skin of the lower leg. True lymphangitis will result in lameness.

Occasionally, heavily pregnant mares will develop swellings on their bellies due to the lymphatic vessels being unable to cope with the increased workload from development of the mammary glands. This usually dissipates quite soon after birth.

# Chapter 6
# The Control Systems

Horses need to respond to their environment. They need fast and efficient internal communication systems in order to survive.

Animals have two coordinating systems, namely the endocrine (hormonal) and nervous systems which work together triggering responses to external stimuli. In horses the flight or fight response to danger is brought about by both nervous and hormonal signals; however, the nervous system is much faster in its reactions and is also responsible for the control of more delicate movements by the horse's body.

The endocrine system is involved with information transfer. It consists of a series of ductless glands and its operation is much slower than the nervous system. It controls the horse's behavioural patterns by releasing hormones which are responsible for numerous body processes including growth, metabolism, sexual development and function.

## The nervous system

This is a highly intricate and organised data processing system. A cubic centimetre of brain contains several million nerve cells. The nervous system of the horse detects and interprets changes in conditions both inside and outside the horse's body, and then responds to them. It is effectively three interconnected systems:

(1) Sensory input
(2) Integration
(3) Motor output.

The sensory input (Fig. 6.1) is the conduction of signals or messages from the sensory receptors such as the nose, eyes, ears, skin, etc., to processing centres in the brain and spinal cord. Integration is the interpretation of all these sensory signals within the processing centres. Motor output (Fig. 6.2) is the conduction of signals to the effector cells such as muscles which move in direct response to the signal. So, information in the form of signals passes from the receptors to processing centres and from there to the effectors.

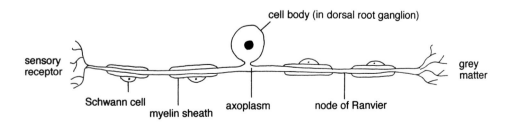

**Fig. 6.1**  Sensory neuron – afferent neuron.

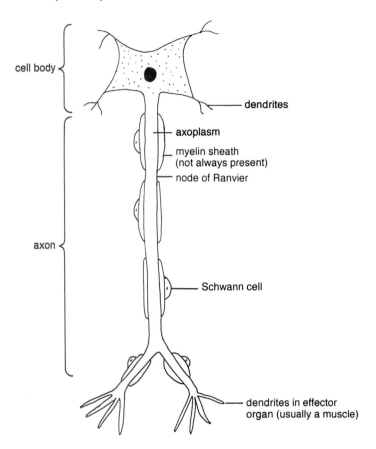

cell body

dendrites

axoplasm

myelin sheath
(not always present)

node of Ranvier

axon

Schwann cell

dendrites in effector
organ (usually a muscle)

**Fig. 6.2**   Motor neuron – efferent neuron.

The cables along which all this information is carried are the nerves. Each nerve consists of a bundle of filaments known as axons which originate from the nerve cell or neuron.

All neurons contain the same basic parts as any animal cell, but they are specially adapted to be able to carry electrical impulses. To enable them to do this they have long thin fibres of cytoplasm stretching out from the cell body. These are the nerve fibres; the longest ones are known as axons which can be more than 1 m long. The shorter fibres are known as dendrites. The dendrites are able to collect messages from other neurons nearby. They pass these messages to the cell body and then along the axon. The axon may then pass the message to another neuron.

The nerve fibres of horses are wrapped in a layer of insulating material called myelin which forms a sheath around the nerve fibre. These insulated fibres carry impulses much more quickly than those fibres without a myelin sheath. The nerve fibres are usually in groups of several hundred and this group is known as a nerve (Fig. 6.3).

For convenience, the nervous system is divided into two main parts, the central nervous system (CNS) and the peripheral nervous system (PNS) (Fig. 6.4). CNS consists of the brain and spinal cord. PNS is made up mostly of communication nerves which carry signals out of the CNS. The PNS also has ganglia. These are clusters of nerve cell bodies belonging to neurons which make up the nerves.

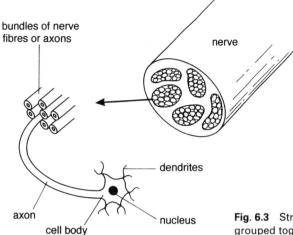

bundles of nerve
fibres or axons

nerve

dendrites

axon

cell body

nucleus

**Fig. 6.3** Structure of a nerve. Many nerve fibres grouped together form a nerve.

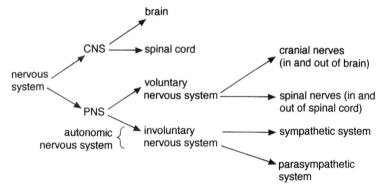

brain

CNS → spinal cord

nervous system

PNS

voluntary nervous system

autonomic nervous system

involuntary nervous system

cranial nerves (in and out of brain)

spinal nerves (in and out of spinal cord)

sympathetic system

parasympathetic system

*Parasympathetic*

- slows the heart
- dilates arteries
- constricts bronchioles
- constricts pupil (iris)
- stimulates tear gland
- stimulates flow of saliva
- speeds up gut movement
- relaxes bladder and anal sphincters
- contracts bladder

*Sympathetic*

- accelerates the heart
- constricts arteries
- dilates bronchioles
- dilates pupil (iris)
- contracts erector pill muscles
- increases sweat production
- slows down gut movement
- contracts bladder and anal sphincter
- relaxes bladder

**Fig. 6.4** Nervous system.

## CNS

The CNS consists of the brain and spinal cord which are protected by the skull and spinal column respectively. The CNS receives input from the sense organs such as the skin, eyes, ears, etc. and sends signals to the muscles and glands via the peripheral nervous system.

## PNS

This system consists of all the nerves which connect the brain and spinal cord to the rest of the horse's body. The nerves and ganglia of the PNS form a vast communications network. The nerves which carry signals to and from the brain are known as cranial nerves whereas those carrying signals to and from the spinal cord are known as the spinal nerves. The horse's eyes, nose, tongue and ears, for example, are served by the cranial nerves whereas the muscles and skin of the limbs are serviced by the spinal nerves.

All spinal nerves and most of the cranial nerves contain both sensory and motor neurons. Hundreds of thousands of signals, both incoming and outgoing, pass each other within the same nerves all the time.

In addition to these anatomical divisions of the nervous system, there are also functional divisions. Two of the most important are the autonomic nervous system which is concerned with the automatic or unconscious regulation of internal body functioning and the somatic system which controls the muscles responsible for voluntary or willed movement.

## Neurons

Neurons or nerve cells are the basic units of nerves. There are three main types of neuron:

(1) Motor neurons carry signals from the CNS to muscles or glands. The axon terminals form a motor end plate.
(2) Sensory neurons carry signals from the sense receptors situated within sense organs along their axons to the CNS.
(3) Intermediate, interneurons or relay neurons form all the complex interconnecting nerves within the CNS itself.

For each sensory neuron in the horse's body there are about 10 motor neurons and 99 intermediate neurons.

A neuron consists of a cell body and several branching projections known as dendrites. Every neuron also has a filamentous outgrowth called an axon or nerve fibre. Axons vary in length from a millimetre to a metre. Dendrites receive stimuli and axons send stimuli. The axon branches at its end to form terminals via which signals are transmitted to the target cells, such as dendrites of other neurons, muscle cells or glands. Axons tend to be grouped together in bundles and these are known as nerves.

Groups of nerve cell bodies within the spinal cord or brain are generally called the nuclei, whereas groups of nerve cells outside of the brain and spinal cord are usually called ganglia. Regions of the brain and spinal cord consist mainly of closely packed nuclei of nerve cells and these form the grey matter. The filamentous axons produce the white matter. If the cell body of a neuron is damaged or dies, it is never replaced. A foal therefore starts life with a maximum number of neurons which continuously decreases throughout the horse's life. However, if a peripheral nerve is damaged the fibres are able to regenerate themselves slowly.

The function of the neuron is to transmit an electrical impulse along its axon under certain very specific conditions. The electrical impulse triggers the release of a chemical known as a neurotransmitter from the axon terminals. This neurotransmitter, once released, may have one of a series of effects. It may:

- make a muscle cell contract;
- make an endocrine gland release a hormone into the blood;
- cause an electrical impulse in a neighbouring neuron.

Different stimuli will excite different types of neurons. For example, sensory neurons may be excited by a physical stimuli such as heat or cold, or pressure on the skin. The activity of most neurons is controlled by the effects of neurotransmitters released from neighbouring neurons.

### Action potential

The ability of a neuron to carry an electrical impulse depends upon a small difference in electrical potential between the inside and the outside of the cell. Under the direct influence of an excitatory neurotransmitter, a sudden change in electrical potential occurs at one point on the cell's membrane. This change is known as an action potential and it flows along the cell membrane, and therefore along the axon of the cell, at up to 250 miles per hour (110 m/s).

The neurotransmitter brings about a change in sodium and potassium ions inside the outside and cell membrane. These changes produce a voltage which leads to an electrical impulse or signal passing through the nerve cell. A neuron is capable of transmitting electrical impulses this way several times per second.

Different neurons are stimulated by different parameters, such as light, temperature, taste, smell, pain, touch, and oxygen, carbon dioxide and glucose levels in the blood etc. Other neurotransmitters are capable of preventing action potentials and therefore have a stabilising effect on the cell membrane of the neuron. A balance of the two – excitatory and inhibitory influences – will determine the impulse firing pattern of the nerve cell.

## Synapses

There is a gap between the junction of two neurons across which a signal has to pass. A single neuron may have thousands of these connections with neighbouring ones. A typical neuron as described previously has one axon that projects from its cell body and this splits into several smaller branches, each ending in a terminal which forms a synapse which is usually close to the cell body of another neuron (Fig. 6.5). At a

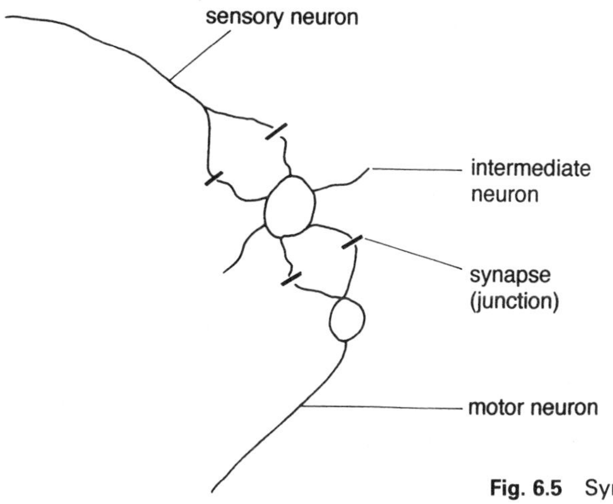

**Fig. 6.5** Synapse.

synapse the two neurons do not actually come into direct contact, because their two surface membranes are separated by a gap known as the synaptic cleft. When an electrical impulse travels along the axon to the synapse, it cannot bridge this gap directly. Instead it causes the release of a neurotransmitter chemical which then bridges the gap and produces a change in the electrical potential of the membrane of the next neuron. An example of a neurotransmitter is acetyl choline.

The axon membrane from which the neurotransmitter is released is known as the presynaptic membrane and the membrane at which the chemical is received is known as the postsynaptic membrane. This is important because signals may pass across a synapse in one direction only, from presynaptic to postsynaptic membrane. This is because the neurotransmitter is produced only by the presynaptic membrane.

An enzyme known as cholinesterase breaks down the acetyl choline making it inactive after the passage of an impulse across the synapse. This is so that an impulse is not continuously generated at the synapse.

As with neurons, a synapse may be excitatory or inhibitory. If a neurotransmitter passes across an excitory synapse the effect is to excite the postsynaptic membrane thus producing an electrical impulse in the receiving neuron. Inhibitory synapses have the function of reducing the excitation of the next neuron.

## Neurotransmitters

There are many different types of neurotransmitters within the horse's body (Fig. 6.6). Many neurotransmitters also act as hormones, such as noradrenaline. These are released into the blood where they are taken to their target cells. Noradrenaline is important in the nervous control of blood flow, heart beat and the horse's responses to stress. This hormone is also produced by the adrenal glands as well as the neurons.

Perhaps one of the most important neurotransmitters is acetyl choline which is released by neurons connected to skeletal muscles, causing these muscles to contract, and also to neurons which are connected to other nerve cells which have an effect on the sweat glands and the heart beat. Acetyl choline is also responsible for transmitting impulses between neurons and the brain and spinal cord.

Dopamine is another neurotransmitter, which plays an important part in the area of the brain which controls movement. Serotonin is another chemical which is found in those parts of the brain which are concerned with conscious activity.

### Neuropeptides

Recently a new group of neurotransmitters has been discovered. These are known as neuropeptides and are small proteins which are larger than the previously known neurotransmitters. Neuropeptides are peptide hormones and they have a regulatory effect, being secreted by cells situated throughout the horse's body. Neuropeptides include renin, glucagon, gastrin and somatostatin. Relatively recently, other neuropeptides have come to light such as the encephalins and endorphins. These are secreted by neuroendocrine cells in the brain in response to severe pain or stress. They have a strong analgesic or painkilling effect and are thought to block pain impulses at specific sites in the spinal cord and brain. The application of a twitch to a horse is thought to result in the secretion of endorphins which reduce the pain felt by the horse.

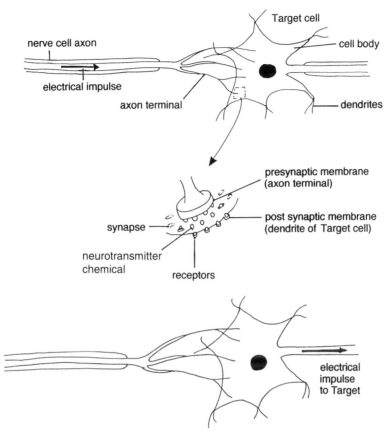

**Fig. 6.6** Function of neurotransmitters.

## The peripheral nervous system (PNS)

The PNS undertakes extremely complex tasks. It has a sensory division and a motor division.

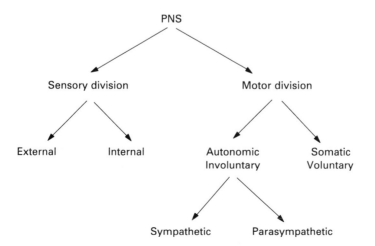

## Sensory division of the PNS

This has two sets of neurons: one set supplies information concerning the outside environment from, for example, the ears, eyes and skin, and the other set supplies information concerning the inside environment, such as the acidity of the blood and body temperature.

## Motor division of the PNS

The body's motor neurons make up this second major division of the PNS. Within the motor division, neurons of the somatic nervous system carry signals to skeletal muscles mainly in response to external stimuli. The somatic nervous system is said to be voluntary in that many of the actions it produces are under conscious control. Conversely, the motor neurons of the autonomic or self-governing system are generally involuntary.

## The autonomic nervous system

This consists of two sets of neurons with opposing effects on most of the internal organs. One set is known as the parasympathetic system and this prepares the body for activities which gain and conserve energy in the body, such as stimulation of the salivary glands and digestive juices and decreasing of the heart and respiratory rates. The other set of neurons is known as the sympathetic system which tends to have the opposite effect, preparing the body for energy consuming activities such as fight or flight. The digestive organs are inhibited, the heart and respiratory rates are increased and the liver releases glucose into the blood. The adrenal glands secrete hormones. It can be seen that the sympathetic and parasympathetic systems are at opposite extremes and the horse's body normally functions at an intermediate level, i.e. somewhere between the two.

Sympathetic and parasympathetic neurons emerge from different regions of the CNS and they use different neurotransmitters. Acetyl choline is the neurotransmitter released by neurons of the parasympathetic system and these neurons emerge from the brain and distal part of the spinal cord.

Norepinephrine is the neurotransmitter released by neurons of the sympathetic system and these neurons emerge from the more central regions of the spinal cord. The sympathetic and parasympathetic systems, carrying command signals, constitute lower levels of the hierarchy of the nervous system as a whole. The CNS is the major site from where these commands originate.

## The brain

The brain is the control centre of the nervous system. It contains millions of highly organised neurons with a large number of supporting cells, all intricately arranged within the skull or cranium.

The brain has a jelly-like consistency and is protected by membranous layers known as the meninges. The skull and the meninges have a highly protective function – to prevent injury to the brain. The meninges consist of three layers: the dura mater (thick and tough), arachnoid layer (contains blood-vessels and fluid) and the pia mater (helps to nourish the brain).

The vertebrate brain has evolved from what were originally a group of bulges at the top of the spinal cord. These three ancestral regions, known as the forebrain, midbrain and hindbrain, can still be seen during embryonic development. As the brain evolved further, these three regions became subdivided into specific regions, with particular responsibilities.

## Intelligence

The forebrain contains the largest and most sophisticated area of the brain known as the cerebrum. The cerebrum is folded to increase the surface area and so the larger the cerebrum and the more folded it is, the better it performs. The horse's cerebrum is highly folded but it is now thought that it is the brain volume to body size ratio that is the most accurate method of intelligence.

The human brain and that of the porpoise are highly folded and these mammals also have the largest brain surface area to body size, making them highly intelligent. The human brain weighs approximately 1.3 kg (3 lb).

The horse's brain is relatively small compared with its body weight and it weighs approximately 0.65 kg (1.5 lb) or about 1% of its body weight. The horse is not considered to be a highly intelligent animal and the cerebrum is much smaller than that of the human. The horse is ultimately an animal of instinct and this shows in its behaviour. Reasoning and conscious thought are not abilities that we associate with horses, although there is no doubt that they can, and do, suffer from depression which is often brought about by poor management.

Figure 6.7 shows the three ancestral brain regions and their subdivisions.

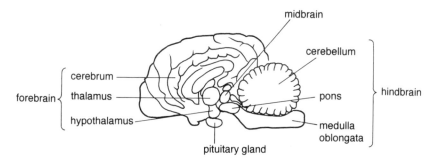

**Fig. 6.7**   Brain of the horse.

## Hindbrain

This consists of three parts: the medulla oblongata, pons and the cerebellum.

### Medulla oblongata and pons

The medulla oblongata and the pons contain all the sensory and motor neurons passing between the spinal cord and the forebrain. These parts are therefore responsible for conducting information. They also control heart rate and breathing and help to coordinate the horse's movements – walking, trotting, cantering, etc.

### Cerebellum

The cerebellum is mainly responsible for fine tuning and balance of movement. The cerebellum of the horse compared with other species is relatively large. This could be expected due to the horse's ability to move fast over most types of ground.

## Midbrain

This relays sensory information to the cerebrum, such as sound and touch. In mammals, sight is dealt with mainly by the forebrain with the midbrain coordinating eye reflexes such as blinking. Part of the midbrain is also associated with sleep and waking.

## Forebrain

The most sophisticated information processing occurs in this region of the brain. The three main centres are the hypothalamus, the thalamus and the large cerebrum.

### Hypothalamus

The hypothalamus, although small, is important in controlling homeostasis, i.e. maintaining the horse's internal environment, such as body temperature and blood chemistry, etc. It also controls the pituitary gland and thus the secretion of many of the body's hormones; and it regulates the fight or flight response which is a strong instinct in horses.

### Thalamus

The thalamus contains most of the cell bodies of the neurons that relay information to the cerebrum, and is able to exert some control over sensory messages, which is receives and then sends, by suppressing some signals and enhancing others.

### Cerebrum

The cerebrum is the largest part of the brain. It consists of two halves, the right and left cerebral hemisphere, which are joined together by a thick band of nerve fibres called the corpus callosum. Beneath the corpus callosum, are large clusters of nerve cell bodies known as the basal ganglia. These are important in motor coordination.

The surface of the cerebrum is folded to increase the surface area. The nerve cell bodies are situated in the outer layer of the cerebrum known as the cerebral cortex, and this area is therefore known as the grey matter, whereas the inner areas which are rich in nerve fibres are known as the white matter.

The cerebral cortex stores information with regard to memory, consciousness and sensory perception, and interprets visual and sound signals. It is able to interpret all the sensory information which it receives and then act upon it. The cerebral cortex does not contain any pain-detecting cells.

## Spinal cord

This is a cylinder of nerve tissue which is as thick as a thumb and runs down the central canal of the spine. It is an extension of the brain and together with the brain makes up the central nervous system (Fig. 6.8).

At the centre of the spinal cord is a region whose cross-section is shaped like a butterfly and this is the grey matter. This contains the cell bodies of neurons and supporting cells. Some of the neurons are motor neurons whose axons pass out of the spinal cord in bundles within the spinal nerves and pass to muscles or glands in the horse's trunk or legs. Others are the intermediate neurons which connect between other neurons. Entering the grey matter are also sensory neurons which have their cell bodies just outside the spinal cord and these connect with the motor or intermediate neurons. The grey matter is surrounded by tracts of nerve fibres running lengthways through the spinal cord and this is the white matter.

Sprouting from the spinal cord on each side at regular intervals are two nerve bundles, the spinal nerve roots which contain the nerve fibres of the motor and sensory nerve cells. These join together to form the spinal nerves which connect the spinal cord to all parts of the trunk and legs.

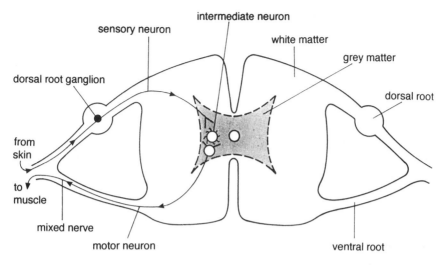

**Fig. 6.8** Section through the spinal cord.

The nerves that make up the white matter act as pathways for sensory information passing upwards to the brain or motor signals passing downwards. The cord is capable of handling some of the sensory information itself and of inducing motor responses without involving the brain itself. These are the reflex actions.

## Reflex actions

These account for only a small part of the behaviour of horses. A reflex is an action which occurs automatically and more importantly, predictably, to a particular stimulus. This reflex action is completely independent of the will of the horse. The stimulus is supplied by one or more senses and an action is initiated by the nervous system in response to the stimulus.

In the simplest reflex, a sensory nerve cell – perhaps at the skin surface of the horse – reacts to pressure or heat. The sensory cell sends a signal along its axon or nerve fibre to the CNS (brain and spinal cord). Here the fibre connects to a motor neuron which initiates a muscle contraction to move the horse away from the heat or pressure. The passage of the nervous impulse from the source, through the sensory neuron to the motor neuron and finally to the muscle is known as a reflex arc (Fig. 6.9). Often, however, the reflex arcs are more complicated than this example.

Many reflexes are present from birth such as shivering in response to cold or the emptying of the bladder when it is full. Other examples of reflex actions include sneezing, coughing, swallowing and blinking and the horse has no voluntary control over these actions. The autonomic nervous system (Fig. 6.10) is responsible for these bodily functions but some autonomic reflexes are under partially voluntary control. For example, an older horse may consciously delay urinating or staling in the field until he is brought in to the stable. Ultimately, however, the reflex is stronger than the will and if the horse is not brought in to the stable until later than normal he may not be able to hold on as the reflex exerts its control.

Other reflexes are conditioned, having been brought about by experience of the horse through its lifetime. These experiences result in the formation of new pathways and junctions within the nervous system itself. These ways in which these processes are acquired is known as conditioning. Learning is a type of operand conditioning in

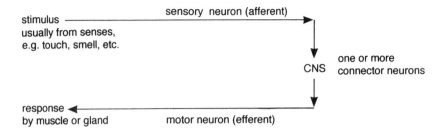

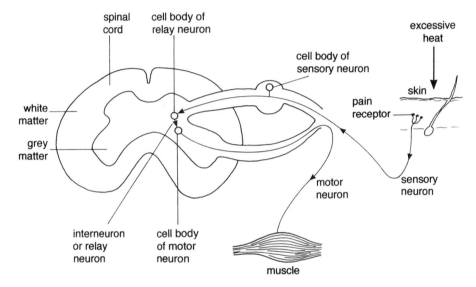

**Fig. 6.9**   A simple reflex action or arc. The lower diagram shows spinal cord involvement.

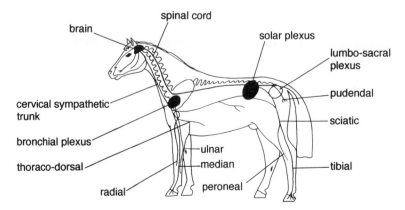

**Fig. 6.10**   The major nerves of the horse.

that once a response to a new situation has been repeated several times, a response becomes automatically initiated next time that stimulus occurs. For example, a horse will learn to move away from the handler when a hand is placed against his side. Eventually he will do this automatically and without conscious will.

## The endocrine system

Nerves carry electrical messages at high speed from one part of the horse's body to another. However, another much slower messenger system exists and this is the endocrine system. The endocrine system controls the horse's behaviour patterns and it sends chemical messages in the form of hormones to target organs.

The word 'hormone' is derived from the Greek word 'hormon' which means to activate. Hormones are manufactured in special glands known as endocrine glands. The most important endocrine glands in the horse are shown in Fig. 6.11. Hormones are responsible for numerous body processes including metabolism, stress responses, growth and sexual development and function. An increase or decrease in the hormone level will produce a change in the process it controls. Unlike exocrine glands which pass their secretions through ducts to the target area, for example salivary glands, endocrine glands do not have ducts and they release their hormones directly into the bloodstream to be transported to the target organs. They are therefore often known as ductless glands. Glands of the endocrine system include the ovaries, testes, adrenal glands, pancreas, pituitary gland, pineal gland, thyroid gland and the parathyroid glands. Hormones are also secreted by the placentas of pregnant mares. These glands control puberty, growth, pregnancy and birth, lactation, aggression etc. All endocrine glands have a good blood supply with capillaries running straight through them so that when the hormones are manufactured they can be released immediately into the blood, where they dissolve in the plasma. Each kind of hormone is specific in its effects on certain target organs.

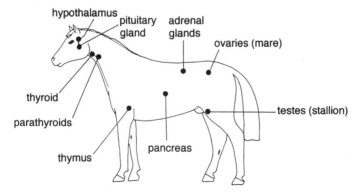

**Fig. 6.11** The endocrine glands of the horse.

There are other differences between the nervous and endocrine systems besides the fact that the nervous system carries messages so much faster. Because hormones are carried in the blood, they are longer lasting than the quick, short acting impulses carried by the nerves.

## Hypothalamus

As mentioned previously the hypothalamus is a region of the brain, which is about the size of a cherry. The hypothalamus exerts overall control over the sympathetic nervous system and it therefore has nerve connections to most other parts of the nervous system. The hypothalamus has a direct contact with the pituitary gland through a short stalk of nervous fibres. It can therefore stimulate the pituitary gland in one of two ways. It may release hormones into the blood which will arrive at the pituitary gland or it may send nerve signals. In this way the hypothalamus can convert nervous signals to hormonal ones. It secretes releasing hormones which stimulate the pituitary gland to produce other hormones (Fig. 6.12).

The hypothalamus has indirect control over many of the endocrine glands including the thyroid gland, adrenal glands, the ovaries and testes.

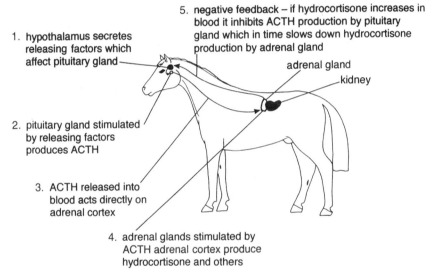

1. hypothalamus secretes releasing factors which affect pituitary gland

2. pituitary gland stimulated by releasing factors produces ACTH

3. ACTH released into blood acts directly on adrenal cortex

4. adrenal glands stimulated by ACTH adrenal cortex produce hydrocortisone and others

5. negative feedback – if hydrocortisone increases in blood it inhibits ACTH production by pituitary gland which in time slows down hydrocortisone production by adrenal gland

adrenal gland

kidney

**Fig. 6.12** The effects of negative feedback on the hypothalamus and pituitary gland.

## Pituitary gland

This is sometimes referred to as the master gland as it regulates and controls the operation of other endocrine glands and many of the important body processes of the horse. The pituitary gland is about the size of a pea and hangs down from the base of the brain. It is attached by a stalk of nerve fibres to the hypothalamus which is inside the brain. The pituitary gland consists of two lobes known as the anterior and posterior lobes, each producing a range of hormones.

The anterior pituitary lobe produces six hormones:

- Growth hormone – responsible for growth;
- prolactin – stimulates milk production from the udder after birth;
- adrenocorticotrophic hormone (ACTH) – stimulates the adrenal glands;
- thyroid stimulating hormone (TSH) – stimulates the thyroid gland;
- follicle stimulating hormone (FSH) – stimulates the ovaries and testes;
- luteinising hormone (LH) – stimulates the ovaries.

The posterior pituitary lobe produces two hormones:

- antidiuretic hormone (ADH) – increases resorption of water by the kidneys and therefore reduces the volume of urine produced (see Chapter 10);
- oxytocin – produces contractions of the uterus during the birth of the foal and stimulates milk secretion from the udder in response to suckling from the foal.

Pituitary adenomas (tumours) may be responsible for laminitis and produce a long and often curly coat even in the summer months.

## Thyroid gland

This gland is situated on either side of the voice box or larynx. It consists of two lobes, one on each side of the trachea. The two lobes are connected by a narrow strip known as the isthmus. Figure 6.13 shows a section through the thyroid gland.

Thyroid tissue is composed of two types of cells:

- Follicular cells – arrange in spherical, hollow follicles these cells are responsible for the secretion of thyroxine (T4) and triiodothyronine (T3). Thyroxine contains iodine. The hollow space is filled with a thick fluid material which is responsible for producing the T3 and T4 hormones.
- Parafollicular cells or C cells – arranged in small groups in the spaces between the hollow follicles and secrete the hormone calcitonin.

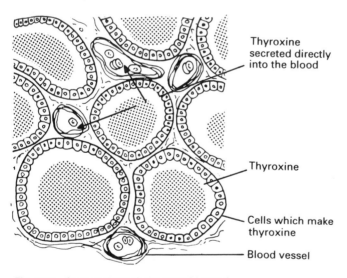

Thyroxine secreted directly into the blood

Thyroxine

Cells which make thyroxine

Blood vessel

**Fig. 6.13** Section through the thyroid gland.

## Thyroid hormones

T3 and T4 are responsible for regulating the horse's metabolism. Calcitonin works in conjunction with parathyroid hormone secreted by the parathyroid glands to maintain the calcium balance within the horse's body.

## Parathyroids

This group of four small glands lies behind the lobes of the thyroid gland in the horse's neck. The parathyroids secrete parathyroid hormone which is released into the bloodstream if the blood level of calcium decreases. This causes the bones to release more calcium into the blood, the gut to absorb more calcium from food and the kidneys to conserve calcium. These effects quickly restore the blood calcium level. If the blood calcium level rises, the amount of parathyroid hormone secreted is reduced and the above effects are reversed, with the horse's body storing more calcium in bone and excreting more calcium in the urine.

## Adrenal glands

These glands lie next to and immediately above the kidneys (Fig. 6.14). Each adrenal gland is divided into two distinct regions, the adrenal cortex and the adrenal medulla (Fig. 6.15).

The adrenal cortex is responsible for the secretion of a group of hormones known as the corticosteroids and each one has an important effect on the horse's body:

(1) Aldosterone – reduces the amount of sodium being excreted in the urine (see Chapter 9). This helps to maintain the blood pressure and volume within a normal range.
(2) Cortisol (hydrocortisone) – controls the metabolism of fats, carbohydrates and proteins within the horse's body. Cortisol together with another hormone, corticosterone, may reduce inflammatory reactions occurring within the body and may inhibit the immune system to a small extent. Cortisone is used as a drug treatment in horses to reduce inflammation and reduce the effects of shock. Cortisone preparations were often used in the horse's joints to reduce pain and inflammation but it was found that it had a deleterious effect on the joint surfaces themselves and so non-steroidal anti-inflammatory drugs (NSAIDs) such as phenylbutazone or 'bute' are now used in preference.
(3) Androgens – responsible for the sexual development and function of the male horse.

The adrenal medulla, on the other hand, is part of the sympathetic nervous system. The adrenal medulla is closely linked with nerves and produces the hormones adrenaline and noradrenaline. The adjacent nerves stimulate the production of these hormones in response to stress and fear.

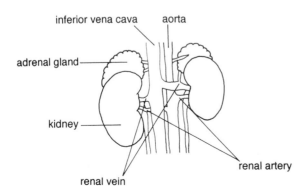

**Fig. 6.14**  Position of the adrenal glands in the horse.

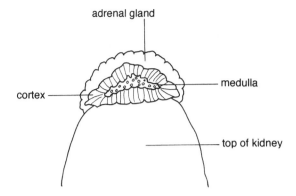

adrenal gland

cortex

medulla

top of kidney

**Fig. 6.15** Section through the adrenal gland.

## Pancreas

This gland, which has an elongated triangular shape, is situated behind the horse's stomach in a loop of small intestine. The pancreas is both an exocrine and endocrine gland. The exocrine cells secrete digestive enzymes through the pancreatic duct directly into the small intestine. The endocrine glands secrete the enzymes glucagon and insulin from small specialised groups of cells known as the islets of Langerhans. Both insulin and glucagon are responsible for maintaining the blood glucose level within a normal range and diverting glucose to and from tissues.

Horses rarely suffer from the common human condition of diabetes mellitus.

## Thymus

The thymus is situated just behind the sternum, between the horse's lungs. It is made up of two lobes joined together in front of the trachea and consisting of lymphoid tissue made up of fat, epithelium and lymphocytes.

The thymus plays a role in the immune system and it is particularly active in foals. It is unusual in that it is active until puberty and then starts to lay down more fat and become relatively inactive. The function of the thymus is to produce the T-lymphocytes (see Chapter 16) which are vital for the horse's defence system in its fight against disease.

## Ovaries

As well as producing eggs, the ovaries are glands which produce the female hormones progesterone and oestrogen. The oestrogens are responsible for the behavioural changes in the mare during her oestrous cycle. Oestrogens include oestradiol, oestrone sulphate, oestrone and two other oestrogens which are unique to horses, equilenin and equinin (see Chapter 12).

Progesterone has a role in the oestrous cycle and is also responsible for maintaining pregnancy in the early days after conception.

## Testes

The testes are responsible for producing the male hormone testosterone which produces the characteristics of the male horse. Testosterone is responsible for the increased musculature of stallions because it has an anabolic effect (body building).

## Pineal gland

This is a tiny structure located within the brain itself. It is responsible for the secretion of the hormone melatonin. The amount of hormone secreted varies with the length of the day, as more is produced during darkness. The pineal gland is thought to have an effect on mares in the spring when oestrous activity begins as the days get longer.

## Neuroendocrine system

It was thought that the endocrine and nervous systems worked independently of one another, but it now seems that they are able to work together. It is now known that many neurons can actually produce hormones within the cell itself.

Many endocrine glands act in direct conjunction with the nervous system. The pineal gland is one example of this. Nervous messages concerning daylight hours are passed from the horse's eye to the pineal gland in the brain. This gland then secretes hormones which act on the pituitary gland stimulating the production of LH and FSH thus beginning the mare's oestrous activity in spring.

Some nerves are also able to produce hormones themselves, albeit in smaller quantities than the endocrine glands. For example, the hormone oxytocin is produced as a prohormone in the neurons of specialised areas of the brain. This prohormone is then transported to the pituitary gland where it is stored for future use.

A summary of the major hormones and their site of production and effects is shown in Table 6.1.

# Common problems associated with the nervous system

## Wobbler syndrome

This syndrome results from a narrowing of the cervical vertebrae in the horse's neck, resulting in compression of the spinal cord in the neck and therefore loss of coordination and abnormal gait. The horse seems to wobble and be unbalanced when walking. It is a progressive disease, but is most commonly seen in young rapidly growing thoroughbreds, particularly colts. It can also occur in older horses of all types. The clinical signs may be sudden and severe or subtle and insidious in onset; the horse may show intermittent hind leg lameness and as the condition worsens the horse will tend to stand with its hind legs in odd positions and become less coordinated.

It is an incurable disease and affected horses are not safe to ride.

Diagnosis is often confirmed by X-ray of the neck to see if a nerve is trapped. In the USA surgery may be attempted to effect some improvement but it does not cure the problem. It has been suggested that the syndrome may be due to nutritional imbalance in rapidly growing animals, but there may be a hereditary factor also. Therefore high planes of nutrition which encourage this rapid growth should be avoided so that the young horse is allowed to grow more slowly, at an even rate.

## Shivering

This poorly understood disease is characterised by involuntary muscular movements of the hindlimbs and tail. Occasionally the forelimbs may also be involved. The cause of this disease is unknown, although some experts believe it is a nervous disorder which may follow other systemic diseases such as strangles. Signs are often difficult to detect because they occur irregularly. They become more evident when an attempt is made

**Table 6.1**  Summary of the major hormones, their site of production and effects

| Position within the horse's body | Hormones produced | Effects |
|---|---|---|
| Hypothalamus | Releasing factors or hormones | Stimulate pituitary gland to secrete hormones |
| Posterior pituitary gland | Oxytocin | Causes uterine contractions during birth |
| Anterior pituitary gland | Antidiuretic hormone (ADH) | Reduces urine production by kidneys |
| | Growth hormone | Stimulates growth |
| | Adrenocorticotrophic hormone (ACTH) | Stimulates adrenal glands to produce hormones |
| | Thyroid stimulating hormone (TSH) | Stimulates thyroid gland to produce hormones |
| | Follicle stimulating hormone and luteinising hormone (FSH and LH) | Stimulates ovaries or testes |
| Brain | Neuropeptides, endorphins and encephalins | Analgesic effect (pain killers) |
| Thyroid gland | Calcitonin | Maintains calcium levels in the blood |
| | $T_3$ and $T_4$ | Affect general metabolism and growth |
| Parathyroid glands | Parathyroid hormone | Maintains calcium levels in blood |
| Thymus | Thymic hormone | Stimulates lymphocyte development |
| Pancreas | Insulin | Both maintain blood sugar levels |
| | Glucagon | |
| Testes | Testosterone | Stimulates male characteristics to develop, physically and in a behavioural sense |
| Ovaries | Oestrogens | Control oestous cycle of mare and maintain pregnancy |
| | Progesterone | |
| Gut | Secretin | Regulate synthesis of some digestive enzymes |
| | Gastrin | |
| Placenta | Equine chorionic gonadotrophin (ECG) (previously known as pregnant mare serum gonadrophin (PMSG) | Contains both FSH and LH |
| | Progesterone and oestrogens | Assist in the maintenance of pregnancy |
| Adrenal glands | Adrenaline/noradrenaline | Released during fear or stress |
| | Aldosterone | Regulates sodium excretion by kidneys |
| | Hydrocortisone (cortisol) | Affects metabolism and reduces inflammation |
| Kidneys | Renin | Controls blood pressure |
| | Vitamin D | Controls calcium and phosphorus metabolism |
| | Erythropoietin | Stimulates the production of red blood cells (erythrocytes) |

to move the horse backwards. As the horse tries to move backwards, he may suddenly hold a hind foot up and away from the body in a flexed position and this will start to shake uncontrollably. At the same time the tail is elevated and shivers.

The prognosis is poor as this is a progressive condition and no efficient method of treatment exists.

Some horses with mild symptoms may be worked for a while.

## Stringhalt

This condition is characterised by the horse hyperflexing one or both of the hocks. This is done when the horse walks and a goose-stepping action can be seen in the hindlimbs. It may disappear altogether at the trot. The condition may remain static or the horse may deteriorate further. The cause is unknown, but horses in Australia have been found to develop stringhalt rapidly after the ingestion of plant toxins following periods of drought. These horses, however, usually make a full recovery. Surgery may be attempted in some cases to remove a piece of the lateral digital extensor tendon, but in most cases stringhalt returns at some stage. Affected horses are still able to carry on jumping, but dressage is not possible.

## Laryngeal paralysis (hemiplegia)

This is more commonly referred to as roaring or whistling and occurs as a result of damage to the nerve that supplies the muscles of the larynx. Affected horses make abnormal sounds when being exercised due to the muscle flapping within the respiratory airway. The nerve cannot be regenerated and so surgical intervention is required. This may be in the form of a hobday operation, a tie-back operation, or a tube may be inserted directly into the trachea, thus bypassing the problem area. These tubes have to be kept very clean; often the surrounding tissue will reject the foreign body and another hole will have to be made. Horses which have been tubed, however, have gone on to perform extremely well. Some disciplines such as eventing do not allow tubed horses to compete.

# Chapter 7
# The Senses

It is impossible to know exactly what a horse feels, hears, sees or smells. Scientists can only observe their reactions to various stimuli under experimental conditions. Certain responses such as the pain response, can vary tremendously between different horses, just as it can between people!

Horses, like all mammals, have certain specialised structures which help to give them an awareness of their environment. These are essential for survival. All mammals have sense organs responsible for sight, hearing (and balance), smell and taste. All these sense organs are extensions of the brain and are directly connected to it by nerve trunks. These special sense organs all differ tremendously from each other in both structure and function.

## Sight

The eye is probably the most highly developed of all the sense organs. It receives stimuli in the form of light and changes these stimuli into nervous impulses which are then sent to the brain. The brain then converts the messages to pictures.

The horse appears to have very good vision, possessing large eyes which are bigger than the eyes of both the whale and the elephant. The horse's eye also has a light intensifying device called the tapetum lucidium, which consists of a layer within the eye which reflects light back on to the retina, allowing the horse to see in dim light. This layer will reflect back the light of a torch at night, in the same way that a cat's eye reflects the glare of car headlights. The ability to see in conditions of poor light indicates that the horse is a nocturnal animal; indeed, studies of feral horses show them to be most active at dawn and dusk.

The horse's eyes are set high up on its head; the head in turn is set on a long flexible neck. The eyes are also positioned on the side of the head, not on the front as in humans. This means that even when grazing the horse has excellent all-round vision.

The positioning of the eyes means that the horse has limited binocular vision, the ability to judge depth and distance, which results when both eyes are set along the same parallel and view the object simultaneously. However, the horse has extensive monocular vision, where each eye observes a semicircle on either side of the body separately (Fig. 7.1). Extreme muscular effort is required to produce converging vision towards the front of the horse. In practical terms the fact that the horse's eyes are set on the side of the head means that the horse cannot see immediately in front of his nose or directly behind his tail. Horses should never, therefore, be approached from behind without speaking to alert the horse to your presence.

Horses do not have a spherical eyeball like humans, but one which is slightly flattened from front to back. The lower part is also more flattened than the upper part. This means that the retinal layer (the area where the image is focused) is nearer to the lens at the bottom of the eye than at the top. This retina is known as a ramped retina (Fig. 7.2). Both near and far images can then be focused at the same time. This allowed

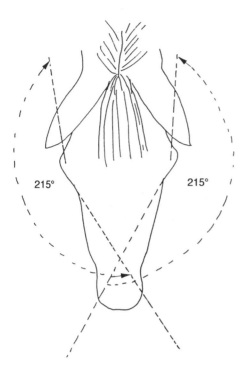

215°          215°

**Fig. 7.1**   Visual field of the horse.

the wild ancestors of the horse to see predators approaching in the distance at the same time as viewing their food while grazing with their heads down (Fig. 7.2b).

If horses become alerted by something in the distance they will stand with their heads held very high and their nose back, so that they can focus on the object of interest. In the horse the ciliary muscles which help to focus the lens and fix images on to the retina are under-developed. The horse therefore has to move his head up or down to bring the image on to the part of the retina at the correct distance to focus the image sharply. The ciliary muscles do provide, however, some assistance to the focusing process. For this reason the horse should be allowed to move his head when approaching obstacles so that he can obtain a sharp image of the fence before he jumps.

Horses also have the added problem of their own muzzles obscuring their view. For this reason a horse's view is indistinct below eye level. By the time the horse is 1.5 m (4–5 ft) away from a fence, he can no longer see it, and all horses therefore are jumping blind from this point! In fact many show jumpers can be seen to ask the horse to move his head from side to side when approaching a fence to improve the horse's vision.

Horses which race over fences are less likely to suffer from this problem because they have a longer take-off distance and can see the fence before jumping.

The eyes are situated in bony sockets or orbits which are positioned in the skull for maximum protection. The orbit is surrounded by a ridged arch of particularly strong bone known as the supraorbital process. The orbit also contains a large pad of fat which lies behind the eye and acts as a cushion if the eye should receive a blow. Horses have excellent reflexes which is why they rarely injure their eyes.

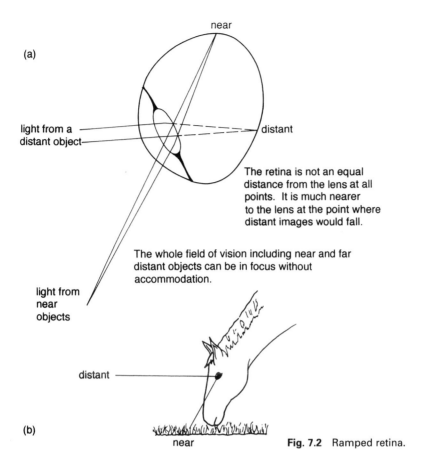

(a)

near

light from a distant object

distant

The retina is not an equal distance from the lens at all points. It is much nearer to the lens at the point where distant images would fall.

The whole field of vision including near and far distant objects can be in focus without accommodation.

light from near objects

distant

near

(b)

**Fig. 7.2**  Ramped retina.

## Anatomy of the eye

The eye consists of the eyeball or globe, the optic nerve and accessory structures such as the eyelids, conjunctiva, cornea, lacrimal apparatus (which makes tears) and the muscles which move the eye (ocular muscles). Fig. 7.3 shows a longitudinal section through the eye.

The eye is essentially a hollow ball, the wall of which is made up of three layers. The outermost layer is called the sclera (more commonly known as the white of the eye) and is composed of tough connective tissue and some cartilage to help hold its shape. At the front, the sclera becomes much thinner and is transparent. This part is known as the cornea. At its outer limits it is continuous with the sclera. The junction between the cornea and sclera is known as the limbus. There are free nerve endings in the cornea which if stimulated cause reflex blinking, tear secretion and pain. The cornea must be transparent so that light can enter the eye.

Immediately within the sclera is another layer known as the choroid. This layer contains many blood vessels and is the nutritive layer. At the front of the eye, the choroid layer has a hole in it (the pupil) and surrounding this hole is the pigmented area known as the iris. The iris itself contains both circular and radial muscles which make the size of the pupil larger or smaller depending upon the amount of light entering the eye. When light is bright, the pupil becomes narrower and more oblong shaped (in the horizontal plane). When dull the pupil becomes dilated and is more round in shape.

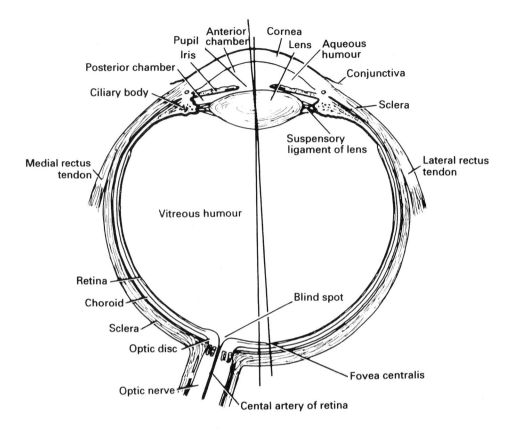

**Fig. 7.3**  Longitudinal section through the eye.

The edges of the iris in the horse are irregular and are not smooth as in the human eye. Projections of dark coloured pigment can easily be seen, particularly lining the upper edge of the iris. These are known as the corpora nigra and they may partially block the pupil particularly when it is contracted.

Just behind the iris lies a circular shelf which arises from the choroid, known as the ciliary body. This forms the attachment for the lens via the suspensory ligament which attaches the lens to the ciliary body around the whole of its circumference. The ciliary body contains muscles (ciliary muscles) which help to change the shape of the lens, so that horses can focus on objects at various distances away, a process known as accommodation. The lens must be transparent so that light can enter the eye. The lens is spherical in shape when viewed from the front, but is biconvex when viewed from the side. It helps to focus light entering the eye on to the sensitive region at the back known as the retina which forms the innermost layer of the eyeball on the inside of the choroid.

### The retina

This is a thin, light-sensitive layer. It is complicated in structure and contains many nerves and blood vessels. The image which the horse sees is caught on the retina where it is converted to nervous messages which are then sent via the optic nerve to the brain for translation. The optic nerve enters the eye from behind, passing through the sclera and the choroid and spreading our nerve fibres over the surface of the retina which they penetrate by turning back on themselves. The area where the optic nerve leaves the eye is known as the optic disc and as it has no light receiving powers it is known as the blind spot. The nerve fibres themselves are not sensitive to light.

The retina contains two types of light sensitive cells called, according to their shape, rods and cones (Fig. 7.4). There are fewer cones than rods and both types of cells cover the general surface of the retina. The rods are extremely sensitive and are able to perceive varying intensities of light (only rods exist at the outer edges of the retina). Both the rods and cones contain pigments which undergo chemical changes in the presence of light. These are called photochemicals.

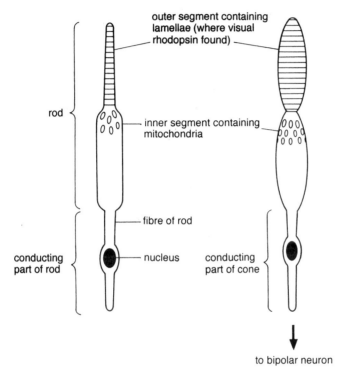

**Fig. 7.4**  Rods (left) and cones (right).

The rods contain a pigment known as visual purple or rhodopsin. This is formed from two chemicals namely opsin and retinene, the latter being derived from vitamin A. This is the origin of the popular theory that carrots help horses and people to see better in the dark!

Rhodopsin decomposes and bleaches in the presence of light (similar to the effect of light on a negative in a camera), and splits it into its constituent parts, i.e. opsin and retinene. This chemical decomposition starts a nerve impulse in the nerve fibre supplying the rod. Rhodopsin then regenerates in the dark. If, however, vitamin A is deficient, rhodopsin cannot regenerate because of the absence of retinene which is derived from vitamin A. It is thought that cones contain a different visual pigment because they show different responses to a given quantity or quality of light.

Only the cones can discriminate colours but they need stronger stimuli than the rods. It is assumed therefore that horses can only see colour in ordinary light and not when it is going dark. Horses were once thought to be colour-blind like cattle and dogs, but recent work has shown that they are most responsive to yellow, then green, then blue and least of all red. Horses are therefore more likely to spook at yellow fences than red ones.

## Accommodation

### Adaptation

The eyes are capable of adapting to high levels of light intensity and low levels of illumination. Light adaptation occurs when the horse is exposed to bright light such as when coming out of a dark stable into bright sunlight. This causes the photochemicals of the rods and cones to be altered in such a way that the amount of photochemical present is reduced. This decreases the sensitivity of the eye to light. At the same time, the pupil is constricted by a parasympathetic reflex constriction of the circular muscle of the iris.

On the other hand, when the horse moves from a light to a dark place or as the sun comes down there is a replenishment of photochemicals, enabling the eyes to detect very low levels of light intensity. Within 30 minutes of entering darkness, the sensitivity of the photoreceptors can increase by about 5000 times and 45 minutes later by 25 000 times. The pupil also dilates to allow more light to enter.

The time taken for the horse to adapt to sudden changes in light conditions, such as jumping into or out of a wood, jumping in an indoor arena and under floodlights, seems to be longer than in humans. This should be compensated for by allowing horses more time to adjust. For example, the horse may be walked into an indoor school and walked for as long as possible before the bell goes to begin the round. Also when jumping the horse into or out of a wood, the horse should be slowed down to give the horse's eyes time to adjust.

## Chambers of the eye

The lens and ciliary body form a partition dividing the cavity in the eye into two parts known as the anterior and posterior chambers. The anterior chamber contains a watery fluid which is known as the aqueous humour, whereas the posterior chamber contains a thicker, jelly-like fluid known as the vitreous humour.

## Eyelids

The horse has two eyelids and an inner one known as the third eyelid. This third eyelid is pink in colour and consists of mucus membrane and cartilage. It assists in lubrication by spreading tears over the eye surface. The third eyelid is also known as the nictitating membrane and usually it can be seen only in the corner of the eye when the eye is open. One of the first signs of tetanus is the protrusion of the third eyelid partially across the eye. This becomes exaggerated if the horse is excited.

The eyelids consist of sheets of cartilage which are covered by skin on the outside and conjunctiva on the inside. The upper eyelid is the most mobile and closes over the eye. The eyelashes help to protect the eye and filter off dust particles.

## Conjunctiva

The conjunctiva is a thin, mucus membrane which is pink in colour and is found on the inside of the eyelids as previously mentioned. From the inside of the eyelids, the conjunctiva folds back on itself to cover the front of the eye as a fine layer of transparent cells which form part of the cornea.

## Lacrimal apparatus

Tears are produced by the lacrimal glands which are situated beneath the supraorbital process. The tears are secreted on to the eye surface and then collected into two tear ducts in the inner corner of the eye. These ducts then run down beneath the nasal bones and empty into the floor of the nostrils. The tears can be commonly seen as a clear fluid running from the nostrils. These openings can easily be seen if the nostril is pulled back slightly. If the tear ducts become blocked for any reason, then tears will overflow the lower eyelid and run down the horse's face. This can be a problem, particularly in the summer when flies become attracted to this fluid. Some horses lose the hair on their face underneath the passage of tears and this can become sore.

## Common conditions of the eye

Some conditions of the eye can easily be seen by the horse owner, but others need specialist diagnosis and treatment by the vet.

### Conjunctivitis

This refers to inflammation of the conjunctiva. The membranes turn a deep red colour and become swollen. It is often quite painful for the horse and he may not open the affected eye fully. There is usually some yellow discharge from the eye. There are several causes of this condition including direct irritation from a foreign body such as a small piece of hay or straw, or infection. The foreign body must be removed and this can be done with the help of local anaesthetic drops which are placed in the eye. It may also be removed by washing the eye with warm saline solution, if the horse will let you!

Infections are treated with antibiotic drops or ointment. Ointment is preferred because although it is more messy, it tends to stay in contact with the eye longer, before tears wash it away. Liquid drops are usually flushed out very quickly by tears.

### Cataract

The lens becomes less transparent and more opaque. Obviously this reduces the amount of light entering the eye, which affects the horse's ability to see. The degree of opacity will determine the degree of sight and some horses may become completely blind.

Cataracts may have been present from birth, i.e. they are congenital. These may vary from small cloudy spots on the lens to the lens being completely opaque. These congenital cataracts rarely progress any further. Some horses, however, develop degenerative cataracts as a result of injury or disease. There is no effective treatment for cataracts.

### Keratitis

This may develop from conjunctivitis or may result from a direct blow or injury to the cornea. As mentioned previously, the cornea contains nerve endings and is very sensitive . When an injury occurs to the cornea the horse will usually not open his eye and tears will run down his face. After the initial inflammation has subsided, a visible grey patch can be seen on the otherwise clear cornea. It is important that veterinary treatment is sought before an ulcer develops, with the possibility of the cornea becoming perforated and the aqueous humour leaking from the eye, causing the eventual collapse of the eyeball itself.

## Hearing

Another equally important sense to the horse is that of hearing. Horses needed their senses to help them survive in the wild situation. Being able to hear helps them to detect anyone or anything approaching, whether it be friend or foe. The sense of hearing in horses is highly developed and acute. Horses are able to hear sounds outside of the human range and can detect sounds from very low to very high frequencies. This sense of hearing does deteriorate as the horse gets older.

The horse's excellent sense of hearing is helped by the highly mobile ears which can each rotate through 180 degrees and are controlled by no fewer than 16 muscles! The horse can also use his head to pinpoint the exact source of sounds.

Sound travels by means of sound waves through air (or water or solids). Sound waves cause the eardrum to vibrate. These vibrations are converted into electrical impulses which are then sent to the brain.

Because the horse's sense of hearing is so acute, they can become distressed when placed in a noisy environment. Horses, particularly young stock, can become highly strung if they are kept near busy roads, railways, airports, etc. It is a well-known fact among horse owners that windy days can turn their normally safe hack into a nightmare, as the horse becomes much more nervous. This is because sounds (as sound waves) are being carried by the wind, and the horse has far greater difficulty in pinpointing the source.

Horse owners should make as much use of the horse's excellent sense of hearing as possible, by talking quietly to them and using their voice as a training aid. Use softly spoken, simple words of command. Also, when moving around horses, particularly in the stable, talk to the horse so that he knows exactly where you are, because as previously mentioned, the horse has two blind spots, immediately in front and behind him. He will not be startled if you let him know where you are!

## Anatomy of the ear (Fig. 7.5)

The ear consists of three parts: the outer, middle and inner ear. The inner ear in particular is responsible for balance and informs the brain of the position of the horse's head at all times.

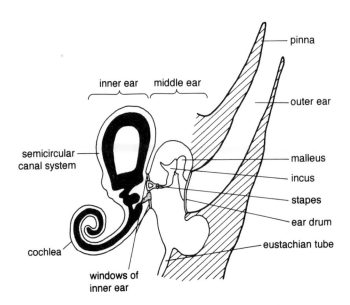

**Fig. 7.5**   Anatomy of the external ear of the horse.

## The outer ear

The horse has large, mobile ears which can move independently from each other through a rotation of 180 degrees. This enables the horse to pick up sounds from different directions without moving its body.

Most horse owners are familiar with the outer ear or pinna, which forms the visible part of the ear. This part of the ear consists of three cartilages. The conchal cartilage is the largest of the three. This cartilage funnels sound waves down into the ear canal towards the tympanic membrane (eardrum) and is funnel-shaped and lined with skin. The scutiform cartilage is a shield-shaped cartilage which acts as a lever for some of the ear muscles. It is located on the surface of the temporal muscle and attaches to the external ear muscles.

The third cartilage is the annular cartilage which is shaped like a tube and connects the conchal cartilage with the external auditory canal.

## The middle ear

The tympanic membrane separates the outer from the middle ear and this is connected to three small bones with 'horsey' names, known (from outside in) as the malleus (hammer), incus (anvil) and stapes (stirrup). These little bones provide a mechanical link with the eardrum and they form a bridge across the middle ear to a small opening in the skull covered by two membranous windows which lead to the inner ear. The stapes bone connects to one of these two windows in the middle ear. These two windows are known as the round (fenestra rotunda) and the oval window (fenestra ovalis). The oscillations (vibrations) of the stapes hit the oval window and act like a miniature piston, setting the fluids of the inner ear and the cochlea into vibration.

The middle ear is an air-filled cavity which connects to the pharynx (throat) by a tube known as the Eustachian tube. This tube allows the adjustment of pressure between the middle ear and the outside. The opening into the pharynx from the tube is protected by a flap of cartilage which opens during swallowing.

The horse is unique in that it has two large sacs connected to each of the two Eustachian tubes (one for each ear!) and these are known as the guttural pouches. They are situated between the pharynx and the skull and have a capacity of about 300 ml. The guttural pouches lie very close to important nerves and arteries and there is a condition known as guttural pouch mycosis (caused by a fungus) which can be life-threatening if the vital nerves and blood vessels become affected.

## The inner ear

The inner ear consists of a series of membranous tubes (labyrinth) which are filled with a fluid known as endolymph. The membranous labyrinth is bathed externally by a fluid known as perilymph, the whole structure being embedded deep in the skull. The membranous labyrinth performs two functions: (1) hearing and (2) balance and orientation. For simplicity's sake, it is easier to describe the inner ear as two groups of tubes, one being the cochlea (associated with hearing) and the other containing the three semicircular canals which are responsible for balance.

### The cochlea

The cochlea is a membranous structure which is wound spirally rather like a snail's shell. The cochlea picks up vibrations from the action of the stapes on the oval window. These vibrations cause the nerves to send impulses via the auditory nerve to the brain. Here they are interpreted as sound, the quality, pitch and loudness of the sound being determined by the way in which the vibrations are picked up by the cochlea.

### Semicircular canals

These all lie at right angles to each other and are continuous with the main membranous tubes of the inner ear, i.e. they share its endolymph. When the horse moves its head from a resting position, the fluid or endolymph within the semicircular canals is set in motion. According to the plane of movement (vertical, horizontal, etc.) so the movement of endolymph is restricted to a particular canal in that plane. Thus if the horse is moving his head sideways then the fluid within the horizontal semicircular canal will be moving the most. So, depending upon the angle of the horse's head, the endolymph moves within the semicircular canals and this results in the sending of impulses to the brain. The brain can then interpret these signals and balance accordingly.

Horses also use their ears to give visual signals to other horses and humans. The position of the ears can give us clues as to the mood of the horse. Pricked ears are typical of horses who are alert, interested or startled. If the ears are pinned flat back, then this is a threat signal. In the wild situation, the pinning back of the ears was a protective measure in the case of attack by a predator. If the ears are pinned back, they are less likely to be torn or damaged.

## Conditions of the ear

### Guttural pouch mycosis

This is a fungal infection of the guttural pouch. It can produce a foul-smelling nasal discharge and cause difficulty in swallowing. Other signs include pain under the base of the ear, swelling of the throat (hence the difficulty in swallowing, stiffness of the neck, colic, patchy sweating). However, the most frequent and potentially disastrous sign of this problem is a nosebleed from both nostrils (bilateral nasal haemorrhage). This haemorrhage may be massive and even fatal. This is because as previously mentioned, the guttural pouch lies very close to important blood-vessels. A fungal infection can weaken the wall of these blood-vessels and therefore cause an haemorrhage. Any horse which has a nosebleed from both nostrils which is not associated with exercise should be seen by the veterinary surgeon immediately as an emergency. If the horse has survived the bleeding, diagnosis of the problem can take place, usually by endoscopic examination. Once the diagnosis is confirmed, the horse will require an operation to mend the blood vessel which has caused the bleeding. The horse will then be treated for the fungal infection.

Many cases of this disease eventually recover although the prognosis is not good if the horse cannot swallow.

### Dentigenous cyst

This is a discharging sinus at the base of the ear. It is a congenital abnormality which may contain a rudimentary tooth which can be surgically removed.

### Ear mites

Ear mites occur in horses and more often than not do not produce any clinical signs of infestation. However, in some horses these mites may be responsible for severe irritation which may cause head shaking. Ear mites may be removed by treating the horse with antiparasitic drugs.

### Swollen parotid gland

The parotid gland is one of the salivary glands and is therefore responsible for the production of saliva. It is situated at the base of the outer ear (pinna) and may become swollen. This particularly affects horses and ponies which are out at grass. The cause of the swelling is not known, but it usually subsides by itself when the horse is taken off the grass.

### Bleeding from the ear

This must be taken very seriously, as it is usually the result of a skull fracture. It may also be caused by guttural pouch mycosis as discussed previously.

## Taste and smell

The senses of taste and smell are very closely linked in horses, so much so that they are often thought to be inseparable. Many horses are renowned for being fussy feeders. They seem readily to go off their feed and this may be partly to do with the fact that horses cannot vomit and they therefore have to be extremely careful in their choice of food. Unlike humans, who can be sick to get rid of an offending substance before it causes too much harm, it will have to pass right through a horse's digestive tract and this could cause quite serious problems.

### Taste

Taste sensations are produced from minute raised areas on the tongue called papillae on which the taste buds are situated (Fig. 7.6). The highest concentration of taste receptors (nervous supply) are situated at the back of the tongue and these specialised receptors are enclosed in the membrane which covers the tongue. These nerve endings send messages to the brain.

The taste buds consist of gustatory and support cells which are arranged in barrel-shaped groups with hair-like projections which protrude through a pore at the top (on

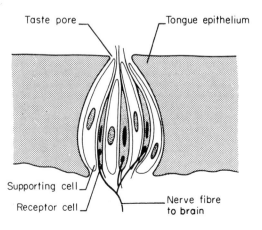

**Fig. 7.6** A taste bud.

the tongue surface). The taste buds of the horse are melon-shaped and slightly smaller than those found in cows and sheep. The dog has the greatest concentration of taste buds at the front of the tongue whereas ruminants such as cows and sheep have the greatest concentration at the back. Taste stimuli also increases gastric secretions in the stomach.

Taste is an important factor in the ability of horses to select their food, particularly when they are deficient in some nutrient. It has been proved scientifically in other animals that, if they are mineral-or vitamin-deficient, they will select foods high in that mineral or vitamin (if it is available to them). This ability to correct dietary deficiencies is lost if the sensory nerves to the taste buds are cut. We know this is particularly true where salt is concerned, and a salt lick should therefore always be made available to horses.

Salt should not, however, be added by the horse owner to the concentrate feed for two reasons:

(1) If it is a compound feed it will already be present in the feed. Salt is a cheap ingredient to add and will therefore not be excluded from the mix.
(2) If the horse is not deficient in salt the feed will taste horrible and I have known horses who have gone off their feed to eat up when the added salt was taken out.

It is important to stress that the taste system in a horse – or any other animal for that matter – would be expected to suit that particular animal's diet and requirements. In other words, grass may taste bitter to humans, but not to horses. This seemingly obvious relationship has not yet been scientifically investigated.

Although it is known that there are four specific tastes in man – sweet, salt, bitter and sour (acid) – there are considerable differences between different species. For example, it has been shown that while cats hate sugars and will avoid them, horses have a sweet tooth, hence their preference for sweet feed or molasses mixtures. It has also been shown that horses cannot distinguish between pure water and highly concentrated sucrose (sugar) solutions which are offensive to man.

Taste can vary considerably within a species, so different horses will show individual preferences to the same taste. It is thought that this has a genetic base. To most horse owners this will not be surprising, as most horses on a yard will certainly make their preferences known.

## Smell

The sense of small (olfaction) is commonly associated with seeking and selecting food and water and is also a communication system within groups of horses. Horses, particularly those in the wild situation, need to be able to smell the presence of predators so they can make their escape. This highly developed sense of smell enables wild *Equidae* to detect blood from freshly killed animals up to two miles away. The sense of smell is also important in horses for their reproductive patterns and social behaviour.

All horses have the ability to hold up their noses and curl the upper lip in a gesture which is known as flehmen (Fig. 7.7). This is often seen when horses are presented with a strange or strong smell, but it is most often seen in stallions in their courtship activity with mares who are in oestrus.

Horses also use their sense of smell to smell droppings on the pasture or a patch of grass which has been staled upon by another horse. Stallions or geldings showing

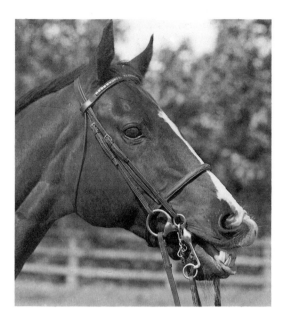

**Fig. 7.7** Flehmen posture. (Courtesy of Joanna Prestwich)

stallion-like behaviour will then dung on top of these smells to mark the territory as their own.

### Olfactory system

The sense of smell is associated with this system. The nasal passages contain two tightly rolled turbinate bones which increase the surface area of the nasal passages. The turbinates divide each nasal passage into three channels known as the dorsal meatus, medial meatus and ventral meatus respectively. The dorsal meatus is closed at the back and it conducts air breathed in to the olfactory region. Olfactory nerve cells are scattered among support cells throughout the mucus membranes within these areas of the nose.

Each olfactory cell bears a tuft of tiny hair-like projections which are the actual receptors for the sense of smell. Because the inside of the nose is moist, it follows that the material to be smelled must go into a solution before it can reach the sensory cells, however some very fine particles may be smelled without actually dissolving first. There are several sinuses in each half of the skull, which fill partly with air during the breathing process but they play no part in the sense of smell.

### Organ of Jacobson

Otherwise known as the Vomeronasal organ, this is an elongated sac which opens into the nose. This organ is well developed in horses. Its lining contains olfactory cells and it is thought that these organs are particularly efficient at detecting scents from other horses. These are chemical signals known as pheromones. This enables groups of horses to recognise one another and individual herds in the wild have their own identification system. When new horses are introduced to a group, they will blow air into the other's nose and a process of recognition or otherwise will be observed. Also, horses are able to smell food in their mouths through the organ of Jacobson.

Mares rely on their sense of smell to bond with their foals. As soon as the foal is born the mare will lick and smell the foal. If she loses her foal and is given an orphan to foster then the orphan is usually covered in the dead foal's skin so that the mare recognises it as her own.

As the sense of smell is so important to horses, they should be encouraged to use it when settling into new pastures or yards. Lead them around their new home and let them have a good smell. This will help them to settle sooner. Try not to keep moving them from one stable to another and try to find a yard where there is a low turnover of horses, so that the horse has time to bond and become friendly with other horses and his environment.

# Chapter 8
# The Skin

The skin is the horse's largest single body organ and a very important defence mechanism. It is also the most visible part of the horse's body and an understanding of its structure and functions helps the horse owner use the condition of the skin and coat as indicators of health and disease.

## The common integument

The term 'common integument' describes the protective covering of the body, consisting of skin, hair and hooves. It acts as a protective envelope, as a secretory and excretory organ, as a sense organ and a temperature regulating device. The functions of the skin and coat include:

- protection against wear and tear by providing a covering of cells which are constantly being replaced;
- maintenance of shape (the elasticity of the skin restores its shape when bent joints are straightened);
- protection from the uncontrolled loss or entry of water;
- protection from the entry of harmful organisms;
- protection from the harmful effects of ultraviolet light;
- formation of vitamin D;
- receiving sensations of the environment, temperature, pain, touch and pressure;
- temperature regulation.

## Structure of the skin (Fig. 8.1)

The skin is tough, resilient and highly elastic. It is attached to underlying tissues by fibrous connective tissue (fascia) and fatty tissue. The skin consists of the three layers; the epidermis, dermis and subdermal layer.

### The epidermis

The epidermis is formed from three horizontal zones of non-vascular stratified epithelial tissue: the inner Malpighian layer, the middle granular layer and the outer cornified layer. The cells of the deeper Malpighian layer are pigmented and undergo continuous division from a basement membrane, this process resulting in the cells being continually pushed to the surface of the epidermis. New cells from this germinative layer pass through the granular layer and a fibrous protein called keratin is deposited in the cells. Keratin waterproofs the cells and prevents water from evaporating from the living tissues underneath. It also stops the skin from absorbing water and gives the cells a horny texture – they are said to be cornified. The change in appearance due to the presence of keratin is marked and the now dead cells move into

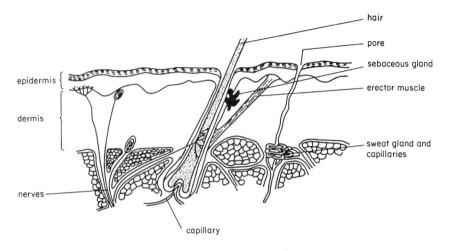

**Fig. 8.1**  Section through the skin.

a clearly defined horny layer and take on a flattened shape. The superficial cells of the horny layer are constantly removed by friction while being replaced from below by the active dividing Malpighian layer. Areas which are subject to a lot of friction are protected by a thicker horny layer; this is illustrated by the calluses soon developed by those mucking out regularly. Similarly the areas of the horse's body in contact with tack must be allowed time to 'harden up' when horses are brought up from grass otherwise rubs and galls will occur. Hair and hooves are heavily keratinised structures.

## The dermis

The dermis is highly vascular, containing capillaries which supply the hair follicles, sweat glands, sebaceous glands and the Malpighian layer of the epidermis. The dermis also contains numerous nerve endings or sense organs which collect information about the surroundings. Another dermal structure is the erector muscle of each hair. When this muscle contracts the hair rises.

## The subdermal layer

The subdermal layer is continuous with the dermis and contains subcutaneous fat and connective tissue which binds the skin to the underlying tissues. In some areas the skin is connected to cutaneous muscle lying in the subcutaneous tissue, contraction of this muscle allows the horse to twitch its skin to rid itself of flies and other irritants.

The skin varies in thickness over the horse's body and is thickest where the danger of injury is greatest, the back, loins and hindquarters. The skin over the face and inner part of the limbs is much thinner. The skin around the muzzle is very sensitive and in conjunction with the whiskers is used like fingertips. There are marked breeds differences in skin thickness with draught breeds and mountain and moorland types having much thicker skin that thoroughbreds. Thin-skinned horses may be sensitive to grooming and tightening of the girth and must be treated with consideration. Healthy skin has great tensile strength and elasticity to help prevent injury; nevertheless the skin is often broken or torn.

## Sensation

The nerves involved with the sense of touch tire quite easily and although there will still be a feeling of general pressure the horse should become unconscious of the presence of a well-fitting saddle. The pain-detecting nerves require greater pressure or injury before they are stimulated. However, the horse is particularly sensitive over the ribs where the rider applies the aids. Sensitive horses are likely to respond to subtle movements resulting in anticipation of the rider's demands. Before giving an intramuscular injection the vet will bang the horse's neck and this discharges the nerve endings making the injection less painful for the horse. Touch is an important means of communication to the horse and they find it pleasurable to have the withers scratched and often indulge in mutual grooming.

## Melanoma

The epidermis produces a skin pigment called melanin which acts as a filter for ultraviolet light. Thus horses with black skin are not liable to sunburn, but horses with pink skin can become sunburned, especially on the face. The melanin can migrate to form tumours known as melanomas. They are most common in grey horses and tend to be found on the underside of the dock, around the anus, vulva or sheath or on the head.

## The hair and coat

The hair is an epidermal structure despite the fact that it penetrates the dermis. Each hair is composed of the visible shaft, set at an oblique angle to the surface of the skin, and a root which lies in the hair follicle projecting into the dermis. Hair is made up of dead cells which are highly keratinised. At the base of the hair there is a bulb of living tissue which is continuous with the Malpighian layer, here cell division and growth take place along with the incorporation of the pigment cells which give the hair its colour.

The coat is the horse's first line of defence against injury and the environment and it covers the majority of the body surface. More hair is found on the parts of the skin exposed to direct sunlight than on less exposed areas such as the inner thigh and the perineal areas.

The skin carries several types of hair:

- permanent hair of the mane, tail, eyelashes and feathers. These long hairs are designed and positioned to help shed rain water;
- tactile hairs of the muzzle, eyes and ears;
- temporary hair which makes up the bulk of the coat.

The coat is shed and changed for a new growth in the spring and autumn. The change of coat is associated with metabolic changes and traditionally horses are never thought to perform at their best when they are changing their coat. The temporary hair consists of longer hairs ($4$–$5/cm^2$) which cover an undercoat of densely packed finer shorter hairs ($620/cm^2$). There are clear differences between breeds and thorough-breds have a finer coat than draught breeds. A thick coat reduces the horse's winter feed requirement because the horse keeps warmer.

The horse changes its coat in response to the environmental temperature, dietary influences and day length, all of which affect the total body metabolism. The response to longer days and higher temperatures is greater on a higher plane of nutrition, thus the stabled rugged horse sheds its winter coat sooner as it is also being better fed than the out-wintered horse.

Connected to each hair follicle is a sebaceous gland which produces an oily secretion called sebum. The sebum keeps the hairs supple and resistant to wetting.

# Temperature regulation

The horse's body temperature is maintained at 38°C. Temperature receptors in the skin sense the external temperature, and there is also a thermoreceptor in the hypothalamus of the brain which monitors the temperature of the blood flowing through it. If the temperature of the blood is too high steps are taken to lose heat; if the temperature is too low heat is conserved.

## Heat conservation

If the body temperature falls too low body heat is conserved by:

- constriction of the superficial blood vessels, reducing the heat lost from radiation and diverting the blood to the core;
- the erector pili muscles contracting so that the coat rises and traps a layer of warm air next to the skin. Air is a poor conductor of heat so losses from the surface of the skin are further reduced;
- reduced sweating;
- shivering, caused by involuntary contraction of the skeletal muscles and resulting in heat production;
- seasonal coat changes.

## Heat loss

If the body temperature rises to too high a level, excess heat is lost by:

- dilation of the superficial blood vessels in the dermis allowing more blood to come close to the surface and lose more heat to the atmosphere by radiation;
- the hairs of the coat lying flat to the skin, so trapping the minimum amount of air;
- increased sweating;
- slowing down the rate of metabolism.

## Sweating

Sweat glands are epidermal structures which extend into the dermis. They consist of a coiled tube which opens on to the surface of the skin. Under temperature stress the adrenal glands produce adrenalin which stimulates the sweat glands. The horse can sweat freely compared to other domestic animals and has sweat glands over the entire body except for the legs. Some areas such as the base of the ears, the flanks and the neck are densely populated with glands. Heat is lost as sweat evaporates from the surface of the skin and coat. Sweating is a continuous process but sweat is only visible on the surface of the skin when the rate of sweating exceeds the rate of evaporation from the skin's surface. Thus the horse becomes wet with sweat when exerting itself. A horse grazing in summer can normally lose six litres of fluid a day without any visible dampness of the skin and coat.

Sweating is influenced by:

- ambient temperature – as the temperature rises so sweating increases;
- humidity – as humidity rises it becomes increasingly difficult for sweat to evaporate into the atmosphere, the horse becomes soaked with sweat but effective heat loss is reduced.
- length of the coat;
- level of exercise;
- fitness;
- insulation by fatty tissue;
- excitement, temperature, pain and fever.

When looking at the weather conditions, it is the effective temperature that is important, i.e. the combination of ambient temperature and relative humidity (how much water the air contains). Table 8.1 shows heat loss ability (effective cooling) at different effective temperatures.

A further important factor affecting the horse's ability to control heat loss is the amount of radiation, i.e. direct sunlight.

There are two types of sweat gland:

(1) Apocrine glands which respond to nervous stimulation and secrete sweat that is higher in organic matter, leading to the sweat having a frothy appearance. Thus excited horses tend to 'lather up';
(2) eccrine glands which are activated mainly by temperature, producing watery sweat promoting evaporative cooling.

**Table 8.1**  Heat loss ability at different effective temperatures

| Ambient temperature and relative humidity | Effective cooling |
|---|---|
| Less than 54°C (130°F) | No problem |
| More than 60°C (140°F) | Increased sweating |
| More than 66°C (150°F) | Effective sweating lowered |
| More than 82°C (180°F) | Cooling from skin ineffective, horse pants |

**Breaking out**

A horse may sweat when it is cold due to stress or fatigue. There is nervous stimulation of the adrenal glands causing increased adrenalin production which stimulates the areas of the brain controlling sweat production. Thus horses can sweat up in anticipation when being transported to a competition.

**Excretion**

Table 8.2 shows the composition of sweat. Horse sweat is very rich in electrolytes, which are mineral salts contained in blood plasma. Electrolytes must be present in the body in the correct proportions so that normal metabolism can continue. Thus it is vital to ensure that the sweating horse is given both water and electrolytes to replace losses during exertion. Horse sweat is also very high in protein, which leaves the coat matted and contributes to lathering up. However, this protein is lost only during the early stages of sweating. The protein is stored in the sweat gland and has detergent-like properties, allowing the sweat to spread along the hair and encouraging more effective evaporation. As horses undergo a fitness programme and sweat more frequently, there is less time for the proteins to accumulate in the sweat gland and fit horses lose less protein in sweat and tend to sweat cleanly with little white lather.

**Table 8.2**  The composition of sweat

|  | Sodium (Na) (g/l) | Potassium (K) (g/l) | Chloride (Cl) (g/l) |
|---|---|---|---|
| Plasma | 140 | 3.5–4.5 | 100 |
| Human sweat | 10–60 | 4–5 | 10–60 |
| Horse sweat | 130–190 | 20–50 | 160–190 |

## Dry coat or anhydrosis

Horses reared in temperate climates and then exported to much hotter and humid countries may lose the ability to sweat, a condition known as dry coat or anhydrosis. The condition rarely develops in horses native to hot climates. It would appear that the apocrine glands lose the ability to respond to adrenalin, the horse is unable to lose heat and will develop heat stroke if exerted. The signs usually appear within 12 months of the horse's arrival in the new environment and include:

- (initially) excessive sweating;
- distressed breathing;
- decreased ability to sweat which may be confined to small areas;
- frequent urination;
- fever.

There is no apparent cure, but the signs will disappear if the horse is returned to a cooler climate.

# The skin as an indicator of health and disease

The skin of a healthy stabled horse should be elastic, smooth, clean and slightly warm. The coat should be fine, smooth, glossy and clean and give the horse a sleek appearance. Horses at grass build up a layer of protective grease which should not be removed by grooming as it helps them withstand cold and wet conditions. It is normal and healthy for a grass-kept horse to have a more greasy skin and coat and to have a longer coat in winter.

The skin can be affected by local problems but it is also the best indicator that the horse owner has of the horse's general health and condition. The coat may become dry and dull (known as staring) if it is not lubricated by normal sebaceous secretions; this is a well-known sign of digestive problems and worm infestation. The horse is said to be hidebound when the skin is tight and does not move freely over the underlying structures. This can be due to dehydration and lack of subcutaneous fat and is also seen in grass sickness and poorly nourished horses.

The colour of the mucus membranes of the eyes, gums and tongues is also used as a guide to health; the membranes should be a salmon pink colour and may be pale if the horse is anaemic or red if the horse is fevered.

Other more obvious signs of disease include wounds, heat, pain, swelling, bruising, blisters, ulcers, abscesses and scabs. These signs may be due to a number of causes – bacterial (mud fever), fungal (ringworm), viral (warts), parasites (warbles), allergy (urticaria), injury (ill-fitting tack) or sunlight (photosensitisation).

Unexplained sweating or evidence of dried sweat may indicate that the horse has been in pain (colic), fevered or perhaps cast in its stable.

It can be seen that a daily inspection of the horse's skin and coat is an essential stable management routine. It should not be confined to visual inspection and the horse owner must also feel for any changes. This is best done during the daily grooming session.

# Care of the horse's skin and coat

The condition of the skin and coat of the stabled horse rely on correct nutrition and adequate grooming.

## Feeding the coat

This is achieved by:

- a balanced diet
- adequate provision of electrolytes
- sufficient fat in the diet.

## Grooming

Grooming removes dead skin cells and clears dried sweat ducts, allowing the skin to function more effectively. Cleaning the skin also helps prevent skin diseases which are encouraged by a dirty condition. For example, careful cleaning and drying of the legs will help prevent mud fever and cracked heels.

Vigorous grooming and strapping (rhythmic muscle stimulation by gently banging the muscles of the neck and quarters) helps to increase blood circulation in the dermis, aiding the supply of oxygen and nutrient and the removal of waste products. The action also helps spread the sebum on to the skin and coat, producing a gloss to the coat. This is said to imitate the natural action of rolling. Close scrutiny of the coat will also reveal injuries and areas of heat, pain and swelling.

## Clipping

Removal of the heavy winter coat enables the horse to work without excessive sweating, avoiding loss of condition. It also allows the horse owner to dry off and clean the horse, effectively reducing the chance of the horse becoming chilled. Adequate rugs must be provided to replace the winter coat and keep the horse warm.

## Bathing

Horses may be bathed to reduce the amount of grooming necessary to clean a horse prior to a competition or to remove dried sweat. Excessive bathing with unsuitable shampoos can be detrimental as it removes too much sebum, leaving the coat dry, dull and unprotected.

# Skin and coat colour

Skin and coat colour relies on the presence of pigment called melanin. Mast cells give rise to melanoblasts which wander throughout the body until the animal matures and eventually migrate to the dermis where they give rise to melanocytes. The cells multiply throughout this migration and eventually reach the epidermis. Here the pigment cells produce pigment (melanin). The horse has two types of pigment:

- eumelanin – black/brown
- phaeomelenin – red/yellow.

Melanoblasts form a continuous layer at the junction of the dermis and epidermis. In the fetus the development of the hair follicle begins as a thickening of epithelial cells, resulting in the hair bulb. Cells migrate from the mesenchyma to the hair bulb and form the follicle. Some melanocytes also migrate to the hair bulb and as differentiation takes place they are incorporated into the hair shaft to give the birth coat of the foal. Melanocytes within the follicle produce pigment granules but this process does not take place in albinos. Melanin production requires the amino acid tyrosine and is controlled by the enzyme tyrosinase. Once formed the melanin moves along the dendrites and is injected into the adjoining tissues and cells to give coloration. Normally this is a continuing process but it may be interrupted if the surface tissue of the body is damaged. Horses with saddle sores and poorly fitting rugs often develop white areas where pigmentation of the hair is not possible.

# Chapter 9
# The Urinary System

The excretory products of the horse are shown in Fig. 9.1. The urinary system is primarily involved in the extraction and removal of waste products from the blood. In particular it is responsible for the removal of nitrogenous waste and together with the digestive system it removes all waste products produced in the body except gaseous carbon dioxide which is removed via the lungs. While removing these waste products, the urinary system is also very closely involved with the water balance of the horse, acid/base and salt balance. These processes are highly complicated and involve the influence of hormones.

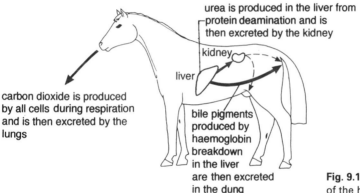

urea is produced in the liver from protein deamination and is then excreted by the kidney

kidney

liver

carbon dioxide is produced by all cells during respiration and is then excreted by the lungs

bile pigments produced by haemoglobin breakdown in the liver are then excreted in the dung

**Fig. 9.1** Excretory products of the horse.

The urinary system itself is composed of two kidneys, two ureters, one bladder and the urethra (Figs. 9.2 and 9.3). Each day approximately 1000–2000 litres of fluid are delivered to the kidneys of the horse. Since only approximately 5–15 litres of urine are excreted daily, the kidneys must remove most of the substances present in them. If the

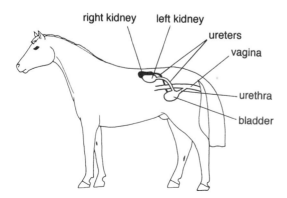

right kidney    left kidney

ureters

vagina

urethra

bladder

**Fig. 9.2** Position of the urinary organs.

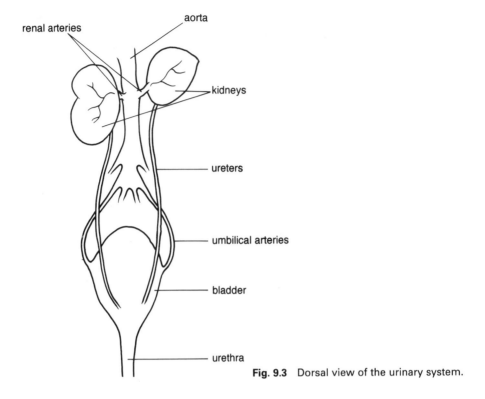

renal arteries

aorta

kidneys

ureters

umbilical arteries

bladder

urethra

**Fig. 9.3**  Dorsal view of the urinary system.

kidneys did not reabsorb fluid entering them, horses would lose their entire water and salt content in less than half a day!

## The kidneys

These are a pair. In the horse the kidneys lie on either side of the body, approximately midway between the withers and the croup underneath the spine. The left kidney lies farther back towards the last rib whereas the right kidney lies under the last three ribs. In this position they are well protected from external injury and it is therefore uncommon for them to become bruised!

The kidneys are situated outside the abdominal cavity but are bound to the upper wall of the abdomen by a layer of peritoneum which prevents the kidneys moving about as the horse moves. There are often large collections of fatty tissue around the kidneys which also help to protect them.

The kidneys are organs that filter plasma from the blood. In other words, they are highly efficient sieves, which allow the passage of smaller particles such as the contents of plasma through, but not the larger blood cells. From the substances which are filtered through, the kidneys can selectively reabsorb water and other useful constituents, so that they are not wasted.

Most of the domestic animals have bean-shaped kidneys similar to humans, but the horse has two different-shaped kidneys; the left is bean-shaped and the right is heart-shaped. In the adult horse each kidney weighs approximately 700 g and measures 15–18 cm in length.

The indented portion of the kidney is known as the hilus. This is where the blood vessels and nerves enter and the thin muscular tube known as the ureter and lymphatic vessels leave.

If the kidney is cut open, it can be seen that the hilus marks the boundary of an area known as the renal pelvis (Fig. 9.4). This is shaped like a funnel and is the origin of the ureter which then takes urine to the bladder. The renal pelvis receives urine from the kidney lobules and has no relationship with the bony pelvis as described in the skeleton.

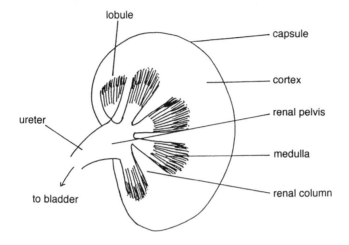

The lobular form of the kidney is partially obliterated in the horse

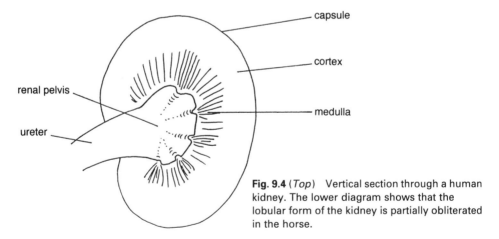

**Fig. 9.4** (*Top*)  Vertical section through a human kidney. The lower diagram shows that the lobular form of the kidney is partially obliterated in the horse.

The portion of the kidney immediately surrounding the renal pelvis is known as the medulla which appears striated or lined because of the radially arranged collecting vessels or tubules. The inner medulla has well marked projections known as pyramids and urine drains from the tips of these pyramids into the renal pelvis and then into the ureter.

The cortex or outer part of the kidney is situated between the medulla and the thin connective tissue capsule which surrounds the whole kidney itself. The cortex is velvety and granular. The granular appearance comes from the large number of filtering capsules otherwise known as glomeruli.

## Nephrons

Apart from blood vessels and a small amount of connective tissue the kidney consists of a mass of tubules known as nephrons (Fig. 9.5). The horse has approximately 2.5 million nephrons, each being a hollow tube which starts in the cortex as a blind-ended thin-walled sac (Bowman's capsule) into which a knot of blood-vessels passes (the glomerulus). Each unit of a Bowman's capsule together with its own glomerulus is known as a Malpighian body (Fig. 9.6). Proceeding from Bowman's capsule the next part of the nephron becomes coiled into a series of loops which again are situated in the renal cortex and this part is known as the proximal convoluted tubule. Following this the nephron loops down into the medulla as a thin-walled tube known as the loop of Henle which returns to the cortex again to end in another series of coils known as the distal convoluted tubule. This empties into a series of collecting ducts which eventually discharge into the renal pelvis.

The blood supply to the nephron is such that most of the blood passes into the glomeruli for filtration before reaching the rest of the kidney. There are two capillary

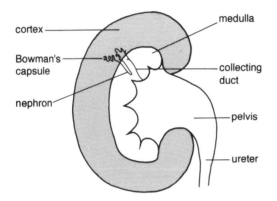

**Fig. 9.5**   Vertical section through a kidney showing the position of a nephron (left) and detail of a nephron (below).

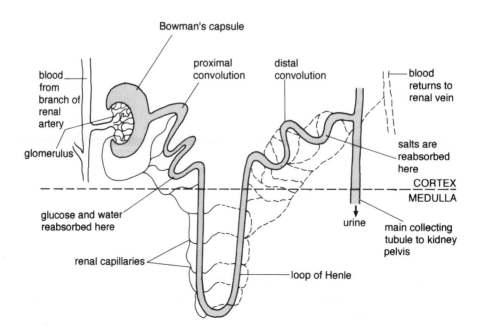

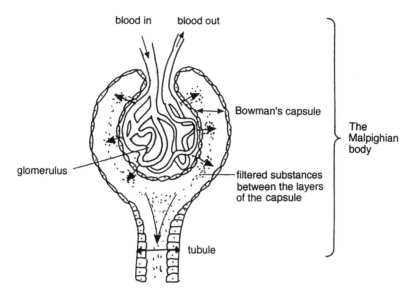

blood in    blood out

Bowman's capsule

The Malpighian body

glomerulus

filtered substances between the layers of the capsule

tubule

**Fig. 9.6**  Malpighian body showing that fluid passes from the glomerular blood vessels into the tubules.

beds (one after the other) – one which surrounds the Bowman's capsule and the other which intermingles with the tubular parts of the nephron. This is to allow the movement of salts, water, etc. back into the blood supply from the nephron. The blood in the glomerular vessels is at relatively high pressure to help the filtering process.

## The formation of urine

Bowman's capsule is the swollen, thin-walled, blind end of the nephron and into this tightly fits the glomerulus, so that the inner layer of the cup is in very close contact with the glomerulus. The layers which separate the plasma in the glomeruler capillaries from the cavity of Bowman's capsule are the capillary wall, a basement membrane on which the capillary wall rests and the visceral layer of Bowman's capsule. Of the three layers that act as the barrier through which filtration takes place, only the basement membrane acts as a barrier to the *free* movement of substances.

In some places the capillary wall has 'holes' in it so that blood plasma is in direct contact with the basement membrane. The cells of the visceral layer of Bowman's capsule have many branched projections which adjoin directly on to the basement membrane. Between these branches are gaps through which water and substances dissolved in it can move from blood plasma into the cavity of Bowman's capsule without having to pass through the cytoplasm of either the capillary cells which make up the wall, or the visceral layer of the capsule itself.

Because the blood in the glomeruli is under such high pressure, there is no tendency for fluid to enter back into the glomeruli blood-vessels. The blood cells and larger substances such as proteins are retained within the capillaries in the glomeruli and only water and smaller substances such as mineral salts, glucose, amino acids, urea, etc. are filtered out of the capillaries. The glomerular filtrate therefore contains water, salts, glucose, amino acids and excretory products such as urea. If there is a fall in blood pressure, for example if the horse is haemorrhaging (bleeding), the filtration process may stop and no urine will be formed.

## The role of the tubules in the formation of urine and in homeostasis

The main role of the tubules is therefore to reabsorb large volumes of fluids and most of the substances dissolved in that fluid. The mechanisms of reabsorption and secretion in the kidney tubules, however, are complicated. Water moves passively through the walls of the renal tubules down an osmotic gradient. Substances dissolved in the filtrate fluid, however, move passively in and out of the tubular fluid down chemical and electrical gradients. But some compounds have to be actively transported against chemical and electrical gradients and this requires the use of energy.

If a substance is removed from tubular fluid to the blood, then it is said to be reabsorbed, whereas if it is moved from the blood to the tubules it is said to be secreted. The tubules may add more of the substance to the tubular fluid (tubular secretion) or may remove some or all of the substance from the tubular fluid (reabsorption) or may do both, a very complicated process.

Most of the dissolved substances filtered off in the glomerular filtrate are reabsorbed in the proximal tubules of the kidney. This reabsorption is accompanied by the passive reabsorption of water. So, all the glucose and amino acids and a great proportion of potassium are reabsorbed in the proximal tubule. This reabsorption takes place against a concentration gradient since as these substances are being reabsorbed into the blood, the concentration in the blood plasma in the capillaries soon becomes higher than in the tubule. This reabsorption is an active process requiring energy which is supplied by the cells of the proximal tubule.

A maximum amount of glucose can be reabsorbed by the proximal tubule. If more than this is delivered by the blood to the tubule, glucose will start to appear in the urine. This situation occurs in the condition known as diabetes mellitus, a common condition in humans but rarely found in horses. All the amino acids will be reabsorbed as long as there is no damage to the proximal tubule or if there is an abnormally high concentration of amino acids in the blood.

Sodium is also reabsorbed actively (using energy) by the proximal tubule. Because the sodium ions are positively charged, negatively charged particles such as chloride move with the sodium to maintain neutrality. Water moves passively with the sodium and chloride ions to maintain osmotic balance (a complicated process). Since both water and the substances dissolved in it are reabsorbed in the proximal tubule, the fluid in the tubules stays at the same concentration (isotonic) with the plasma in the blood, even though its volume is considerably reduced. Bicarbonate is also conserved by the proximal tubule.

## The regulation of body water

The kidneys play a vital role in the control of body water, by altering the amount of water excreted in the face of large variations in water intake. When horses are deprived of water, the quantity of urine produced is low and the concentration of that urine is high. Of the water that enters the tubule, about 85% is reabsorbed in the proximal part and the remaining 15% is passed on to the further parts of the tubule. It is this fraction of the filtered water that is modified by the kidney according to the state of the body's water balance (hydration).

If the body is dehydrated, most of the water in the distal end of the tubule will be reabsorbed, whereas if the body is over-hydrated almost all of this water will be excreted in the urine. This is the body's way of maintaining water balance. How does the kidney regulate and absorb this water?

## The mechanism of urine concentration

The ability of mammals to conserve water by producing highly concentrated urine varies between species. Some animals such as desert-living mammals need to produce a much more concentrated urine because water is scarce.

A mechanism known as the sodium pump which is situated in the ascending loop of Henle (see Fig. 9.5) is responsible for the addition or removal of water (and therefore the concentration of urine). Here, sodium is forced out from the tubular fluid into the tissue fluid between the tubules making the tissue fluid hypertonic (i.e. more concentrated) in the region of the kidney medulla. The collecting ducts draining all the nephrons have to pass through this medullary region of hypertonic fluid in order to reach and empty into the pelvis of the kidney. This osmotic gradient causes water to move out of the urine in the collecting ducts and into the more concentrated tissue fluid. As the tissue fluid becomes even more concentrated, the greater the osmotic gradient and movement of water, producing a more concentrated urine. In order that the urine concentrating ability may be regulated according to the water balance of the horse, the permeability (or leaking ability) of the collecting ducts and the distal convoluted tubule can be adjusted. So, if the horse is dehydrated, the distal tubules and collecting ducts will allow water to pass through into the tissue fluid thereby conserving water. This results in the production of a smaller quantity of more concentrated urine.

If the horse is over-hydrated, i.e. has too much body water, the distal parts of the tubule and collecting ducts will not allow water to pass through. Thus this water cannot be removed from the collecting tubules and is consequently evacuated in the urine. This results in a copious, dilute urine being produced.

The regulation of permeability in the distal convoluted tubules and the collecting ducts and therefore the control of urine concentration is controlled by a hormone known as ADH (anti-diuretic hormone).

## The regulation of permeability of the collecting ducts by ADH

The permeability of the distal parts of the nephron to water is controlled by a hormone, ADH, which is secreted by the posterior lobe of the pituitary gland. The term diuresis refers to the condition when large volumes of dilute urine are produced. Anti-diuresis means the opposite and applies when water is reabsorbed and smaller amounts of a concentrated urine are produced.

The name of the hormone ADH therefore describes its effect on the nephrons in the kidney. The release of ADH from the pituitary increases the permeability of the distal parts of the nephrons to water, allowing more water to diffuse out into the tissue fluid and making a reduced volume of urine which is more concentrated. In the absence of ADH, the collecting tubules remain impermeable to water and no concentration of urine occurs.

In the condition known as diabetes insipidus which occurs in horses (as well as humans), the posterior pituitary gland either does not secrete ADH or secretes insufficient amounts of the hormone. This means that the urine is not concentrated and affected horses will pass large quantities of pale, thin, dilute urine. These horses will also need to drink more to replace these losses in the urine and therefore may show excessive thirst as one of the symptoms of the condition. Other signs include weight loss, weakness and exercise intolerance.

Frequently, this condition in horses is the result of a tumour in the pituitary gland. It can be treated, but this is often not practical.

In addition to regulating the body water, the kidneys are responsible for regulating the plasma concentration of body salts (electrolytes) such as sodium and potassium. This regulation takes place by an exchange mechanism in the distal convoluted tubule between sodium and potassium.

The regulation of this exchange is undertaken by another hormone, aldosterone, which is secreted by the adrenal gland. An excessive secretion of aldosterone results in a loss of potassium (in the urine) and a retention of sodium in the body. A deficiency in the amount of aldosterone results in the opposite, i.e. a net loss of sodium from the body (in the urine) and a retention of potassium. When sodium is excreted in the urine in this way, water is also lost (water is secreted to maintain osmotic balance). This leads to progressive shrinking of the amount of fluid circulating in the body and eventually circulatory collapse will occur.

If a horse is deficient of salt (i.e. sodium), aldosterone will be secreted to conserve sodium in the distal convoluted tubule.

The horse is able to self-limit his salt intake and if he needs extra salt, a salt lick should be available to him at all times, so that he can help himself. I do not like the addition of salt by horse owners to the concentrate feed. My view is that horses should be allowed to help themselves unless they are ill.

## Acid/base balance

Large amounts of chemical reactions take place in the body and acids are being continuously produced by cells as a result of metabolism. Also, a large number of these potential acids may come from the horse's diet. However, in spite of all this acid production, the pH of the blood plasma and other body fluids must remain constant. The normal average pH of arterial blood is 7.4, whereas the venous blood is 7.35 due to the extra carbon dioxide being carried back to the lungs. The pH within cells in the body varies from 4.5 (very acid) to 8.0 (alkaline) depending upon the type of cell. The kidney has an important role to play in acid/base balance by controlling the excretion of bicarbonate in the urine thereby making it more or less acidic and compensating for alkalosis or acidosis in the horse's body.

## Urea

Urea is the main nitrogenous waste product found in mammals. It is soluble in water and fairly toxic. Urea is manufactured in the liver in a cyclical chemical reaction known as the ornithine cycle, from ammonia (Fig. 9.7).

## Micturition or urination

This is the term used for the evacuation of urine from the bladder. The urine produced in the kidneys in the collecting tubules is then transferred to the renal pelvis where it enters the ureter and is carried to the bladder. The bladder acts as a storage vessel for urine.

Micturition is a reflex activity stimulated by the fullness of the bladder itself. The bladder adjusts to the gradual inflow of urine from the ureters until the pressure becomes too high and reflex centres in the spinal cord are stimulated. This causes contraction of the muscles in the bladder wall and evacuation of the urine. Horses tend to urinate (stale) at rest when on grass or bedding. Many horses will wait to urinate (if

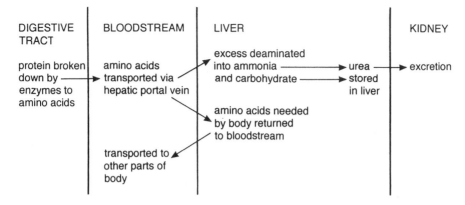

**Fig. 9.7** Summary of the formation of urea.

the bladder is not too full) until they are brought into the stable, particularly when the bedding is clean and deep.

Horses adopt a typical posture when urinating, with the hind legs separated, the horse leaning slightly forward. There is contraction of the muscles of the abdominal wall and the tail is raised. Often horses will grunt and groan when urinating. This is normal! Horses produce about 5–15 litres of urine per day (depending upon water intake and diet) and will urinate approximately 4–6 times in that period.

Horse owners should be vigilant in watching their horses' urinating habits. Early recognition of abnormal signs will allow prompt veterinary attention if something is wrong.

Horse owners should watch out for:

- any signs of pain when the horse is urinating. Is there continual straining and excessive grunting?
- how frequently the horse urinates and whether he is producing an excessively large or small volume of urine. Is he more thirsty than usual? Is he not drinking enough?
- The colour of the urine. It should be light yellow to amber in colour and this darkens on standing (i.e. if left in a bottle to show the vet). If it is dark coloured or bloodstained the vet should be called immediately.

## Conditions of the urinary system

Diseases of the urinary system are relatively rare in horses. The kidney is an unusual organ in that it can continue to function even when it is quite considerably damaged (up to 70%). Even though this is the case, conditions of the urinary system must always be taken seriously as they can be life-threatening.

### Acute renal failure

There are many causes of acute renal failure. The causes tend to be split into groups depending upon the area of the urinary system which is affected:

(1) Pre-renal causes. Pre-renal causes encompass those which affect the blood supply to the kidney by a drop in blood pressure such as seen in severe dehydration, haemorrhage (blood loss), shock, or heart failure.

(2) Post-renal causes. These occur when there is an obstruction to urine flow after the kidney part of the urinary tract, e.g. blockage of the urethra or neck of the bladder by stones known as calculi.
(3) Other causes that affect the kidney tissue itself such as poisons (nephrotoxins). These include some plants, heavy metals (e.g. mercury) and drugs such as some antibiotics and sulphonamides. Myoglobin, the pigment from muscle which is released into the bloodstream following a severe attack of azoturia can also cause renal damage.

Most often there is a reduction in the volume of urine which becomes very concentrated. The kidneys become swollen and tender (which may be detected by rectal palpation by the veterinary surgeon). If the horse survives this initial acute phase, then it is often followed by diuresis where the volume of urine increases dramatically and the urine is very dilute.

The prognosis depends upon the cause and the severity of the condition.

## Polynephritis

This condition tends to occur in mares after foaling. An infection of the pelvis of the kidney occurs after infection passes up the urinary tract. The mare will show symptoms of cystitis (i.e. pain and straining when urinating).

Polynephritis may also result from infections picked up from the bloodstream (pyaemic nephritis). This may occur in foals with infected umbilical stumps after birth. Signs include weight loss, depression and weakness and considerable swelling of the underbelly and legs. The horse is very thirsty. Accurate diagnosis requires blood and urine samples which may show anaemia, severe body salts (electrolyte) imbalance and increased blood levels of urea.

Prognosis depends upon the extent of renal failure by the time a diagnosis is made. Some cases may respond to antibiotic therapy and correction of the electrolyte imbalance. Also, good sick nursing of the equine patient is essential.

## Cystitis

Cystitis, meaning inflammation of the bladder, is relatively rare in horses. The problem may result from passage, e.g. bacteria up the urethra. If the bladder cannot empty itself properly, infection is more likely to result. Conditions which may cause this are bladder stones or bladder paralysis.

Signs include frequent attempts to urinate and severe straining on urinating. Sometimes the condition may be chronic (long lasting) and signs include urine dribbling and caking of the vulval lips of mares. The urine may also be bloodstained.

Treatment depends upon the initial cause which must be identified. Antibiotic therapy will be given depending upon the organism which has caused the problem. This can be found by culture of urine samples to grow the bacteria. An antibiotic is used which will be excreted at high levels in the urine and therefore kill the bacteria in the urinary tract.

## Bladder stones (cystic calculi)

Stones may develop anywhere in the urinary tract, but the bladder is the most common site. Substances dissolved in the urine precipitate out on to bladder cells. If the urine pH increases in alkalinity this will aid the precipitation of carbonate dissolved in the urine to form a carbonate stone. If the water consumed by the horse has a high mineral content, then this will increase the chances of the condition occurring. Usually only one stone forms at a time normally made up of calcium carbonate. Affected horses strain to urinate and dribble urine. This may be accompanied by mild colic.

The stone has to be surgically removed. The horse's management, particularly with regard to mineral intake and water sources, should be investigated to prevent recurrence of the stone.

# Chapter 10
# The Teeth and Ageing

The horse has developed a system of cutting and grinding teeth that is both effective and simple, allowing the horse to survive on its grazing diet. The horse owner must pay regular attention to the teeth as they can become sharp and cause the horse discomfort during eating or when being ridden. The horseman also uses the horse's teeth to determine its age.

The horse has two sets of teeth during its life – temporary and permanent. Temporary or milk teeth are smaller and whiter than the permanent teeth. There are no temporary molar teeth. From the age of two-and-a-half years the milk teeth are gradually replaced so that by the time the horse is five-years-old it has a full set of permanent teeth which are larger, more yellow adult teeth.

The horse has three types of tooth (Fig. 10.1):

- incisors or biting teeth in the front of the mouth. The incisor teeth are called the centrals (the pair top and bottom in the centre), laterals (the teeth next to the centrals) and the corners;
- molars or grinding teeth lining each side of the jaw bone – the cheek teeth. These in turn can be divided into molars and premolars with the molars at the back of the jaw. Unlike the human the horse's premolars and molars are very similar in shape;
- tushes or canine teeth.

As the horse evolved the organisation and structure of its teeth became different to that of carnivores and omnivores. Two major changes allowed the horse to cope with a diet of tough fibrous herbage without wearing its teeth down prematurely. Firstly, the

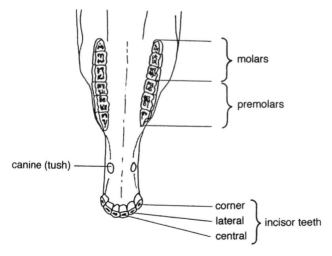

**Fig. 10.1**  Dentition of the horse.

# Chapter 11
# The Digestive System

The horse evolved as a grazing animal and the anatomy and physiology of the digestive system as well as feeding behaviour reflect this. Many horses are stabled for all or part of the time and only have access to limited areas of grazing, preventing them from following their natural feeding patterns.

The horse's gut is designed to take in small amounts at frequent intervals, with wild horses spending up to 14 hours a day grazing. This is known as trickle feeding and the horse's digestive system has evolved over millions of years to suit this way of feeding. In the wild the horse is also able to select from a wide variety of grasses, herbs and shrubs. Domestication of horses has led to increased stresses on the horse's gut due to 'abnormal' feeding patterns which humans have imposed on their horses.

The natural diet of herbivores consists of grasses and vegetation containing large amounts of the insoluble, or complex carbohydrate known as cellulose. No mammal has the ability to secrete the enzyme cellulase, which breaks down cellulose, in its digestive tract and the horse therefore has to rely upon a large number of micro-organisms in its hindgut to perform this task.

## Nutrients

Horses need to eat food to provide nutrients for them to grow, live and reproduce and to follow an athletic career. To have a healthy existence horses must obtain over forty important nutrients from their food.

For horses to develop a high level of physical fitness and performance, a basic understanding of nutrients and their effects on the body is required, and diets for horses should be thought of in terms of nutrients provided and not just the ingredients themselves.

## Composition of food

Food serves a number of purposes:

- to provide fuel for the horse's body in the form of energy;
- to provide material for the building and maintenance of body tissues;
- to supply substances which act to regulate the wide range of body processes.

Food consists of six basic categories of nutrients. They are classified by their actions in the body and not by their chemical composition. These are carbohydrates, fats, proteins, vitamins, minerals and water.

## Carbohydrates

These are an important source of energy for the horse's body cells and tissues. Within this class fall the sugars, starch, glycogen and cellulose. All carbohydrates are characterised by being made up of the elements carbon, hydrogen and oxygen with the hydrogen and oxygen almost always present in the $2 : 1$ ratio found in water, hence the name carbo-(carbon) hydrate (water). In fact the name 'carbohydrate' is derived from the French *hydrate de carbon.*

The majority of carbohydrates are derived from plants where they are formed from carbon dioxide, water and energy from the sun, by the process of photosynthesis.

## Monosaccharides

The simplest carbohydrates are the simple sugars such as glucose or fructose. Glucose and fructose consist of single unit sugars and are therefore known as monosaccharides from the Greek *mono-*, single and *sacchar*, sugar. The chemical formula for glucose, an important monosaccharide, is $C_6H_{12}O_6$. Glucose is the main fuel for cells, providing energy for them to work.

Glucose is absorbed into the blood following digestion, where it is maintained at a steady concentration. It may then either be transported directly to the body cells for energy or converted to another polysaccharide, glycogen and stored in the liver and muscles. Other monosaccharides include arabinose and xylose which are five carbon sugars known as pentose sugars. Also glucose, fructose, galactose and mannose which contain six carbons and are therefore known as hexose sugars.

## Disaccharides

Cells are able to build disaccharides or double sugars from two monosaccharides, for example, maltose is built from two glucose molecules. Perhaps the most common disaccharide is sucrose which is obtained from a glucose and a fructose. This is the main carbohydrate found in plant sap and is the sugar extracted from sugar beet roots or sugar cane. Other disaccharides include lactose and cellobiose.

## Trisaccharides

Trisaccharides can also be built up in the same way from three sugar molecule units. An example is raffinose.

## Polysaccharides

These are long chains of sugar molecules, which may contain from a few hundred to several thousand units. Starch is a polysaccharide and is made of a number of glucose units linked together to form long chains. Starch is the storage form of sugar in plants (and therefore grass). Plant cells need sugar for energy and horses make use of this plant starch, by breaking it down during the digestive process and absorbing the glucose units. Cereals are major sources of starch.

Horses store excess sugar in the form of glycogen, another polysaccharide, which is identical to starch in being built up of glucose units, but containing more branches to the long chain. The long chains in both starch and glycogen molecules are coiled in to a helical shape.

Many polysaccharides are structural in that they provide strength, for example cellulose. More generally known as fibre, cellulose forms the fundamental structure of all plant cell walls which is why it is the most abundant organic compound found on Earth. Cellulose is also similar to glycogen and starch in that it is made from many glucose units, but these are linked together differently to form long rods with no branches rather than the coil shape of starch and glycogen. Unlike the glucose links in starch and glycogen those in cellulose cannot be broken down by enzymes produced by the horse. All herbivores need micro-organisms which produce the enzyme cellulase to break down the cellulose. In the horse this process takes place in the caecum and colon, where a huge microbial population are housed in order for the cellulose to be broken down. The end products of cellulose digestion are not single sugar units, but substances known as volatile fatty acids – the most common being acetic, propionic and butyric acids – which are then absorbed and used as an energy source by the horse. They can provide at least 25% of the energy required.

Several different substances are now thought to contribute to fibre in the horse's diet including cellulose and the hemicelluloses. Hemicelluloses contain many different sugar molecules in their chains forming a mixed polysaccharide which is easier to digest than cellulose, but less easily digested than starch. Hemicelluloses are abundant in pasture and therefore conserved forages. The structure of cellulose is shown in Fig. 11.1.

To summarise, carbohydrates can be found with a number of different chain lengths (Fig. 11.2). They are broken down by the body's digestive system to simple sugars, e.g. glucose, before being absorbed into the horse's body.

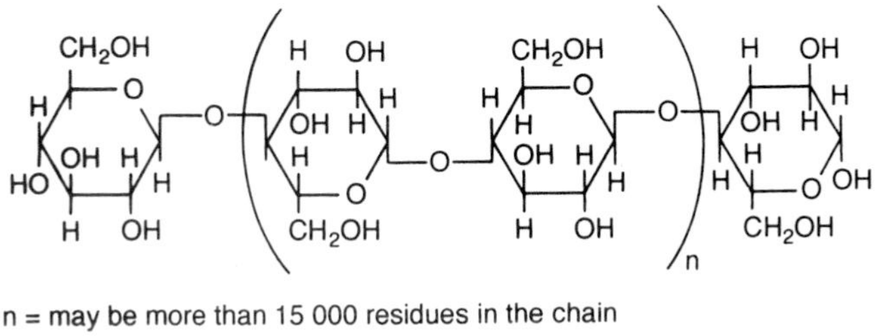

n = may be more than 15 000 residues in the chain

**Fig. 11.1**   Structure of cellulose.

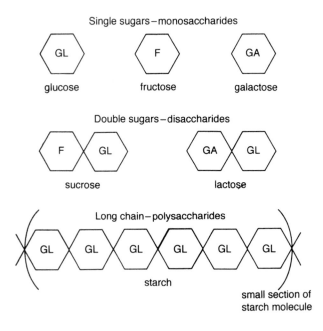

**Fig. 11.2**   Hexose carbohydrates showing the formation of monosaccharides, disaccharides and polysaccharides.

## Lignin

Lignin, which is not a carbohydrate, but is closely associated with this group, gives mechanical strength to plants particularly when plants age. Lignin refers to a number of closely related compounds. It is indigestible. Wood, mature pastures, hays and straw are all high in lignin. Because it is indigestible it remains in the gut longer and causes the characteristic hay belly. It is of no nutritional value to the horse.

## Lipids or fats

Fats and oils are essential and like carbohydrates are made up from carbon hydrogen and oxygen, but the proportion of oxygen is much lower in fats. Fats are a concentrated source of energy and can be stored in the horse's body as an energy reserve. Fats and oils contain two-and-a-quarter times more energy than carbohydrates.

Fats and oils both have the same basic structure, but different physical characteristics. The melting point of oils is such that at room temperature they are liquid, whereas most fats such as butter are solid. The term fat is frequently used to include both groups.

True fats are made up of a glycerol molecule combined with one, two or three fatty acids to give mono, di or triglycerides respectively. The differences between fats are largely the result of different fatty acids being attached to the glycerol molecule. The basic structure of a fat molecule is shown in Fig. 11.3.

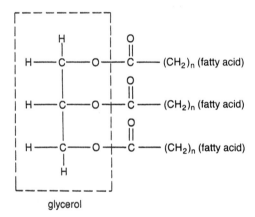

glycerol

triglyceride = 1 glycerol unit + 3 fatty acids          **Fig. 11.3**   Basic structure of a fat molecule.

The term lipid is often interchanged with fat, but while all fats are lipids, *not* all lipids are fats. Also in addition to fats, the group of lipids also includes related substances such as waxes, cholesterol and lecithin.

There are many fatty acids but the most important one is linoleic acid. This is an essential fatty acid in that it is required in the diet of the horse to maintain normal health. It is thought that polyunsaturated fats are important in the horse to maintain the health of the skin. Fats, therefore, are of value in the diet for a number of reasons. They are:

- a source of the essential fatty acid, linoleic acid;
- a concentrated energy source;
- carriers for fat soluble vitamins.

Fats and oils are now being used extensively in the diets of hard working horses including long distance, endurance horses and racehorses.

## Protein

Protein was one of the first nutrients to be discovered. It was recognised in the first half of the nineteenth century. The name protein is derived from the Greek word *proteios* meaning 'to come first', which suggests the importance of this nutrient.

All living matter discovered to date contains protein as it forms a vital part of every cell. Each horse has tens of thousands of different types of protein each with its own three-dimensional structure corresponding to a specific function. There are seven major classes of proteins:

(1) Structural proteins, e.g. those in hair, tendons and ligaments.
(2) Contractile proteins, e.g. those proteins which result in muscle contraction.
(3) Storage proteins, e.g. ovalbumin which acts as a source of amino acids for the developing embryo.
(4) Defence proteins, e.g. antibodies.
(5) Transport proteins, e.g. haemoglobin which carries oxygen around the body.
(6) Signal proteins, e.g. hormones.
(7) Enzymes. These promote and regulate most of the chemical reactions which occur in the horse's body.

A protein is a large molecule made up of many units known as amino acids. The amino acids are put together in various combinations to form the body proteins. Each protein has a different amino acid composition and no two proteins are the same.

Proteins are composed of larger and more complex molecules than those of either fats or carbohydrates. They contain the elements nitrogen, carbon, hydrogen and oxygen and sometimes also contain sulphur, iron and phosphorous. The nitrogen is present in the form of an amino group ($NH_2$) and this gives the amino acid its name.

### Amino acids

There are twenty-two different amino acids (Table 11.1). Some of these amino acids are known as essential or indispensable in that they must be provided in the diet as the horse cannot make them in the body. Others are known as non-essential or dispensable in that they can be made by the horse and therefore they do not have to be provided in the horse's diet. It is not known how many indispensable amino acids are required by horses, due to a lack of research, but it is known that lysine is indispensable. The other twenty-one are dispensable to the horse. However, horses under stress, such as racehorses, may not be able to make all the dispensable amino acids they need and some may need to be added to the diet. It is thought that methionine is indispensable during growth, and work in the USA has implicated the possible importance of methionine and threonine, particularly for growing horses.

Protein obtained from food cannot function in the horse's body until it is broken down into its constituent parts, the amino acids. Figure 11.4 shows the general basic structure of amino acids. The R group is the variable part of the amino acid.

### Polypeptides

Cells are able to link amino acids together. Two amino acids linked together form a dipeptide; a chain of amino acids linked together is known as a polypeptide. Polypeptides may contain more than a thousand amino acids and are capable of forming three-dimensional shapes within a protein.

**Table 12.1**  Amino acid classification for the horse

**Essential or indispensable**
Lysine
Methionine

**Non-essential or dispensable**

| | | |
|---|---|---|
| Glycine | Threonine | Hydroxyglutamic acid |
| Tryptophan | Arginine | Cystine |
| Valine | Serine | Citrulline |
| Histidine | Alanine | Proline |
| Phenylalanine | Norleucine | Hydroxyproline |
| Leucine | Aspartic acid | Tyrosine |
| Isoleucine | Glutamic acid | |

Total = 22

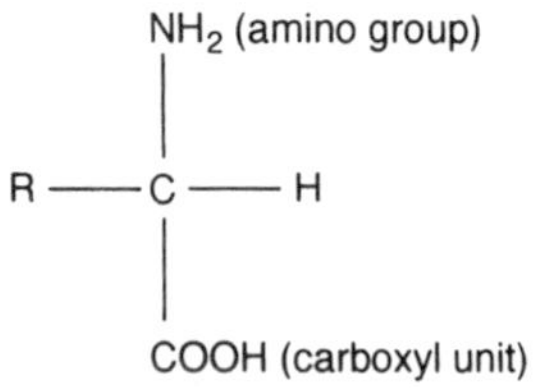

NH$_2$ (amino group)

R ——— C ——— H

COOH (carboxyl unit)

R varies between the different amino acids     **Fig. 11.4**  General formula for amino acids.

It has been shown that horses are more prone to infections when they are fed inadequate protein. Alternatively, if excess protein is fed to the horse it cannot be stored for later use unlike other nutrients. The excess must be broken down in a process known as deamination and the nitrogen part of the molecule is removed as ammonia or urea and excreted. The remainder of the protein molecule (carbon skeleton) serves as an energy source, but it is an expensive source and horses use energy to break the protein down in the first place.

## Protein quality

Feeds that supply the correct proportion and amount of indispensable amino acids are known as 'good quality' proteins, whereas those containing a high quantity which are dispensable are considered 'poor quality' proteins. All grains are lacking in lysine and therefore contain 'poor quality' protein. Soya bean meal however is a good source of lysine.

## Energy: protein ratio

There is an optimum calorie to protein ratio for each stage of growth of the horse. If this ratio is correct it maximises the energy utilisation, and as the energy amount in the diet increases, there is an increased need for amino acids.

# Vitamins

A vitamin is an organic nutrient which is required in much smaller amounts than the indispensable amino acids. Most vitamins have functions in metabolic reactions, where they are used over and over again. Even though vitamins are required in tiny amounts they are still absolutely vital for life. Deficiencies of vitamins can result in severe ill health in the horse but some vitamins are also dangerous if taken in excess. Some vitamins can only function after undergoing a chemical change and these are known as provitamins or vitamin precursors. An example of this is beta-carotene which is converted to vitamin A.

Vitamins are normally divided into two groups, fat soluble and water soluble. Fat soluble vitamins include A (retinol), D, E (tocopherol) and K. Vitamin D is known as the sunshine vitamin because it can be made in the skin in the presence of sunlight. This is a good reason to keep horses' rugs off in the spring and summer and to turn them out as much as possible. Horses which are stabled or rugged will not be able to make enough vitamin D to meet their needs. Water soluble vitamins include B complex ($B_1$ thiamine, $B_2$ riboflavin, $B_3$ niacin, $B_5$ pantothenic acid, $B_6$ pyridoxine, folic acid, $B_{12}$ cyanocobalamin, $B_{15}$ pangamic acid and biotin) and vitamin C, ascorbic acid.

The water soluble vitamins are particularly important in cell metabolism for example, vitamins $B_1$, $B_6$, folic acid, biotin and $B_{12}$ are coenzymes used in the metabolism of amino acids, sugars, nucleic acids and fats. Vitamin C has many roles but it is now thought to have a mainly antioxidant role, preventing cell damage occurring as a result of toxic substances produced normally during respiration.

Fat soluble vitamins are stored in the horse's body, mainly in the liver, and fresh green herbage is rich in these vitamins. Therefore the horse can take in plenty of these vitamins during the summer when pastures are richer and store them for later use in the winter when grass growth ceases. Because these vitamins are stored, feeding excessive amounts may result in toxicity and care should be taken when feeding large quantities of supplements. Water soluble vitamins on the other hand, are mainly produced by the micro-organisms in the horse hindgut. For this reason storage is not necessary and these vitamins if produced or fed to excess will be broken down and excreted through the urine.

A list of the vitamins, their function and dietary sources is shown in Table 11.2.

**Table 11.2** Functions, sources and deficiencies of vitamins and minerals in horses

| Vitamin | Required for | Source | Deficiency signs |
|---|---|---|---|
| **Fat soluble vitamins** | | | |
| A<br>B<br>Carotene | Healthy eyes<br>Immune system<br>Growth and<br>  maintenance, of<br>  body tissues | Grass<br>Green forage | Lack of appetite<br>Night blindness<br>Poor growth<br>Keratinisation of eyes<br>Hoof and skin in poor<br>  condition<br>Infertility |
| D<br>Sunshine vitamin | Aids absorption of<br>  calcium and<br>  phosphorous<br>  absorption in the gut<br>Bone formation<br>Joint integrity | Horses synthesise<br>  vitamin D in their skin<br>  in the presence of<br>  sunlight<br>Sun dried hay<br>(Stabled horses may<br>  need supplementing) | Bones fail to calcify<br>  leading to rickets in<br>  young horses and<br>  osteomalacia in older<br>  ones<br>Swollen joints<br>Fractures |
| E<br>Tocopherol | Muscle integrity<br>Fat metabolism<br>Acts with selenium as<br>  an antioxidant<br>Reproduction | Alfalfa<br>Green forage<br>Cereals | Muscular disorders<br>Infertility |

**Table 11.2**   Continued

| Vitamin | Required for | Source | Deficiency signs |
|---|---|---|---|
| K | Blood clotting | Produced by healthy hindgut microbial population<br>Leafy forage | True deficiency is rare<br>Levels can be assessed by measuring blood clotting time |
| **Water soluble vitamins** | | | |
| C<br>Ascorbic acid | Immune system<br>Antioxidant<br>Muscle and blood capillary integrity | Made in body tissues from glucose | Bleeding, ulcerated gums<br>Internal bleeding<br>Interacts with copper and iron |
| $B_1$<br>Thiamine | Fat and carbohydrate metabolism, particularly glucose | Produced by healthy hindgut microbial population | Deficiency may be caused by eating bracken<br>Loss of appetite<br>Incoordination<br>Staggering |
| $B_2$<br>Riboflavin | Carbohydrate, protein and fat metabolism | Produced by healthy hindgut microbial population | Reduced growth rate<br>Reduced utilisation of feed<br>Possibly involved in periodic ophthalmia |
| $B_6$<br>Pyridoxine was known as Vit H | Carbohydrate, protein and fat metabolism<br>Enzyme systems | Grass<br>Green forage | In absence of $B_6$, tryptophan and niacin cannot be utilised<br>Poor growth, dermatitis<br>Nerve degeneration |
| $B_{12}$<br>Cyanocobalamin | Carbohydrate, fat and protein metabolism | Produced by healthy hindgut microbial population, but requires cobalt to do this | Poor growth<br>Infertility<br>Poor appetite<br>Rough coat |
| Folic acid<br>Folacin | Maturation of red blood cells<br>Interacts with $B_2$, $B_{12}$ and C | Grass<br>Green forage<br>Synthesised in hindgut by healthy microbial population | Not described in horses |
| Biotin | Hoof horn production<br>Carbohydrate, protein and fat metabolism | Maize, yeast, soya<br>Green forage | Poor hoof condition, hoof crumbles at ground surface |
| Niacin<br>Nicotinic acid | Enzyme systems in all body cells<br>Cell integrity and metabolism<br>Carbohydrate, protein and fat digestion | Can be synthesised from the amino acid tryptophan<br><br>Cereals | Never been produced in the horse |
| Pantothenic acid<br>Calcium pantothenate | Part of coenzymes<br>Carbohydrate, fat and protein digestion | Synthesised in hindgut by healthy microbial population | No specific deficiency signs seen in horses. |

**Table 11.2** Continued

| Mineral | Required for | Source | Deficiency signs |
|---------|-------------|--------|-----------------|
| **Major minerals** | | | |
| Ca<br>Calcium | 98% of body Ca is<br>  found in skeleton and<br>  teeth<br>Blood clotting<br>Nerve and muscle<br>  function<br>Lactation | Alfalfa<br>Limestone flour<br>Green forage<br>Sugar beet | Bone problems<br>Rickets (young)<br>Osteomalacia (old)<br>Nutritional secondary<br>  hyperparathyroidism<br>  (big head disease)<br>Enlarged joints<br>Tying up |
| P<br>Phosphorus | 85% of body P is found<br>  in skeleton and teeth<br>Energy production<br>Enzyme systems | Cereals | Bone problems<br>Rickets (young)<br>Osteomalacia (old)<br>Reduced or depraved<br>  appetite<br>Decreased growth |
| Mg<br>Magnesium | 60–70% of body Mg<br>  found in skeleton and<br>  teeth<br>Enzyme systems | Alfalfa<br>Linseed | Weakness in limbs<br>Muscular tremors<br>Ataxia<br>Sweating |
| Na (Sodium)<br>Cl (Chloride)<br>K (Potassium) | Body fluid regulation<br>Muscle and nerve<br>  function<br>Acid base balance | Grass<br>Hay<br>Salt lick (NaCl only)<br>Horses have a specific<br>  appetite for salt | Sweating<br>Dehydration<br>Muscular weakness<br>  fatigue<br>Exhaustion<br>Depraved appetite |
| S<br>Sulphur | Amino acid synthesis<br>Hoof and horn growth<br>Enzyme systems<br>Present in insulin | Grass | Poor hair and skin<br>  growth including<br>  hooves |
| **Trace minerals** | | | |
| Fe<br>Iron | Haemoglobin<br>  syntheses<br>60% of body Fe is in<br>  haemoglobin<br>Enzyme activation | Most natural feeds | Anaemia<br>Weakness<br>Pale mucus<br>  membranes<br>Fatigue<br>Reduced growth<br>Mares' milk is low in Fe |
| Cu<br>Copper | Haemoglobin synthesis<br>Pigmentation of hair<br>Cartilage and elastin<br>  production<br>Bone development<br>Interacts with S and Mo | Depends upon soil Cu<br>  content from which<br>  feed is grown<br>High Mo reduces Cu<br>  availability | Developmental<br>  orthopaedic disease<br>Intermittent diarrhoea<br>Loss of pigment in hair<br>Poor performance<br>Reduced growth |
| Zn<br>Zinc | Cell metabolism<br>Enzyme activator<br>High Zn interferes with<br>  Cu utilisation<br>Immune system | Yeast<br>Cereals | Hair loss<br>Skin lesions<br>Reduced appetite<br>Reduced growth |
| I<br>Iodine | Required for thyroxine<br>  hormone<br>Controls metabolic rate | Most feeds<br>Seaweed products | Infertility<br>Goitre |

**Table 11.2**   Continued

| Minerals | Required for | Source | Deficiency signs |
|---|---|---|---|
| Mo Molybdenum | Enzyme activator | Often excessive in soils and therefore pasture Forage High Mo affects Cu availability | Deficiency symptoms not seen |
| Se Selenium | Antioxidant Interacts with vitamin E | Pasture Soil content varies depending upon area Deficient areas are common USA has many areas where Se toxicity is common | Muscle disease Impaired cardiac function Respiratory problems Tying up |
| Mn Manganese | Carbohydrate, protein and fat metabolism Bone formation Lactation | Bran Grass (depending upon soil content) | Bone abnormalities Poor feed utilisation |
| Co Cobalt | Required for synthesis of vitamin $B_{12}$ | Trace levels present in most feeds | Anaemia Weight loss Reduced growth |

## Minerals

In addition to amino acids and vitamins, which are organic nutrients, the horse's body requires a number of minerals. These are chemical elements which must be supplied in the diet. Minerals are placed in one of two groups depending upon their concentration in the body. Macrominerals are present in much larger amounts than the trace minerals and include calcium, phosphorus, magnesium, potassium, sulphur, sodium and chloride. Trace minerals are present in concentrations of less than 50 mg/kg, but they can still cause severe problems if they are deficient. They include copper, zinc, selenium, iron, fluorine, iodine, manganese, cobalt, chromium and molybdenum.

Relatively large amounts of calcium and phosphorus are required for the horse's skeleton and calcium is also important for the normal functioning of muscles and nerves. Phosphorus is an ingredient of ATP (one of the major compounds in energy production) and nucleic acids. Sulphur is a component of several amino acids. Iron is required for haemoglobin and other molecules important in cellular respiration. Magnesium, manganese, zinc, copper, selenium and molybdenum are components of various enzymes. Copper and zinc have been implicated in developmental orthopaedic disease, if deficient in the diets of young horses. Horses need iodine to make the hormone thyroxin which regulates metabolic rate.

Sodium, potassium and chlorine are important in nerve function and also help to maintain fluid balance in cells. Sodium chloride otherwise known as common salt, is often in limited supply in some pastures and feral horses will regularly return to salt rich areas to get salt. Horses have a specific appetite for salt and for this reason a salt lick should always be available. A list of minerals, their requirements, sources and deficiency signs is shown in Table 11.2.

## Water

Water is the most important nutrient required by horses and it is frequently neglected.

If a horse finds water freely available, then it will consume enough to meet its needs. The body of the adult horse is 70% water and the foal is 75–80%.

Water has several functions in the body including:

- temperature regulation;
- transport medium for various compounds in the body;
- constituent of all body fluids and cells;
- to lubricate joints;
- to maintain water balance;
- milk production.

Fresh grass contains 80% water and horses will consume a large amount of water when eating fresh herbage.

## The digestive system

The entire digestive system is completely unique to the horse and can be split into two parts:

- the foregut
- the hindgut.

The foregut is similar to that of simple stomached animals such as pigs and humans and the hindgut is somewhat similar to the rumen of the cow (Table 11.3).

**Table 11.3** The digestive system of the horse

| Foregut (similar to human or pig) | Hindgut (some similarity to ruminant) |
| --- | --- |
| Mouth | Caecum |
| Pharynx | Large colon |
| Oesophagus | Small colon |
| Stomach | Rectum |
| Small intestines | Anus |

The microbial population breaks down the fibrous part of the diet in the hindgut. However, the amount of microbial digestion is much smaller than that which occurs in ruminants and the absorption of nutrients is not as efficient. This is because the small intestine which is the major site of absorption of nutrients is situated before the fermentation area in the horse. In ruminants, the small intestine is sited after the rumen, and ruminants are therefore far more efficient at removing and absorbing nutrients from their food than horses (Fig. 11.5).

The digestive tract of the horse therefore tends to be slotted mid-way between that of ruminants and simple stomached animals in the way it is treated by scientists and some nutritionists. It is quite possible that because the horse is so unique, work done on other animals cannot always be simply extrapolated back to halfway between ruminants and simple stomached animals for horses.

In simple terms the horse's digestive tract (Fig. 11.6) is a tube beginning at the lips and ending at the anus, the role of which is to break down food into substances which can be absorbed into the bloodstream and utilised by the horse. This breakdown is accomplished by the digestive juices which are secreted by glands housed within the tract. The digestive tract is approximately 30 m (100 ft) long and in order to fit into the horse's abdomen it is coiled and looped and loosely held in place by sheets of

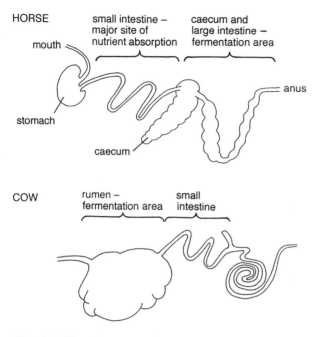

HORSE

mouth

stomach

small intestine –
major site of
nutrient absorption

caecum and
large intestine –
fermentation area

caecum

anus

COW

rumen –
fermentation area

small
intestine

**Fig. 11.5** Digestive system of the horse compared with the cow. Rumen fermentation produces nutrients that can be absorbed by the small intestine, increasing the efficiency of digestion in the cow compared with the horse.

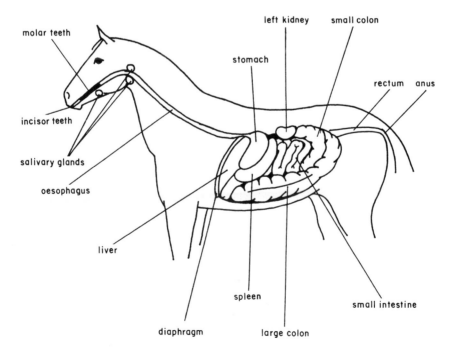

molar teeth

left kidney   small colon

stomach

rectum   anus

incisor teeth

salivary glands

oesophagus

liver

spleen

small intestine

diaphragm   large colon

**Fig. 11.6** Structure of the digestive system of the horse.

mesentery tissue. Throughout its length there are several changes in direction and diameter which partially explains the horse's susceptibility to blockages of the gut which manifest themselves as colic.

# Mouth

The upper lip is strong, mobile and sensitive and the horse uses it to sort through the feed on offer, before manoeuvering the food between its teeth. The incisor or biting teeth can bite off pieces of food in a selective fashion and, if necessary, can graze a pasture very closely. The tongue then moves the food to the molar teeth for grinding, through a series of up-and-down and side-to-side chewing movements, which pulverise the food into smaller pieces suitably lubricated by saliva for swallowing. Horses have evolved as forage eaters and rely on their teeth for 'processing' this fibrous food. All the food has to be ground down to less than 1 mm in length before swallowing – obviously this will take much longer for hay than for concentrates. Indeed it has been estimated that horses will chew 1 kg of concentrate feed 800–1200 times but need 3000–3500 chews to get through 1 kg of hay.

During chewing saliva is produced at a rate of about 10–12 litres (3 gallons) a day. While the saliva has no digestive activity it acts to wet and lubricate the food so that it is turned into an easily swallowed 'porridge', which is passed via the pharynx into the oesophagus on its way to the stomach. The pharynx helps to guide food into the oesophagus which is a muscular tube about 1.2–1.5 m (4–5 ft) long. Food or water cannot return to the mouth from the oesophagus because the soft palate blocks its return. The epiglottis (a muscular flap) also closes over the top of the trachea to prevent food going into the lungs.

The horse has three salivary glands:

(1) parotid
(2) sublingual
(3) submaxillary.

Saliva also contains bicarbonate which is alkaline and helps to neutralise or buffer the acid in the horse's stomach.

The bolus of food, after it has been swallowed, moves along the digestive tract by waves of muscular contractions known as peristalsis (Fig. 11.7). These waves are

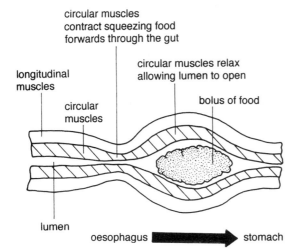

circular muscles contract squeezing food forwards through the gut

circular muscles relax allowing lumen to open

longitudinal muscles

circular muscles

bolus of food

lumen

oesophagus ➡ stomach

**Fig. 11.7** Peristalsis. (Adapted from Jones, G. and Jones, M. (1987), *Biology GCSE Edition*, Cambridge University Press.)

usually irreversible. Occasionally, food becomes lodged in the oesophagus and this is known as choke.

## Stomach

A muscular valve called the cardiac sphincter controls the passage of food from the oesophagus into the stomach. The valve is particularly powerful and does not allow food to be regurgitated, i.e. vomited, indeed the walls of the stomach will burst rather than allow digesta back into the oesophagus. This means that unlike the dog or human the horse has to take care not to consume any food that is likely to cause digestive upset. In the horse the soft palate hangs like a curtain across the back of the horse's mouth and this would cause food to be forced out of the nose rather than the mouth. The presence of food in the nostrils may indicate a ruptured stomach.

The empty stomach of a 16 hh horse is about the size of a rugby ball and can stretch to accommodate about 13–23 litres (3–5 gallons).

The J-shape of the horse's stomach allows water drunk during or after a feed to pass over the top of the food in the stomach, rather than washing the food contents out. This is a common misconception amongst many horse owners who withhold water during and after feed times in the mistaken belief that a drink will wash the feed out of the stomach before the digestive process is complete (Fig. 11.8).

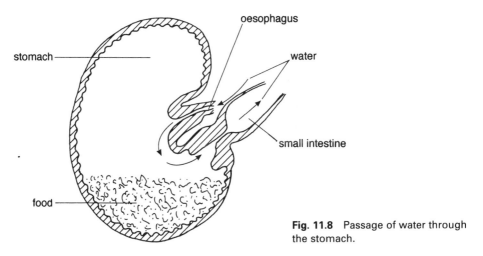

**Fig. 11.8** Passage of water through the stomach.

On a relative basis the stomach of the cow has the capacity to hold 10 times as much food as that of the horse. This is because the horse has evolved as a trickle feeder eating small amounts often. It simply did not need a large stomach. Feeding large concentrate feeds to a horse can lead to severe problems such as laboured breathing and fatigue or worse still, laminitis, colic or a ruptured stomach. The small stomach simply does not have the capacity, nor is it designed, to handle a large feed. The stomach tends to act as a holding vessel for food and it is then passed from here to the small intestine. If too much feed is given at one time, it will be pushed out of the stomach too quickly, before it has time to mix thoroughly with the gastric secretions which help to begin digestion.

Feeds begin to break down due to enzymic and microbial digestion in the stomach. The stomach does have a small microbial population which allows a small amount of digestion to take place.

The stomach can be divided into four regions (Fig. 11.9):

(1) Oesophageal region – no digestive glands, acting as a holding area for food.
(2) Cardiac region – named because it is closest to the heart. The glands in this region produce mucus to help protect the stomach lining from the effects of acid.
(3) Pyloric region – contains the pyloric glands which secrete mucus and small amounts of protein digesting enzymes. This region does not contain any parietal cells.
(4) Fundic region – the main body of the stomach, containing the fundic glands or true gastric glands. These glands contain three types of cells: (a) parietal or border cells which produce hydrochloric acid and 'intrinsic factor), (b) neck chief cells which secrete mucus; and (c) body chief cells which produce enzymes. Intrinsic factor, which is secreted by the parietal cells, is necessary for the absorption of vitamin $B_{12}$ (Fig. 11.1).

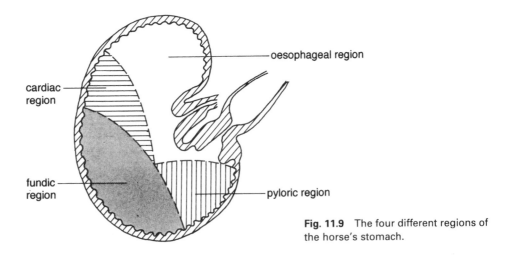

oesophageal region

cardiac region

fundic region

pyloric region

**Fig. 11.9** The four different regions of the horse's stomach.

The acid secretions help to kill any bacteria which may have been eaten with the food. As feed arrives in the stomach, the fundic glands in the stomach wall are stimulated to secrete gastric juice, which contains mucus, the enzyme pepsin and hydrochloric acid. Enzymes are organic catalysts which simply speed up the rate of chemical reactions within the gut in this case. All the digestive enzymes have so far been found to be proteins themselves.

## Gastric juice

Some 10–30 litres of gastric juice are produced daily, containing:

- Pepsin. This enzyme is initially secreted as a substance called pepsinogen which is activated to form pepsin by the presence of hydrochloric acid. Pepsin then begins to break down proteins in the food into intermediate substances called peptones and proteoses. Most of the protein digestion takes place later on in the small intestine.
- Hydrochloric acid. This is produced by parietal cells and is responsible for the conversion of pepsinogen to pepsin. It also has a strong antibacterial function.

There is much controversy about the presence or otherwise of an enzyme known as gastric lipase. This enzyme has a minimal effect on fats in the stomach. It is

STOMACH

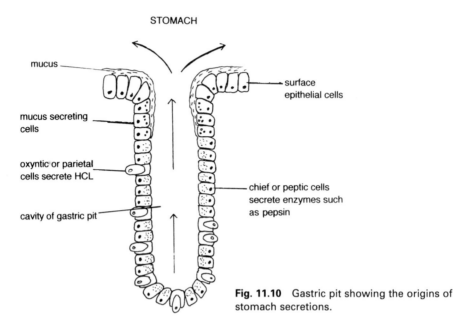

mucus

mucus secreting cells

oxyntic or parietal cells secrete HCL

cavity of gastric pit

surface epithelial cells

chief or peptic cells secrete enzymes such as pepsin

**Fig. 11.10**   Gastric pit showing the origins of stomach secretions.

thought to be abundant in the digestive tract of carnivores (meat eaters). Chewing of food results in the production of large quantities of saliva being produced. This is alkaline and helps to neutralise the acidic environment of the stomach, as the saliva is swallowed. This results in marked variations in the acidity of the food in various regions of the stomach.

Near the entrance to the stomach, i.e. the oesophageal and cardiac regions, the material is neutral; in the fundic region it is slightly acidic; and in the pyloric region it is highly acidic. This is where protein digestion begins. However, food material is only in the stomach for a short time and this limits the amount of digestion which can take place. It is the less acidic regions of the stomach that some bacterial breakdown of food (or fermentation) occurs, resulting in a small amount of lactic acid.

The secretion of gastric juice in horses is thought to be continuous but the rate of secretion increases when food is present in the stomach.

The food material produced by the stomach is now known as chyme and is poured into the first part of the small intestine.

## Small intestine

The length of the small intestine in the horse is approximately 20–27 m (65–88 ft) with a capacity of 55–70 litres (12–16 gallons). It runs between the stomach and the caecum. The small intestine is split into three different parts:

- the duodenum
- the jejunum
- the ileum.

The duodenum is about 1 m long. It forms an S-shaped bend which contains the pancreas. The pancreatic and bile ducts enter the duodenum approximately 150 mm (6 in) from the pyloric sphincter of the stomach.

The jejunum is 20 m (65 ft) long. The ileum is 1–1.5 m (3–5 ft) long. Both the jejunum and the ileum lie to the left side of the horse's abdomen between the stomach and the pelvis. The small intestine can move quite freely except at its attachment to the stomach and the caecum. It lies in several coils with the small colon.

The small intestine is the major site of breakdown of concentrate food such as starch and protein and absorption of the resulting nutrients. The fibre part of the diet is digested mainly in the large intestine.

The digestion of food in the small intestine is similar to that which occurs in simple stomached animals such as humans and pigs.

In order to increase the contact area with the food and the wall of the intestine (the mucosa) the wall is thrown into folds. Furthermore, the entire mucosa is covered in fine finger-like projections known as villi (similar to a carpet with a fairly close pile). Opening between the bases of the villi are the glands known as the crypts of Lieberkuhn. Opening into the crypts are the glands which, in the duodenum, take the form of highly branched and coiled structures.

There are three types of gland in the small intestine which are responsible for the production of many different enzymes:

- intestinal glands (crypts of Lieberkuhn)
- duodenal glands (Bruner's glands)
- Peyer's patches.

The intestinal glands or crypts of Lieberkuhn and Peyer's patches are found throughout the small intestine, but the duodenal or Bruner's glands are found in the first part of the small intestine.

Peyer's patches are accumulations of lymphoid tissue and their function is to control bacterial populations and produce antibodies.

Although the enzymes in the stomach need an acidic environment, the opposite is true of the small intestine. Here the enzymes require alkaline conditions. This alkalinity is produced mainly by the pancreatic juice from the pancreas and the bile from the liver.

## Bile

Bile is produced within the cells of the liver and is a product of red cell destruction. It is a greenish-yellow colour, alkaline, mucus fluid containing bile salts, bile pigments, cholesterol and salts. The bile pigments biliverdin and bilirubin result from the breakdown of haemoglobin and are excretory products. Bile neutralises the chyme and emulsifies fats. Emulsification is the breaking down of fat globules which are emulsified to form smaller globules to increase the surface area for action by the fat digesting lipase enzymes. The horse does not have a gall bladder in which to store bile, instead bile trickles continuously into the duodenum from the liver via the bile duct.

## The pancreas

The pancreas is a lobulated gland which lies alongside the duodenum and empties into it by means of one or more pancreatic ducts. The pancreas has two main functions and contains two different types of tissue. The main bulk of the pancreas consists of glands which discharge their alkaline fluid (sodium bicarbonate) and digestive enzymes via the pancreatic duct into the duodenum. The sodium bicarbonate neutralises the acid content of the duodenum.

The other component, the islets of Langerhans, produce the hormone insulin which passes into the bloodstream.

The production of pancreatic juice is continuous, but the rate of secretion increases five-fold when food is present in the stomach.

## Digestive enzymes

These include those secreted by the pancreas and those secreted by the crypts of Lieberkuhn in the small intestine.

Pancreatic juice contains several protein-digesting enzymes. Trypsin and chymotrypsin are both secreted in an inactive form (trypsinogen and chymotrypsinogen) and are not activated until they reach the duodenum where a substance from the duodenal mucosa, called enterokinase, activates trypsinogen to form trypsin which in turn activates chymotrypsinogen to form chymotrypsin. Like pepsin, these enzymes are able to break down the large protein molecules into smaller fragments. Once these enzymes have begun to break down protein, further enzymes act upon the protein fragments resulting in amino acids. These enzymes are carboxypeptidase and aminopeptidase.

Table 11.4 shows the different digestive enzymes, their origins, substrate (i.e. the substance they act upon) and end products. The rate of passage of food through the small intestine is relatively rapid and food will reach the caecum in just over an hour. Non-fibrous, soluble foods will be substantially digested in this short period through the action of digestive enzymes.

**Table 11.4**   The digestive enzymes, their origins, substrate and end products

| Origin | Enzyme | Substrate | End product |
|--------|--------|-----------|-------------|
| Mouth (salivary glands) | Salivary amylase | Starch | Maltose, dextrins |
| Stomach (body chief cells) | Pepsin | Proteins | Proteoses, peptones |
| Small intestine (crypts of Lieberkuhn) | Erepsin (a mixture of peptidases) | Peptides, proteoses, peptones | Amino acids |
| | Aminopeptidases | Peptides | Amino acids |
| | Sucrase | Sucrose | Glucose, fructose |
| | Lactase | Lactose | Glucose, galactose |
| | Maltase | Maltose | Glucose |
| | Nucleosidase | Mononucleotides | Nucleosides, pentoses |
| | Enterokinase (activates only) | Trypsinogen | Trypsin |
| | Intestinal lipase | Fats | Fatty acids, glycerol |

## Large intestine

This is made up of the caecum, large colon, small colon and the rectum. The large intestine is approximately 8 m (25 ft) long. Although the foregut of the horse is similar to other simple stomached animals, the hindgut is remarkably different. It is in the horse's hindgut that the complex insoluble carbohydrates (cellulose and hemi-cellulose) are digested. Cellulose and hemi-cellulose are substances which make up all plant cell walls. The horse itself does not have any enzymes such as cellulase which could break down these complex substances. Another common component of plant material ingested by the horse is lignin. This is the woody type material which supports the growth of grass stems. Even the micro-organisms are unable to digest this material and poor quality forage will be high in lignin. Lignin tends to stay around in the hindgut for a longer time and it is this which gives the horse a characteristic 'hay-belly' appearance.

Some micro-organisms, however, are able to break down cellulose and hemi-cellulose by a process of fermentation. The horse has a greatly enlarged large intestine which accommodates a vast number of micro-organisms and these are able to release the 'locked' energy providing nutrients to the horse. In return the micro-organisms are provided with a safe environment in which to live.

More than half the dry weight of faeces produced by the horse is bacteria. The amount of micro-organisms in the digestive tract of the horse is huge and number more than ten times all the tissue cells in the horse's body.

## Caecum

This is a large blind-ended, comma-shaped sac situated at the end of the small intestine. The entrance to the caecum lies near the horse's right hip bone and runs forwards and down 1 m (3 ft) to finish midway along the horse's belly, lying on the floor of the abdomen. The capacity of the caecum is approximately 25–35 litres (6–8 gallons).

The caecum acts as a large fermentation vat where fibrous parts of the food are mixed with the micro-organisms.

## Large colon

This is approximately 3–4 m (10–13 ft) long and has a capacity of 90–110 litres (20–24 gallons). In order to fit into the horse's abdomen, the large colon is folded into four regions (Figs 11.3 and 11.4). The first part is known as the right ventral colon and runs forward from the top of the caecum until it reaches the sternal flexure. Here, there is a narrowing of the diameter of the colon and it turns back on itself to continue backwards as the left ventral colon, running along the left side of the horse to the pelvic region. The colon then turns again into the pelvic flexure, the diameter reducing to as little as 9 cm (2.5 in), before it rapidly expands again to continue towards the diaphragm as the left dorsal colon. The colon makes a final turn at the diaphragmatic flexure and the right dorsal colon runs backwards, narrowing to become the small colon.

The large intestine is only held in place by its bulk. The flexures are points where there is a change in direction and a narrowing of the gut. They are, not surprisingly, vulnerable to blockages.

The digesta reaches the caecum approximately three hours after a meal and remains in the large intestine for 36–48 h.

## Small colon

This is 3–4 m (10–13 ft) long but is narrower than the large colon. The small colon lies intermingled with the jejunum and as it is fairly free to move it can lead to abdominal crises such as a twisted gut.

## Rectum

This is a relatively short, straight tube connecting the small colon to the anus. It acts as a storage area for faeces before it is evacuated as dung.

## Digestion in the large intestine

Water is absorbed, throughout the large intestine, from the digesta. By the time it reaches the rectum the waste material is of a firm consistency.

The main function of the caecum and large intestine, as already stated, is to provide a safe environment for the millions of micro-organisms which digest cellulose and hemi-cellulose for the horse. More than half of the dry weight of the horse's faeces is actually bacteria. These micro-organisms ferment the fibrous part of the diet, but they also synthesise some of the essential amino acids and some of the water-soluble vitamins, namely those of the B vitamin group. How much of these products are actually absorbed by the horse is still under great debate.

The micro-organisms consist mainly of bacteria but there are also some protozoa which are much larger than bacteria. The number and types of bacteria in the gut depend to a large extent on the ration being fed to the horse. Numbers of specific micro-organisms may change drastically over a 24-hour period, if the horse is, for example, receiving only two small concentrate feeds per day. These changes reflect the changes in availability of nutrients and subsequent changes in pH within the large intestine. To summarise, the micro-organisms in the hindgut are extremely susceptible to sudden changes in the diet. A change in the ratio of hay to cereal will have a large effect and will influence the types of bacteria which can survive in the large intestine. It is important to maintain a consistent diet so that the population of micro-organisms is not disrupted unnecessarily. Sudden changes in the diet will result in digestive upset and it is vital that changes are made slowly over a period of at least seven days. The number of micro-organisms found within the horse's gut is shown in Table 11.5.

**Table 11.5**  Microbiology of the horse's gut

| Site | Protozoa | Total bacteria/g |
|------|----------|------------------|
| Stomach | 0 | $200 \times 10^6$ |
| Small intestine | 0 | $36 \times 10^6$ |
| Caecum | 567/g ingesta | $482 \times 10^6$ |
| Large intestine | 567/g ingesta | $363 \times 10^6$ |

The micro-organisms ferment insoluble carbohydrate such as cellulose to energy-producing substances known as volatile fatty acids (VFAs). The principal VFAs produced are acetic, propionic and butyric acid. These are absorbed into the blood-stream and converted to energy. This allows the horse to thrive on its natural forage diet.

A change in the diet of the horse will lead to a change in the proportions of VFAs produced. For example a ration which is high in starch will result in a higher proportion of propionic acid.

There is a very delicate balance existing between the bacteria which produce lactic acid and those that convert this lactic acid to VFAs. If soluble carbohydrate arrives in the caecum (most of this should have been digested in the small intestine) as a result of ingestion of too much hard feed, for example, then this is rapidly broken down by bacteria known as lactobacilli to give lactic acid. If other bacteria which can rapidly reduce this lactic acid to VFAs are not present then the pH will drop and serious metabolic problems (e.g. laminitis) may result.

# Summary of digestion (Table 11.6)

## Carbohydrate digestion

The water-soluble carbohydrates (also known as the simple carbohydrates) such as sugars and starches are broken down in the small intestine by enzymes secreted by the digestive tract. The insoluble carbohydrates such as cellulose and hemi-cellulose are broken down by the micro-organisms in the large intestine. Figure 11.11 shows the major energy sources in the horse's diet.

**Table 11.6**  Summary of digestion in the horse

|  | Secretion | Digestion products | Absorbed | Material passed on |
| --- | --- | --- | --- | --- |
| Stomach | Hydrochloric acid Intrinsic factor Mucus | Lactic acid | Minimal | All ingesta and gastric secretions |
| Small intestine | Sodium bicarbonate Pancreatic enzymes Bile Mucus | Amino acids Glucose and other simple sugars Triglycerides Fatty acids | Amino acids Simple sugars Fatty acids Vitamins Minerals Ca, K, Cl, Zn, Cu | Fibre Water |
| Caecum | Water | VFAs B vitamins Microbial protein | VFAs Vitamins* Amino acids* | Fibre |
| Large colon |  | VFAs B vitamins | VFAs Thiamin Amino acids Water P | Indigestible components Waste material |

* It is unclear how much of these end products are actually absorbed.

## Fat digestion

Fat is emulsified (broken down into smaller fat droplets) by bile in the small intestine. It is then hydrolysed by enzymes known as lipases. The end results are fatty acids and glycerol which are absorbed from the intestine into the lymphatic system, which then transports them to the blood stream.

Horses can digest fats very efficiently. This is surprising, as their natural diet is low in fat. Many feeds for competition horses now contain higher amounts of fat to increase the energy density of the feed. (Fat contains 2.25 times more energy than carbohydrate.)

## Protein digestion

This is extensive in the small intestine, where the action of the protein-digesting enzymes result in the production of amino acids. These are then absorbed into the bloodstream. Some amino acids of microbial origin are absorbed from the caecum and large intestine, but it is thought that they are not utilised efficiently by the horse. Young horses which have under-developed caecums must be fed the appropriate balance of non-essential amino acids in the diet as they cannot rely on the small amounts produced by the caecum.

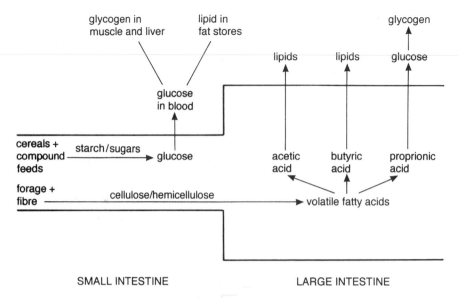

**Fig. 11.11**  Energy sources in the horse's diet.

# The liver

The liver is the largest gland in the body and is one of the accessory glands of the digestive system, the others being the pancreas and salivary glands. It is situated immediately behind the diaphragm and in front of the stomach and it is held in position by six ligaments and the pressure of surrounding organs. The horse's liver weighs from 5 to 9 kg (12 to 20 lb) depending upon the size of the horse. It is reddish-brown in colour and is covered with connective tissue. It has two surfaces and four borders.

The liver is supplied with blood from two sources. The major source (about 75%) is by way of the hepatic portal vein which drains the stomach and small intestine. This blood contains the products of digestion. As the hepatic portal vein enters the liver, it breaks up into a series of branches which supply a capillary bed in the liver tissues. From there the blood drains into the hepatic veins which eventually discharge into the inferior vena cava and is taken back to the heart.

The blood passing into the hepatic veins has therefore passed through two capillary beds, one in the gut wall and one in the liver tissues. This special arrangement reflects the function of the liver as a regulator of the products of metabolism. The liver is therefore able to regulate the blood, bringing products of digestion and some toxic materials before it passes into the general circulation.

The second smaller blood supply (about 25%) to the liver is from the hepatic artery, which delivers oxygenated blood from the dorsal aorta.

The liver tissue is made up of many smaller units known as liver lobules (Fig. 11.12). Running through the centre of each lobule is a branch of the hepatic vein and blood drains across the tissue of the liver lobule from branches of the hepatic portal vein situated around the boundary of the lobule into the central vein. As blood drains across the lobule it bathes the liver cells. At the boundary of the lobule, in addition to branches of the hepatic portal vein, are branches of the hepatic artery and accessory branches of the bile duct which drain away the bile produced by liver cells.

The tissue of the liver lobule is arranged in vertical plates or sheets, separated by blood spaces (the sinusoids) through which blood flows inwards towards the central

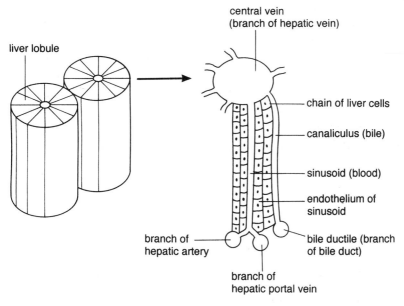

**Fig. 11.12**   Structure of a liver lobule.

vein. The sinusoids are lined by special cells, known as the reticulo-endothelial system, which are capable of phagocytosis, i.e. can engulf bacteria or cell fragments. The vertical plates are two cells thick and between these cells run fine canals which drain the bile produced by the liver cells. These are known as bile canaliculi and they drain outwards towards the boundary of the lobule where they join the larger bile ducts.

## Functions of the liver

It is thought that the liver has over 100 different functions which can be divided into three basic types:

(1) Regulation of the products of metabolism (metabolites). These include proteins, carbohydrates and fats.
(2) Production of bile.
(3) Detoxification of toxic materials absorbed into the body.

### Regulation of metabolites

#### *Proteins*
When amino acids produced from digestion are absorbed into the body they join the quantity of circulating amino acids in the blood. This is known as the amino acid pool and from this tissue take up amino acids in the process of growth and/or repair. The quantity and types of amino acids in this amino acid pool will vary depending upon the dietary protein intake by the horse. In well-fed horses, the protein intake may greatly exceed the requirements of the horse. This is often the case with mature horses who are being over-fed for the amount of work they are doing. Also, some amino acids can be made by the body itself and these are known as non-essential amino acids. The liver is then able to break down the unwanted, excess amino acids and the non-essential amino acids. The liver breaks down the amino acid and removes the amino group

(nitrogen part) and this is excreted as urea, through the kidneys. The remaining organic part can be used as a source of energy, but this is a wasteful process – protein should not be used in the horse's diet as a major energy source. The liver can also synthesise proteins which are dissolved in the blood plasma, such as prothrombin, fibrinogen and the plasma albumens and globulins.

*Carbohydrates*
The liver takes excess glucose absorbed from the intestine and diverts it into storage as either glycogen or fat. The liver cells provide the main storage area for glycogen although the muscles also store glycogen. Liver glycogen is rapidly mobilised and converted to glucose when blood sugar levels become low. The deposition and mobilisation of glycogen in the liver is under the influence of the hormones insulin and adrenaline.

*Fats*
The liver is also involved with the metabolism of lipids. When the horse is using its fat stores as a major energy source, for example in times of starvation or when energy requirements exceed energy intake, large quantities of fat appear in the liver. Accumulation of fat in the liver is a sign of rapid fat mobilisation in preparation for its metabolism to provide the required energy.

## Production of bile

The liver is primarily involved in bile production. Bile salts are required for the emulsification of fats in the digestive system. After they have been used in the small intestine the bile salts, sodium taurocholate and glycocholate, are actively re-absorbed into the hepatic portal vein and taken back to the liver to be re-used again in the bile. These pigments are breakdown products of haemoglobin and are responsible for the green/yellow colour of bile.

Bile does not contain any digestive enzymes.

## Detoxification

This includes the detoxification of products which have been taken into the body, for example drugs, or substances already produced in the body which are then inactivated such as hormones.

## Vitamin storage

Significant quantities of the fat-soluble vitamins, A, D, E and K together with iron and copper are found in the liver. Vitamin $B_{12}$ is also stored here.

## Reticulo-endothelial system in the liver

The reticulo-endothelial tissue lines the liver sinusoids as previously described. The phagocytic cells engulf particles from the blood, including dead bacteria and blood parasites.

# Common problems associated with the gut

## Colic

Colic is a common digestive disorder of horses and must always be treated as potentially fatal. Colic is not a disease but a generic term for abdominal pain which may be caused by a wide variety of disorders. The primary cause of this pain is distension of the stomach or intestines which may be due to an accumulation of gas, fluid or feed caused by a blockage or improper movement of the gut. Generally, the vet should be called as soon as colic is suspected; hay and feed should be removed and the horse left alone, unless it is so violent as to be in danger of injuring itself, in which case it should be walked and kept warm. Most cases of colic will recover within one to two hours, but those do not require urgent veterinary attention.

Colic is characterised by the following early signs:

- reluctance to eat
- few or no droppings
- lethargy
- looking at flanks
- kicking at belly
- pawing the ground.

As the pain grows the horse may show:

- patchy sweating
- acute uneasiness
- getting up and lying down
- rolling (Fig. 11.13)
- increased respiration rate
- increased heart rate.

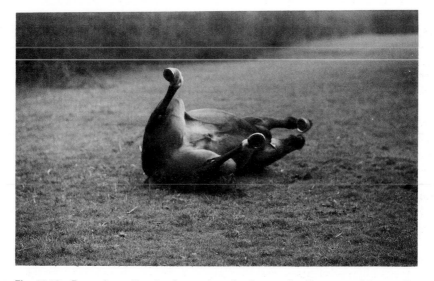

**Fig. 11.13**  Excessive rolling is often a sign of pain or colic. (Courtesy of Joanna Prestwich)

### Spasmodic colic

Spasmodic colic is caused by spasm of the muscular wall of the intestine. There may be several reasons for this including damage to the intestinal wall by migrating strongyle larvae or feeding and drinking too soon after fast work. Affected horses are usually moderately distressed, showing signs of sweating and constantly going down and getting up. They may look at and kick at their flanks and roll, often getting cast. The pulse rate may rise to 68–92 beats per minute and will be over 100 in severe cases; similarly, the respiration rate will increase up to 80 per minute and the temperature will rise. They usually pass few droppings but the condition may come and go quite quickly. If it persists treatment with a relaxant drug usually relieves the problem rapidly.

### Impactive colic

Impactive colics account for about 30% of all colics and are caused by impaction of food material in the large intestine. This often occurs at the pelvic flexure where the intestine narrows near the pelvis to turn back towards the chest. It may occur because the horse has eaten its bedding or when it is brought in from grass, going onto a hay ration. Affected horses are not usually in a great deal of pain and tend to look dull and off-colour, getting up and down in an uncomfortable manner and rolling more than usual. The vet will insert his hand into the horse's rectum to try and feel where the blockage is; he may administer painkillers and also large amounts of liquid paraffin or a similar agent via a stomach tube to lubricate the blockage and stimulate gut movement.

### Gas, flatulent or tympanic colic

This is caused by a build-up of gas in the gut and is usually very painful. Horses will sweat and roll violently, often hurting themselves in the process. Gas build-up may occur in front of an impaction, may be due to a twist in the gut or be caused by fermentation of food in the stomach or small intestine caused, for example, by eating grass clippings or gorging on grain which results in the excessive fermentation of soluble carbohydrate in the large intestine. The vet should be called immediately and if the horse is in danger of hurting itself it should be quietly walked. The gas build-up is dispersed by inserting a tube into the gut and an exploratory operation under anaesthetic may be necessary to discover the site of the distension.

### Sand colic

Horses grazing on sandy soil may take in large quantities of sand which may accumulate and become impacted in the gut, resulting in colic. Large doses of liquid paraffin by stomach tube are used to remove the sand.

### Intestinal catastrophe

Commonly known as twisted gut, this is the most dramatic and serious form of colic. The intestine becomes twisted, telescoped into itself or rotated about the mesentary, all of which obstruct the blood supply. Horses become uncontrollably violent in their agony and immediate veterinary attention is vital if the horse is to survive, as abdominal surgery is necessary.

## Diarrhoea

Horses will often have loose droppings and this can sometimes turn into diarrhoea. Diarrhoea is often seen after a sudden change in diet or when horses are turned out onto lush green pastures in the spring. This grass is very high in moisture and low in fibre so horses should be given access to hay to allow adequate fibre intake. Pastures rich in clover also tend to cause diarrhoea.

Antibiotic treatment will always upset the gut microflora by causing many of the species to die, resulting in the release of endotoxins which irritate the bowel wall. Antibiotics may result in the overgrowth of clostridial bacteria as their main competitors are killed off.

Diarrhoea will not be caused by feeding wet concentrate feeds. Probiotics may be beneficial in some cases.

# Chapter 12

# Reproduction

Reproduction is a vital part of any mammalian life, the horse being no exception. The survival of any species depends on the success of generations which follow. Genetic material (genes) is passed from one generation to another at the time of conception (conception being the fusion of a sperm with an egg).

All mares are naturally seasonal breeders, i.e. they come into oestrus regularly during the season which in their case is spring to autumn. Some mares, however, come into oestrus throughout the year, particular if they are housed and receiving a high plane of nutrition, but this can sometimes be a sign that something is wrong.

In the breeding of thoroughbred horses extra demands are placed upon the mare as an artificial breeding season is used to encourage mares to foal as near as possible to 1 January. All thoroughbred foals in the northern hemisphere are officially aged from this date irrespective of their actual date of birth. Those foals born nearer to 1 January will be bigger, stronger and faster when they are raced as two-year-olds than others born later in the year. As a result the artificial breeding season for mares has been determined by the authorities as running from 15 February to 15 July (in the southern hemisphere, the thoroughbred breeding season runs from 12 August to 15 January). The natural breeding season of the mare begins around mid-April until September, with maximum ovarian activity occurring in mid-July. It is therefore quite obvious that a large number of thoroughbred mares will have difficulty conceiving when their fertility is at its lowest ebb (Fig. 12.1).

## Reproductive anatomy of the mare

The reproductive system of the mare consists of two ovaries and the genital tract, which is composed of the Fallopian tubes, uterus, cervix and vagina. All these are suspended within the body cavity by a sheet of strong connective tissue known as the broad ligament (Fig. 12.2).

### The ovaries

The two ovaries of the mare contain many thousand eggs or ova. Each mare is born with several hundred thousand immature eggs and no more will appear through her lifetime. There is little activity in the ovaries until puberty, which in the mare takes place between her first and second year. Fillies are often seen in oestrus or on heat during their yearling spring/summer, but under natural conditions it is unusual for them to foal until they are over three-years-old. After puberty, mature eggs are released from the ovaries at regular intervals under hormonal control.

The ovaries are situated between the last rib and the point of the hip and they are also responsible for the secretion of the female hormone oestrogen. The ovaries are bean-shaped and will vary in size and shape depending on the stage of the oestrous cycle. For example, the ovaries of maiden mares throughout the winter months are

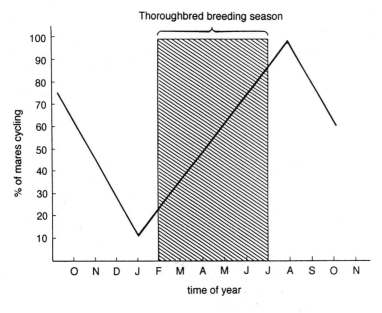

**Fig. 12.1**   The Thoroughbred breeding season does not coincide with the mare's natural breeding season.

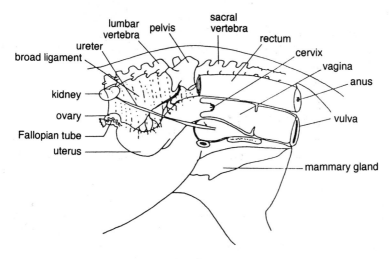

**Fig. 12.2**   Reproductive system of the mare.

approximately 2–4 cm (1–1.75 in) long and 2–3 cm(1–1.5 in) wide, whereas in spring the ovaries may be double this size. The utero-ovarian artery and utero-ovarian nerve, respectively provides the ovaries with a blood and nervous supply.

The ovaries are covered by a lining of smooth membrane known as the peritoneum except at the attached border known as the hilus where nerves and blood vessels enter. The point of attachment of the hilus has a convex border. The opposite free border has a narrow indent known as the ovulation fossa through which the eggs are shed.

The ovaries are composed of a central portion or medulla and a dense outer section known as the stroma (or cortex). The stroma and medulla are not separated by a distinct line but blend together at an indistinct cortico-medullary border.

The stroma is the region in which the immature eggs grow and the development of follicles and the resultant corpus lutea takes place. Each egg begins as a primordial germ cell and is surrounded by a gradually enlarging fluid-filled sac known as the Graafian follicle (see Fig. 12.3). At oestrus this mature follicle ruptures and the egg is expelled through the ovulation fossa into the dilated end of the Fallopian tube. This process is known as ovulation.

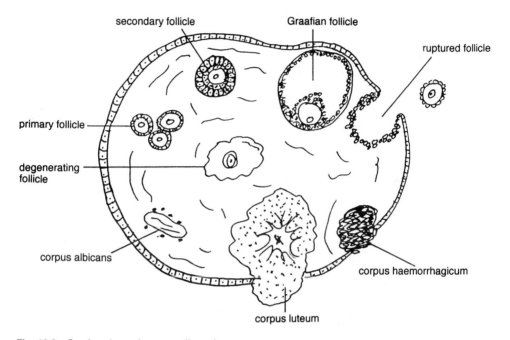

**Fig. 12.3**  Section through a sexually active ovary.

The ruptured follicle then undergoes three separate stages known as the corpus haemorrhagicum (red body), corpus luteum (either of oestrus or pregnancy) and corpus albicans (non-functional).

Immediately after the egg has been released, the remaining follicle collapses and bleeding occurs into its centre, forming a clot called the corpus haemorrhagicum. Blood vessels and specialist cells known as fibroblasts enter the tissue to form the corpus luteum which then begins to secrete the hormone progesterone. The corpus luteum does not project from the surface of the ovary as in the cow and pig, but is embedded in the main body. Eventually the corpus luteum becomes non-functional if a pregnancy does not establish itself, and the active luteal cells are replaced by scar tissue.

## The Fallopian tubes

Otherwise known as oviducts, these tubes carry the ovulated mature egg to the uterine horn. They are coiled and are approximately 20–30 cm (8–12 in) long, and 2–3 mm (0.08–0.12 in) in diameter. The ovarian end of the Fallopian tube is funnel shaped and is known as the infundibulum. This has irregular finger-like projections known as fimbriae which completely surround the part of the ovary where the egg is released without being in direct contact. The sperm, if present will fertilise the egg in the Fallopian tube before the resultant embryo passes into the uterus.

## The uterus

The uterus of the horse is a muscular sac which consists of two horns, a body and a neck (cervix). This is known as a bipartite uterus. Humans have a simplex uterus which consists of no horns, one body and one cervix (Fig. 12.4). In horses, the embryo will develop in the horn of the uterus, whereas in humans the embryo develops in the body. The horns of the equine uterus are about 25 cm (10 in) long and the body 18–20 cm (7–8 in) in length and 10 cm (4 in) in diameter.

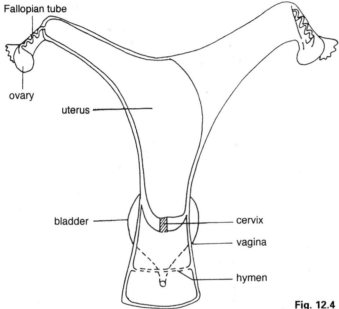

**Fig. 12.4**   Uterus of the mare.

The wall of the uterus consists of three layers, an outer layer which is continuous with the broad ligament, a muscular layer called the myometrium which contains a layer of longitudinal muscle fibres and a layer of circular muscle fibres and a mucus membrane known as the endometrium. The endometrium comprises epithelial cells, connective tissue and glands.

## The cervix

The uterus is separated from the vagina by a neck or cervix. This is a constricted part of the uterus and is usually about 7 cm (3.5 in) long and 4 cm (1.75 in) in diameter. The cervix is normally tightly closed except during oestrus and at parturition (birth). The cervix plays a vital role in protecting both the foetus and the mare by being tightly closed when the mare is pregnant or not in season. This prevents the entrance of infection to the womb.

## The vagina

The vagina consists of a muscular tube which is approximately 20 cm (8 in) long and 12 cm (5 in) in diameter and extends from the cervix to the vulva. The terminal end of the vagina is known as the vestibule and this is separated from the main body of the vagina by a thin fold known as the hymen (Fig. 12.4).

A vestibular seal is formed by the posterior vagina and by the pillars which support the hymen and this helps to prevent the entry of dirt and bacteria into the uterus. Although the vagina plays this protective role it is frequently liable to infections itself.

On the floor of the vagina at the junction with the vestibule lies the urethral opening which allows urine to drain from the bladder. The vagina forms a channel for the entrance of the stallion's penis and for the birth of the foal. It follows therefore that it has to expand a great deal to allow a foal through and it is consequently composed of a thick muscular layer and an elastic mucus coat, which secretes mucus.

## The vulva

This is the external opening of the mare's genital tract. The lips of the vulva are arranged vertically on either side of the vulval opening and are situated immediately below the anus. They are normally held fairly tightly together to form the vulval seal (Fig. 12.5). The vulval lips are covered by thin pigmented skin which contains sweat and sebaceous glands. Beneath the skin lie muscles which also fuse with the anal sphincter.

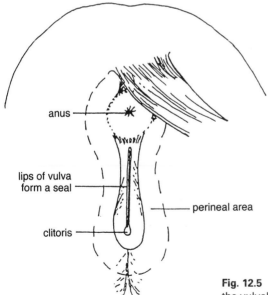

**Fig. 12.5**  External genitalia of the mare showing the vulval seal.

Immediately inside the vulval lips is the clitoris. This lies in a pouch or fossa. The clitoris contains three sinuses which may become a reservoir of infection, particularly for some of the venereal disease-producing organisms. The central sinus is the largest. A swab is often taken from the clitoral fossa to test for contagious equine metritis (CEM), a bacteria renowned for causing infertility. Mares must have a certificate showing they are free from this highly contagious disease before they will be accepted by a stud.

## The oestrous cycle

The oestrous cycle or sexual cycle describes alternating periods of sexual activity in the mare (Figs 12.6 and 12.7). It is controlled by hormones which are initially secreted by the pituitary gland. Mares being oestrous cycles at puberty which is usually around one-and-a-half years of age. As mentioned before, mares are seasonally polyoestrus, which means that they come into oestrus many times during the breeding 'season' and only during this time will they accept the stallion. In the mare this season is spring through summer to autumn. In the winter they are in anoestrus which means there is no cyclical activity and the ovaries lie almost dormant. This is nature's way of ensuring that a foal will not be produced too early or late in the year when its chances of survival in the wild would be less. This winter anoestrus is then followed by a period of change over to regular cyclical activity or seasons. During this transitional phase the oestrous periods may be irregular or very long, up to a month or more. The mare's behaviour during this time is often not typical of a mare in season and therefore it may be difficult to assess accurately. During the first oestrus after the winter period, there is often a poor correlation between sexual behaviour and ovarian activity. Sometimes these early heats do not show palpable follicles when the mare is investigated. However, once ovulation has occurred the mare will usually follow the regular oestrous cycles.

The oestrous cycle has two phases, that of oestrus ('heat', 'in season') when the mare is receptive to the stallion and ovulation takes place and that of dioestrus (between oestrous periods) when the mare is unreceptive. The cycle typically lasts 21 days in the mare, oestrus lasting for approximately 5 days and dioestrus for 15–16

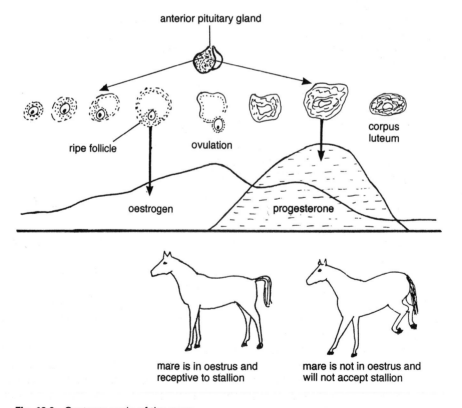

**Fig. 12.6**  Oestrous cycle of the mare.

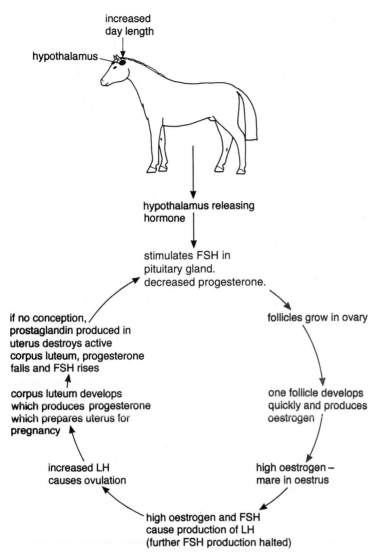

increased
day length

hypothalamus

hypothalamus releasing
hormone

stimulates FSH in
pituitary gland.
decreased progesterone.

if no conception,
prostaglandin produced in
uterus destroys active
corpus luteum, progesterone
falls and FSH rises

follicles grow in ovary

corpus luteum develops
which produces progesterone
which prepares uterus for
pregnancy

one follicle develops
quickly and produces
oestrogen

increased LH
causes ovulation

high oestrogen –
mare in oestrus

high oestrogen and FSH
cause production of LH
(further FSH production halted)

**Fig. 12.7** Diagrammatic representation of the oestrous cycle (FSH = follicle stimulating
hormones; LH = luteinising hormone).

days. However, there is considerable individual variation in the length of oestrous
cycles in mares.

Ovulation typically occurs on the last but one or last day of the oestrous cycle and
this is fairly constant no matter what the length of oestrus is.

The diameter of the ripe follicle is approximately 3–7 cm (1.5–3.5 in). A few hours
before ovulation the tension in this follicle usually subsides. The presence of a large
fluctuating follicle in the ovary is a sure sign of imminent ovulation.

After foaling the mare should come into oestrus some 5–10 days later. This is
known as the 'foaling heat' and usually only lasts for 2–4 days. Traditionally mares
have been covered on the ninth day post foaling, but they often will not be very fertile
at this time. The uterus usually has not had time to return to the normal 'non-pregnant'
state and sometimes infection may be present after foaling. Some studs will therefore

avoid this time for covering but in the thoroughbreds where time is vital the mares will often be covered.

## Oogenesis

The process of production of eggs and sperm is known as gametogenesis (Fig. 12.8). Oogenesis is the name given to egg production and spermatogenesis to sperm production (see later). The end result of gametogenesis is to produce the eggs and sperm which have half the number of chromosomes of other body cells. This is required so that at fertilisation when the sperm fuses with the egg, the resultant embryo will have the full number of chromosomes (half from each parent). The process of gametogenesis involves a special type of cell division known as meiosis. Spermatogenesis and oogenesis vary slightly from each other in that during oogenesis only one egg and two polar bodies are formed. The polar bodies are simply by-products of the egg production process and as far as we know, serve no useful function.

Spermatogenesis on the other hand produces four sperm from one primary spermatocyte. There are, therefore, many more sperm produced than eggs.

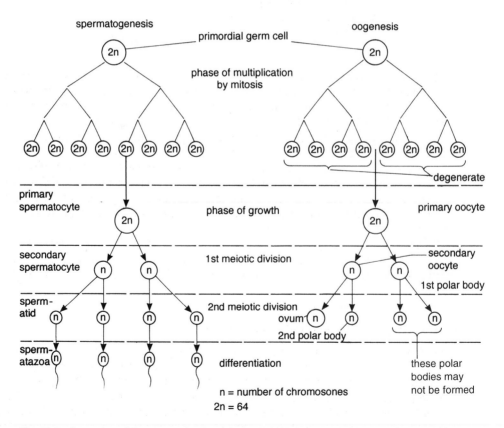

**Fig. 12.8**   Summary of the sequence of events involved in gametogenesis (production of egg and sperm).

## Twins

During oestrus a single egg (Fig. 12.9) is released from the ovary during ovulation. In the mare there is a slight increase in ovulations from the left ovary. However, twin ovulations occur fairly commonly in mares from both the left and right ovaries and some breeds are more prone to it. Thoroughbred mares are very susceptible to this whereas many other mares rarely show it. This is of particular concern to the thoroughbred industry because of the economic implications. The problem occurs because the twin embryos compete for placental space, and a mare's uterus is not really designed to hold two fetuses. One twin will often not survive and this may lead to spontaneous abortion of one or, more significantly, both fetuses. Or, one twin may undergo mummification in the uterus and will appear at birth with the surviving twin. However, the mummified twin will still have been taken up space from the maternal placenta and the chances are that the other twin will not grow to its full potential size.

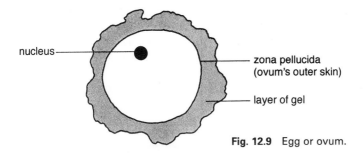

nucleus

zona pellucida
(ovum's outer skin)

layer of gel

**Fig. 12.9**  Egg or ovum.

If twins are detected early on in the pregnancy by ultrasound scan, an attempt may be made to 'pinch' one embryo out. If this is not successful an injection of prostaglandin may be given to abort both embryos. The mare will then be left until she comes back into season before a further covering takes place.

Only fertilised eggs will pass into the uterus; normally the non-fertilised eggs will remain in the Fallopian tubes where they eventually disintegrate.

As oestrus approaches, some changes occur in the genitalia of the mare. The cervix becomes very relaxed and its protrusion can be seen lying on the floor of the vagina. The cervix becomes a deep red colour and the vaginal walls glisten with clear mucus which lubricates the genital passages. After ovulation, the cervix closes and the vagina becomes drier and paler in colour.

The uterus also undergoes cyclical changes; as the corpus luteum grows and secretes progesterone, the uterus increases in tone and thickness, ready to accept an embryo if fertilisation occurs. During dioestrus and during the first few days of oestrus the uterus is flaccid.

## Ovarian changers during the oestrous cycle

Just before the onset of oestrus, several follicles enlarge to approximately 1–3 cm (0.4–1.2 in) in size. By the first day of oestrus one of the follicles will be considerably larger than the others, having a diameter of approximately 2.5–3.5 cm (1.–1.15 in). During oestrus this follicle matures and enlarges to about 3–7 cm (1.5–3.5 in). It contains follicular fluid. At this point ovulation takes place and the other follicles in the ovary begin to regress or reduced in size down to about 1 cm (0.4 in) in the following dioestrus period.

The egg is released and the follicle then fills with blood, hence it is known as the corpus haemorrhagicum. This blood-filled follicle then undergoes further changes over the next three days to become the corpus luteum, otherwise known as the yellow body. The corpus luteum is responsible for secreting the hormone progesterone. It reaches its maximum size approximately 4–5 days after ovulation and it begins to regress at about twelve days after ovulation. As it regresses there is a corresponding fall in blood progesterone concentration.

## Behavioural signs of oestrus in the mare

As oestrus approaches, the mare will often become restless and irritable. She will frequently adopt the urinating posture known as micturition and ejects urine while repeatedly exposing or 'winking' the clitoris. Mares can often be seen doing this to geldings in neighbouring paddocks. When the stallion or teaser is introduced, then the mare will tend to exaggerate these postures and she will raise her tail and lean her hindquarters towards the stallion. A clear mucus discharge may also be seen. The stallion will often exhibit 'Flehmen' where he rolls up his upper lip and stretches his neck outwards and upwards when the mare is in season (Fig. 7.7). This is in response to pheromones present in the mare's urine. A mare which is not in oestrus will react violently towards the stallion's advances and will often kick out. This is the reason why a teaser is often used first, to prevent injury to a valuable stallion.

## Hormonal changes during the oestrous cycle

The physical and behavioural changes which occur in the mare throughout each cycle are controlled by chemical messenger substances called hormones. A hormone is usually described as the product of an endocrine gland which is carried in the bloodstream to some other part of the body where it exercises specific and observable effects. These effects may be inhibitory or stimulatory depending upon the hormone and the target organ involved. The 'master gland' of the body is known as the pituitary gland. This is a small body situated just below the base of the brain where it has a close association with the hypothalamus. The pituitary gland is divided into two parts known as the anterior pituitary and the posterior pituitary. The pituitary gland tends to be known as the 'master gland' because the hormones it produces regulate many other endocrine glands. Despite its broad-ranging control, it is not essential for life as animals can survive for long periods of time when it has been removed.

The hormonal changes associated with oestrus are as follows:

(1) Environmental factors such as increasing day length, nutrition and warmth stimulate the hypothalamus to secrete the hormone GnRH (gonadotrophin releasing hormone), which in turn initiates the onset of oestrous activity in spring after the winter anoestrous period.
(2) GnRH causes the release of FSH (follicle stimulating hormone) from the pituitary gland which causes the development of follicles within the ovary. As these follicles develop they secrete oestrogen. These hormones are responsible for the changes in the mare's behaviour and physical changes in the genital tract of the mare as she comes into season and will accept the stallion.
(3) Rising levels of oestrogen then stimulate the pituitary gland to produce LH (lutenising hormone) and to reduce the amount of FSH being secreted. Ovulation then occurs under the influence of LH and the ovum is released through the ovulation fossa into the Fallopian tube ready for a possible fertilisation. A corpus

luteum is then formed in place of the burst follicle in the ovary. This corpus luteum, otherwise known as the yellow body, is responsible for the production of another important hormone, progesterone. This hormone has the opposite effect of oestrogen. Progesterone prepares the uterus to receive a fertilised egg and is essential for maintaining pregnancy.

(4) Once ovulation has occurred, and the follicle has burst, oestrogen production from the follicle falls. This, combined with the rise in progesterone from the corpus luteum, is responsible for the change in the mare's behaviour and genital tract which occur after ovulation. The mare then goes out of season (generally 24 hours post ovulation).

(5) If fertilisation takes place, the corpus luteum continues to produce progesterone to maintain the pregnancy. If fertilisation does not occur, then the uterus produces a substance known as prostaglandin (PGF$_2\alpha$) which effectively kills off the corpus luteum in the ovary. As a result progesterone secretion falls and this causes the anterior pituitary to secrete FSH and the cycle starts all over again.

The hormonal changes which occur in the bloodstream during the oestrous cycle are shown in Fig. 12.7.

## Artificial control of the oestrous cycle

In the management of horses there are times when some manipulation of the oestrous cycle is required. This is particularly likely in the breeding of thoroughbreds. Because of their artificial breeding season which begins on 15 February in the northern hemisphere, artificial means are often used to encourage the mare to come out of the winter anoestrous period and start coming into season early.

### Light

The onset of cyclical activity in the mare is dependent upon the hours of daylight. The mare is stimulated into activity as the number of daylight hours increase. If mares are stabled at the end of December and are subjected to artificial light, preferably of increasing duration, it is possible to advance the onset of normal cyclical activity so that there is oestrous and ovulation.

Both tungsten and fluorescent lights have been used successfully, although the former seem to give better results. The provision of a minimum 150 watt bulb in each loose box is adequate.

Daylength should be increased from 1 October in a stepwise manner, i.e. the light should be switched on at a later time each day, effectively increasing the day length by 30 minutes per week. A peak of 16 hours effective daylength should be reached by 15 January and maintained for the rest of the winter. The lights do not have to be left on – it has been shown that a flash of light is all that is required to stimulate the pineal gland in the brain.

### Nutrition

There is some evidence that improved nutrition can exert an effect upon ovarian activity. If the mare is kept upon a low plane of nutrition or a maintenance ration for a few months prior to the artificial breeding season, then the energy content of the diet is increased, the ovaries should be stimulated to begin cycling early.

### Hormonal methods

A large number of different hormones have been used to manipulate the oestrous cycle of the mare. These include:

(1) Preparations which stimulate the release of anterior pituitary hormones.
(2) Preparations which replace or supplement anterior pituitary hormones.
(3) Oestrogens – to induce oestrus in mares that are in anoestrus.
(4) Progestagens (progesterone) – to prevent oestrus occurring in mares.
(5) Prostaglandins – to reduce the length of the inter-oestrous cycle. Particularly useful after an oestrous cycle has been missed for some reason e.g. twins conception.

## Reproductive anatomy of the stallion

The male genitalia consists of the testes (within the scrotum), the epididymis, the vas deferens, the accessory glands and the penis (Fig. 12.10). The functioning of these depends upon both hormonal and nervous stimulation.

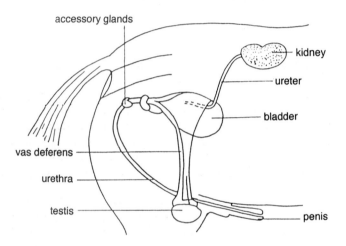

**Fig. 12.10**   Reproductive anatomy of the stallion.

## Scrotum

The testicles are carried in a sac known as the scrotum which is situated between the hind legs of the stallion. This is situated outside the body as the temperature inside the body is too high for sperm development. The temperature in the scrotum is approximately 4–7°C cooler than that in the body. The scrotum is designed to lose heat when the external temperature is warm. When it is cold, a muscle known as the cremaster muscle retracts the testis against the body to reduce heat loss.

## Testes (testicles) (Fig. 12.11)

The stallion normally has two testes. They are egg-shaped and covered with a layer of heavy fibrous connective tissue known as the tunica albugenia. The mature testes are about 6–12 cm (2.4–5 in) long, 5 cm (2 in) wide and 4.7 cm (1.75–3.5 in) high.

In the fetus, the testes develop near the kidneys and well inside the body cavity. Approximately one month before birth, these testes begin their descent into the scrotum, although they are very small at this stage. Hence newborn foals normally

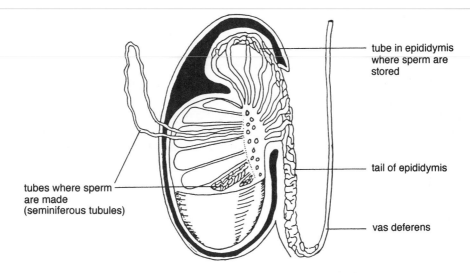

**Fig. 12.11** Section through a testis.

have both testes in the scrotum at birth or very soon after. The testes are guided in their journey by a fibrous cord known as the gubernaculum which extends from the testis through the inguinal canal to the scrotum. This cord is quite thick to begin with, but becomes narrower once its function is complete. The testes have to descend through an opening in the abdominal wall before they reach the scrotum. This is known as the inguinal ring. The testes are held fairly close to the abdominal wall in the horse near to the inguinal ring. Sometimes one or both testes fail to descend and remain within the horse's abdominal cavity; such horses are known as cryptorchids or rigs.

By the time the horse is two-years-old, the testes have reached their full size. The growth of the testes is, however, controlled by hormones which also control sperm production. Once the testes are mature, the male hormone testosterone is produced.

The testis consists of a mass of tiny tubes known as the seminiferous tubules. These tubules are surrounded by a heavy fibrous capsule called the tunica albuginea (see above). A number of fibrous divisions known as traberculae divide the testis into sections called lobules which pass inward from the tunica albuginea to form a stroma (framework) to support the tubules. Within these small tubules are the cells which divide to form the spermatazoa or sperm (Fig. 12.12). These cells also produce testosterone. The seminiferous tubules all join up and converge towards the front of the testis where they pass through the outer covering to merge into the epididymis.

## Epididymis

This is a U-shaped, long convoluted tube which collects the sperm produced by the seminiferous tubules and connects with the vas deferens. The head of the epididymis attaches to the same end of the testes that the blood vessels and nerves enter. The epididymis serves a place for sperm to mature prior to ejaculation. Sperm are immature when they leave the testis and must undergo a maturation period within the epididymis before they are capable of fertilisation.

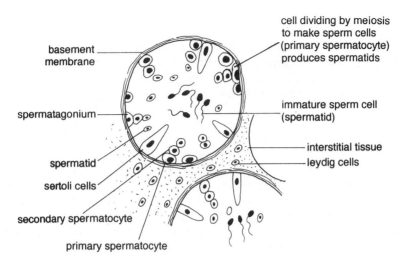

**Fig. 12.12** Section through a seminiferous tubule showing the site of sperm production.

## Vas deferens

This is a muscular tube which at the time of ejaculation propels the sperm and associated fluids from the epididymis to the urethra, a tube which carries urine from the bladder to the end of the penis. The vas deferens passes through the inguinal canal as part of the spermatic cord (which connects the testes with the rest of the body) and then it separates from the vascular and nervous parts of the cord and runs backward to enter the pelvic cavity. As the vas deferens approaches the bladder, the walls enlarge to form the ampulla (which is well developed in the stallion), after which it decreases in size to unite with the urethra.

## Accessory sex glands

During ejaculation these glands secrete approximately 60–90% of the total ejaculate volume. These glands produce a favourable medium for the carriage and nourishment of mature sperm. The accessory glands consists of the vesicular gland (seminal vesicles), the prostate and the bulbo-urethral (Cowper's) glands.

### Vesicular gland (seminal vesicles)

In the stallion this consists of a pair of hollow, pear-shaped sacs which lie either side of the bladder. The contraction of smooth muscles during ejaculation empties the secretions into the urethra.

### Prostate gland

The prostate gland of the horse is a bilobed discrete structure, shaped like a walnut. It is situated near the beginning of the urethra and it releases a milky alkaline secretion into the urethra through a series of ducts.

### Bulbo-urethral gland (Cowper's gland)

These two glands lie on either side of the urethra and release a clear fluid that flushes the urethra prior to ejaculation.

## The penis

This is the male organ of copulation. It is composed of three general areas, the glans (free extremity), the main portion (body) and the two roots (crura) which attach to the ischial arch of the pelvis. The internal structure of the penis contains erectile (or cavernous) tissue. Erection occurs when the penis becomes engorged with blood when the stallion is sexually stimulated. More blood enters the penis through the arterial supply than leaves through the veins. This increased blood volume enlarges the penis. On erection the penis of the horse doubles in length and thickness. The end of the glans penis is surrounded by a prominent margin or rose. This enlarges to three times its resting size after ejaculation. The end of the urethra projects through this rose. The free portion of the non-erect penis is covered by the sheath or prepuce which consists of a double fold of skin, so that two concentric layers surround the penis. This can be quite voluminous and may cause a sucking noise when the horse is trotting. Large glands in this area produce a fatty cheese-like substance called smegma. This can often become foul-smelling and irritating to the horse if allowed to accumulate.

## Sperm

Sperm are produced within the seminiferous tubules. The germinal epithelium which makes up the boundary of the seminiferous tubules contains the primary sex cells, otherwise known as germ cells. These cells are called spermatogonia and are attached to the wall of the tubule and are nursed by other cells known as Sertoli cells. These cells are constantly dividing and as new cells are formed they move gradually from the outside to the inside, or the lumen of the tubule being continuously nourished by the Sertoli cells. As they migrate towards the centre, they undergo changes and develop tails. They are then known as spermatazoa. This process of the multiplication and development of the spermatogonia to form spermatazoa is known as spermatogenesis. During this process the number of chromosomes is reduced by half to 32, so that the resultant sperm have half the number of chromosomes found in the nucleus of other body cells (e.g. muscle cells, brain cells, etc.) which have 64. The egg also has half the number of chromosomes so that when fertilisation takes place, the resultant embryo gains half the chromosomes from the mare (egg) and half from the stallion (sperm). The embryo should thus have the full complement of chromosomes. Chromosomes are the structures in the nucleus of each cell. They are composed of genes, which determine the hereditary information such as coat colour, height, etc. which are transmitted from generation to generation. The extent to which each gene is inherited depends on several factors such as position of the gene on the chromosome and dominance of that particular gene.

### Spermatogenesis

As previously mentioned, the sex cells undergo several changes (Fig. 12.8).

(1) *The spermatogonia.* These increase in number by multiplying through a process called mitosis. The resultant cells all have the same number of chromosomes as the cell from which they derived and these are known as primary spermatocytes.

(2) *Primary spermatocytes.* These travel inwards and undergo a type of cell division known as meiosis where the chromosome number of the resultant cells is reduced by half. One primary spermatocyte produces two secondary spermatocytes each with half the number of chromosomes. The two secondary spermatocytes produced then divide again by mitosis (so they still retain the same chromosome number) to form four spermatids.

(3) *Spermatids*. Each spermatid then undergoes a series of changes from a non-moving cell to a cell capable of movement by the development of a tail (flagellum). This is now known as a spermatozoon. The spermatozoon becomes active after a maturation process which takes place in the epididymis. These spermatozoa then become capable of fertilising the egg in the mare after they undergo a further process called capacitation in the mare's genital tract (see 'Fertilisation' below).

Of the four sperm cells produced from each primary spermatocyte, two cells will contain the X or female sex chromosome and two will contain the Y or male sex chromosome.

The whole cycle of sperm development takes approximately 50–60 days in the stallion. The mean daily production of sperm is in the order of $7 \times 10^9$. The more a stallion is used, i.e. the higher the frequency of ejaculation, the faster the sperm are produced. Each sperm consists of a head, mid-piece and a tail (Fig. 12.13). The head contains the nucleus and is capped by a structure known as the acrosome. This structure plays an important part in fertilisation.

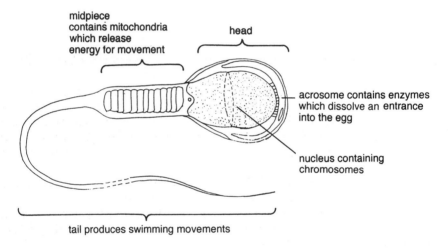

**Fig. 12.13**   Sperm or spermatoazoa.

During spermatogenesis, the cytoplasm of the cell is pushed down the tail length leaving the head mainly composed of the nucleus containing half the number of other body cells. The mid-piece, or the neck, contains a large number of mitochondria which are responsible for producing energy to move the tail quickly from side to side. The tail itself is made up of muscle fibrils.

Semen – the ejaculate – is made up of sperm and seminal fluid produced by the accessory sex glands. The seminal fluid nourishes the sperm on their journey to the egg. In experimental conditions sperm taken from the epididymis (i.e. in the absence of seminal fluid) when mixed with artificial medium, were still capable of producing fertilisation.

## Fertilisation (Fig. 12.14)

The egg enters the Fallopian tube down the funnel shaped fimbriae in the mare. It then travels to a small enlargement called the isthmus. Here, if the mare has been covered by a fertile stallion, it will be met by millions of sperm. These sperm, by whipping their

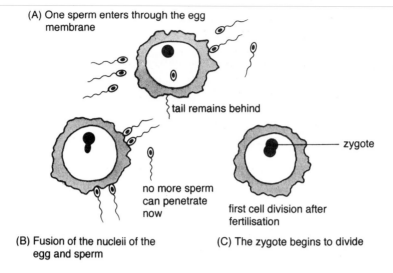

(A) One sperm enters through the egg membrane

tail remains behind

zygote

no more sperm can penetrate now

first cell division after fertilisation

(B) Fusion of the nucleii of the egg and sperm

(C) The zygote begins to divide

**Fig. 12.14** Fertilisation.

tails, force themselves into the outer gelatinous layer of the egg and then on to the zona pellucida.

As previously mentioned, the sperm must undergo a change after they have been deposited in the mare's genital tract, so as to enable them to actually penetrate the egg to fertilise it. This process is known as capacitation. This process enables the acrosome – a structure in the head of the sperm – to form small holes through which an enzyme called acrosin can be released. This enzyme is capable of breaking into the zona pellucida region of the egg.

Once the sperm has penetrated the egg, it injects its own genetic material into it. Remember that both the egg and sperm have half the required number of chromosomes, i.e. 32 each, which are present in other cells of the body. Consequently, at fertilization, when the genetic material of sire and dam meet, the resulting fetus will have the full complement of 64 chromosomes.

Once fertilisation has occurred, the egg will not allow any more sperm to enter it.

# Pregnancy

The term 'pregnancy' applies to the condition of the mare while a fetus is developing within her uterus, as an individual being capable of surviving independently from the mother (after birth). The period of pregnancy from fertilisation to birth is known as the gestation period and the average gestation period of the mare is 333–336 days (eleven calendar months from the date of last service). There is a range in thoroughbreds of 310–384 days. In other breeds a range of 322–345 days has been suggested. The fetus determines its own gestational life as it approaches full term. The genetic makeup and environmental factors, such as nutrition of the fetus, all have a bearing on the length of gestation.

All mammals nurture their young in a womb, the mother providing nourishment for growth and development and security while removing waste products which would otherwise become highly poisonous to the fetus.

## The uterus

The fetus is surrounded by fluids which cushion and protect against the effects of movement and gravity. The wall of the uterus also allows protection and the fetus cannot lose fluids or heat except through its immediate surroundings, i.e. the mother. The mother is therefore responsible for controlling the heat and water balance.

The uterus is a highly muscular organ. This allows the fetus to expand as it grows in size. This is very important. First pregnancies often result in smaller foals than expected, because the uterus is being stretched for the first time. In subsequent pregnancies, the uterus is able to expand more easily.

The fetus contains genetic material foreign to the mother (i.e. the genes inherited from the sire). The fetal and maternal tissues are therefore foreign to each other. Normally when a foreign body is present, the body will do its utmost to reject it, as it does with parasites, bacteria and viruses. In the mare a mechanism must exist which is able to switch off this response to the 'foreign' fetus. Otherwise all pregnancies would be rejected.

The uterus is also kept very effectively closed by the cervix. This prevents the entrance into the uterus of harmful micro-organisms which may harm the developing fetus.

## Placenta

The function of the placenta is to allow exchange between the mother and the fetus. The placenta is attached to the wall of the uterus and is connected to the fetus by the umbilical cord. This cord contains the blood vessels which allow the circulation of blood to and from the fetus from the mother. It is important to note that the fetal and maternal blood never mix, but instead come into close contact. There are six layers of cells between the maternal and fetal blood supplies. The way in which the placenta attaches itself to the uterine wall differs according to the species of mammal.

The placenta develops from a part of the embryo known as the trophoblast. The first identifiable junction between the mother and fetus occurs at about day 25 of pregnancy. This is, however, a temporary attachment. At day 38, fetal cells migrate into the maternal endometrium (uterine lining). These invading fetal cells form structures called endometrial cups which are unique to the horse family. The endometrial cups secrete a hormone known as PMSG (pregnant mare serum gonadotrophin) which is essential for the maintenance of pregnancy in the early stages. At about day 90, the endometrial cups begin to degenerate and eventually they slough off.

The concentration of oestrogens vary during pregnancy. For the first 35 days, the levels are similar to those of a non-pregnant mare who is not in season. They then rise sharply by day 40 of pregnancy and remain at this level until day 60–70. By day 85, the oestrogen level in the mare's blood is higher than for non-pregnant mares in season and this can be used as a pregnancy test. After day 80 the continued rise in oestrogen levels is due to two unique equine oestrogens called equilenin and equilin which are produced by the fetus and placenta together. It is these unique oestrogens which are used in the production of human drugs for HRT (hormone replacement therapy) and there has been much debate about the ethics of the production of these drugs, because pregnant mares are 'farmed' for this purpose in large numbers in Canada and the USA.

The equine placenta covers the entire uterine surface. Early in pregnancy, the placental surface is smooth, but by day 70 it develops minute finger-like projections called microvilli. These give the placental surface a velvety appearance. Bundles of microvilli invade into receiving depressions in the uterine endothelium. These bundles of microvilli are known as microcotyledons. They increase the surface area of the placenta which increases the area for passage of nutrients, oxygen and waste products both to and from the fetus. Within each microcotyledon, the fetal and maternal blood supply come into very close contact to allow efficient exchange.

By day 150, a strong attachment is formed between the mother and the fetus. This consists of six layers of cells. Three of these are on the maternal side (epithelium, endometrium and wall of the blood vessel) and three on the fetal side (endoderm, mesoderm and ectoderm).

## Embryology (Fig. 12.15)

After fertilisation has taken place in the Fallopian tube and the head of the spermatazoan has fused with the ovum a single cell is formed which, as mentioned previously, now contains 32 chromosomes from the stallion and 32 from the mare to make the full complement of 64. This new cell is known as the zygote. Once the zygote is formed, it becomes resistant to the entry of further sperm. The zygote has to develop into a foal by three types of activity: growth, cell division and differentiation. This is a highly complex process. The zygote firstly divides (by mitosis) to form two daughter cells. These cells then divide to form four, then 16, then 32, etc., all joined together in a mass of protoplasm to become a ball-shaped clump of unspecialised cells. After it passes the 16-cell stage it is known as the morula. The morula then swims down the Fallopian tube and attaches itself to the uterine lining (endometrium) at about day 6 after fertilisation. Soon the morula undergoes a process known as differentiation or organisation whereby the mass of cells can be seen to form three distinct areas. These are the trophoblast (which will form the placenta), the blastocoel (the yolk sac which

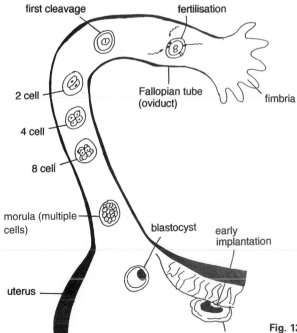

first cleavage
fertilisation
2 cell
Fallopian tube
(oviduct)
fimbria
4 cell
8 cell
morula (multiple cells)
blastocyst
early implantation
uterus
embryo

**Fig. 12.15** Events occurring immediately after fertilisation.

nourishes the young embryo) and the embryonic shield (which will form the true embryo). The cells in each of these areas will undertake different functions in the development of the embryo. At this point the morula becomes known as the blastocyst. The blastocyst then undergoes further differentiation and multiplication which results in growth of the embryo. By day 40 most of the main equine features can be seen such as the tail, nostrils, eyes, ears, elbows, limbs, etc. The embryo can now be regarded as a fetus. After this time most of the development relates to growth or increase in size of the fetus.

A summary of the development of the fetus is shown in Table 12.1.

**Table 12.1**   Summary of fetal development in the horse

| Day of pregnancy | Primary development |
| --- | --- |
| 1 | 24 hours after conception, the zygote (fused egg and sperm) has divided into two cells by mitosis. This cell division continues into 4, 16, 32, 64, etc. cells. |
| 4 | The bundle of cells is now known as the morula and is surrounded by a smooth outer layer. |
| 6 | The morula arrives in the uterus and at the same time breaks open its outer layer and 'hatches' |
| 8 | The blastocyst has now differentiated into the trophoblast embryonic shield and blastocoel. |
| 18 | The fetus now takes on 'C' shape. The gut tube is developing and the umbilical cord is identifiable. |
| 23 | All the basic body structures, neural tube (CNS and brain) pharynx, gut tube and major muscle blocks are present in an elementary state. |
| 26 | The forelimb bud and eye are now evident. |
| 40 | The nostrils are seen, the ears are forming, all limbs are present and the elbow and stifle joints are discernible. |
| 45 | External genitalia present. |
| 55 | Eyelids closing. |
| 63 | Eyelids fused while eye development continues. |
|  | Sole and frog areas of hoof evident. |
| 112 | Long fine hairs growing on muzzle. |
| 120 | Chin hair and eyelashes growing. |
| 180 | Tail and mane present. |
| 240 | Hair growing on head. |
| 270 | Whole body covered in fine hairs. |
| 320 | Testis may drop through the inguinal canal from now onwards. |
| 320–355 | Birth of a well-developed fetus which is capable of walking 20 minutes after birth. |

# Preparation for birth

The foal needs to be mature enough before he is born. Development takes place throughout the pregnancy in preparation for the drastic change in the foal's environment which takes place at birth. The foal grows a good coat of hair while in the uterus and the lungs and nervous system should be fully developed by the end of the gestational period. The heart and circulation are already working while the foal is in the uterus, although after birth they will need to work harder. All the body systems including those of the glands, hormones, digestive and liver enzymes must be in place before birth and most of the organs are working (although not necessarily fully developed). Foals which are premature will be under-developed and face an uphill struggle to survive.

A normal pregnancy should last for more than 320 days. Any foal born before this will be classed as premature. Foals born between 320 and 355 days are considered to be 'full-term'. Any foals born after 355 days are post-mature and some problem may have occurred in the uterus whilst the fetus was growing. They may be born normally, but some may have problems.

Birth, then, should take place only when the foal is mature enough and ready to enter its new environment. It is commonly thought that the foal begins the birth process by sending some kind of signal (probably hormonal) to the mare that it is mature. But, although the foal determines the length of pregnancy, the mare is able to determine the exact time of foaling. Most mares foal at night because, in the wild situation, it would be more difficult for predators to see them.

## Lactation

In the weeks leading up to foaling, the mare's udder (mammary glands) develop and enlarge. The mammary glands are modified sweat glands and the mare has four, in two pairs. Each pair of glands exit through a central teat, i.e. there are two teats supplying the four glands.

The mare's mammary glands are situated between the hindlegs. Each of the four mammary glands is completely separate from the other, i.e. there is no mixture of milk between the four quarters. They are supported by the medial and lateral suspensory ligaments.

The tissues of the mammary glands are made up of millions of alveoli with connecting ducts or branches, rather like a bunch of grapes. Milk is formed in the epithelial cells of the single alveolus. The alveoli are grouped together in units known as lobules. These lobules are, in turn, grouped together in larger units known as lobes. The alveoli are surrounded by myoepithelial cells (muscle cells) which are capable of contraction. These muscle cells are also found in the smaller ducts and they contract as part of the milk ejection or 'let down' reflex. During the gestational period, the hormone progesterone, which is responsible for the maintenance of pregnancy, stimulates lobular and alveolar development, leading to an increase in size of the udder, particularly in the last three months of pregnancy. It is only in the two to four weeks before foaling that milk is produced. This is known as lactogenesis.

## Lactogenesis

The milk is made from components either directly or indirectly from the blood. Milk contains much more sugar, fat (lipid), calcium, phosphorus and potassium, but less protein, sodium and chlorine than blood. The protein in milk is primarily casein with small amounts of albumins and globulins. These albumins and globulins are the principal proteins of blood most of the milk fat is in the form of triglycerides, whereas phospholipids and cholesterol are the blood fats. Table 12.2 gives average composition of milk for some species.

The composition of milk reflects the needs of the young of the species. Colostrum which is known as the first milk, contains a high concentration of immunoglobulins, which confer immunity to the foal. The high level of these proteins in the colostrum falls drastically after about 12 hours and the foal also loses the ability to absorb them

**Table 12.2**    Composition of milk from various species (%)

| Species | Fat | Protein | Lactose | Ash |
|---|---|---|---|---|
| Horse | 1.9 | 2.5 | 6.1 | 0.5 |
| Donkey | 1.3 | 1.8 | 6.2 | 0.4 |
| Zebra | 4.8 | 3.0 | 5.3 | 0.7 |
| Dog | 9.5 | 9.3 | 3.1 | 1.2 |
| Whale | 33.2 | 12.2 | 1.4 | 1.4 |
| Jersey cow | 5.5 | 3.9 | 4.9 | 0.7 |

'whole', i.e. without digesting them first, after about one or two days. Many of the vitamins are present in substantially higher levels in colostrum compared with normal milk. The transfer of vitamin A across the placenta to the fetus is known to be poor in many mammals and consequently the newborn will have very low levels. The high levels in colostrum are therefore extremely important.

Some species, e.g. humans and rabbits, can transfer antibodies across the placenta before birth, but this is not the case in horses. The newborn foal is therefore dependent upon the colostrum as a vital source of antibodies or passive immunity until it is able to build its own immunity.

## Lactation curve

The amount of milk produced by individual mares varies considerably. In general, however, the milk yield increases during the first three months of lactation (Fig. 12.16). The actual amount of milk produced depends upon the requirement by the foal, so smaller pony breeds will produce less milk than thoroughbreds.

Thoroughbreds produce approximately 4–8 litres/day in the first two weeks and this increase to 10–18 litres/day at three months. After three months, the foal's demands begin to decrease as it is beginning to graze with the mother. Consequently, the milk yield starts to drop and continues to fall until the mare stops producing milk after about a year. In the natural state the mare will dry up a few weeks before she is due to foal the

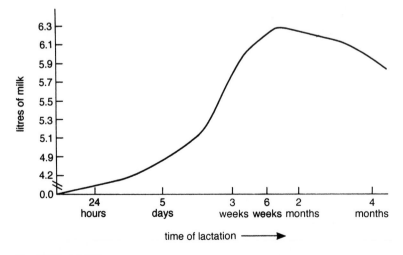

**Fig. 12.16**    Lactation curve.

following year. Human intervention leads to the weaning of foals at about six months of age, and consequently the foal will not be receiving as much nutrition from the mother. Foals weaned later at 10–11 months of age will derive more nutrients from the mare and will be less likely to suffer setbacks at weaning, as the mare is naturally weaning the foal herself.

# Part II
# Science in Action

# Chapter 13
# Conformation and Soundness

Our concept of the ideal equine will be affected by several factors:

- previous experience (having had a good horse of a certain type is likely to predispose towards that type);
- present knowledge;
- the intended use of the horse

It is important to try and view the horse as objectively as possible, taking into account the horse's conformation, temperament, movement and breeding.

## Conformation

Conformation is what the horse looks like, how it is 'put together' and it consists of two aspects:

- skeleton
- muscle and fat, i.e. development.

Ideally a horse should be skeletally correct with correctly developed muscles, adequate subcutaneous fat, covered by healthy skin and a glossy coat. Minor skeletal imperfections can be disguised by well-developed muscle and a covering of fat. It is important to train the eye to assess the horse's skeletal conformation as this has a direct bearing on the horse's ability to withstand work and stay sound.

Assessment of a horse's conformation will also depend on the activity that the horse is to pursue; each activity calls for different levels of speed, strength, stamina and suppleness, perhaps indicating differences in conformation. Although opinion may vary depending on the discipline the horse is intended for, there is no doubt that equal proportions and symmetrical development are essential. The horse's centre of mass must be correctly place; if it is too far forward the horse will be on the forehand, if it is too far back there will be strain on the lumbar region.

Before getting involved in a detailed assessment of the horse's conformation it is important to stand back and look at the overall impression the horse gives:

- Are the forehand and hindquarters balanced in relation to each other?
- Are the feet in proportion and balanced?
- Observe the length of the ribcage and loins.
- Observe the position and shape of the pelvis.

### Ideal conformation

### The head

The horse should be alert with presence – the temperament will show in the horse's face. Observe the ears, eyes, nostrils and head movements. The head should be attractive and in proportion to the rest of the body. The eyes should be kind, bold, large and set well apart; good eye placement means that the horse has wide vision and the ears should be level and equally mobile. The mouth should also be assessed for abnormality and also suitability to take the bit. There must be ample room at the poll and jaw for the degree of flexion needed in dressage (Fig. 13.1), the horse must not feel pain or discomfort from tissues being compressed. The horse's temperament and state of mind is expressed by ear, eye, nostril and head movements. Ideally the horse stands calmly while showing a keen interest in the surroundings. A dull eye and unpricked ears may indicate an unhealthy or ill horse. The head is very important in determining the weight distribution of the horse by altering the centre of gravity. If the head is raised the centre of gravity moves back which helps the horse maintain its balance when landing over a fence, for example.

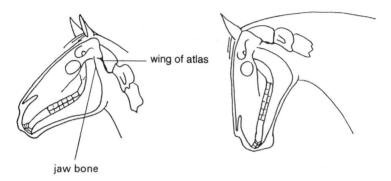

— wing of atlas

jaw bone

It should be possible to lay two
fingers between the wing of atlas
and the jaw bone

**Fig. 13.1**   There should be room at the poll and jaw for flexion.

## The topline

The horse should have a good topline running from between the ears, along the back and to the top of the tail. The head should be well set onto the neck and the withers, the withers should be defined but not prominent, the back should be fairly short and strong, the rump rounded and the tail well set on.

## The neck

The head should be well set onto the neck so that the horse looks elegant at the poll. The neck should be long, elegant and well set onto a sloping shoulder. It should also flow smoothly into the chest with the muscle under the neck not overdeveloped. The seven cervical vertebrae of the neck should give two equal curves (Fig. 13.2); if the curve at the head end of the neck is too steep the horse will be 'peacocky' while a steep curve at the shoulder end gives 'ewe-necked' conformation. Both result in problems in bit communication and supporting self-carriage. The length of the neck should be in proportion to the rest of the body; a long neck may be weak and throw the horse onto his forehand while a short neck can shorten the stride. In general the larger the head the shorter the neck needs to be. A weak neck can be strengthened but if it carries a heavy head it may be difficult to lighten the forehand. The way the horse's neck is placed in relation to the shoulders is very important; the dressage horse needs an elevated set of the neck which will compensate to some extent for the weight and length of the head. Many thoroughbreds have a more horizontal neck set which makes

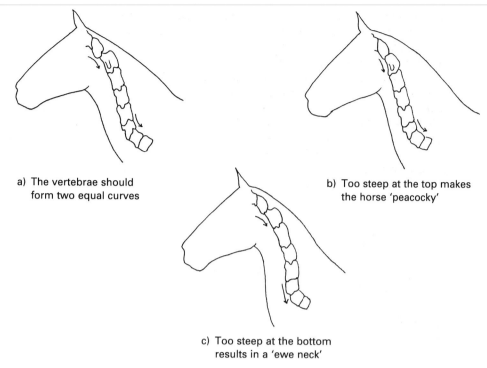

a) The vertebrae should form two equal curves

b) Too steep at the top makes the horse 'peacocky'

c) Too steep at the bottom results in a 'ewe neck'

**Fig. 13.2** Conformation of the neck

it hard to develop the necessary lightness although it is advantageous for the long stride needed for winning races.

## The withers

The withers need to be well defined and to finish as far back as possible; there should be a continuous line to the neck with no dips. Well-defined withers allow plenty of room for muscle attachment and help keep the saddle in the correct position. If the withers are higher than the croup this will compensate for some limitations.

## The chest

The horse needs plenty of depth of chest to allow for heart and lung room. The chest should not be too narrow with 'both legs coming out of the same hole', nor should it be too wide or too open in front, making the horse stable but slow.

## The shoulder

Traditionally the ideal shoulder should have a 45° slope to the horizontal. The hoof pastern angle (HPA) should be the same as the shoulder (Fig. 13.3) so that the concussive forces are absorbed equally by all the components of the limb. However, an HPA of 45° would tend to give a horse the long toe, low heel conformation associated with poor feet and soundness problems. As long as the shoulder is flat and long enough to ensure a good stride length it does not matter if it is a little upright. The angle of the humerus (shoulder joint to elbow joint) is also important and should be about 60° to the horizontal, which is fairly upright. The slope of the shoulder should balance the pelvis and hip articulation; it is to no advantage if the forehand can move excessively but the hind limbs cannot match that movement. The gait will not be balanced and fluid and

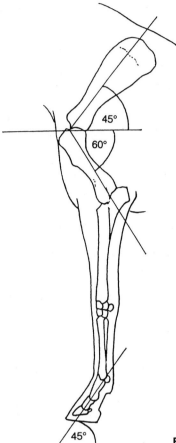

45°

60°

45°

**Fig. 13.3**   Angulation of the scapula and humerus.

the hindquarters will fatigue and suffer performance stress; eventually the horse will become unlevel due to long-term injuries caused by over use. At the walk the knee is usually carried as far forward as the point of the shoulder; at trot the knee reaches a line dropped from the poll, while at the gallop the point of the toe reaches a line dropped from the nose. If the point of the shoulder is less prominent it is possible that the walk stride may be shorter.

### The elbow

The elbow should be 'free' and allow a fist between it and ribs. A 'tied-in' elbow limits stride length. The point of the elbow should be in the same plane as the point of the shoulder, i.e. does not turn in or out. The measurement from the withers to the point of the elbow should be roughly the same as from the point of the elbow to the ground, ensuring adequate depth and 'heart and lung room'.

### The forelimb (Figs. 13.4 and 13.5)

The forearm should be long and well muscled and the cannon bone short with adequate good, flat bone. Seen from the side and front the forelimbs should be straight and not slope backwards, forwards or be angled in or out. From the front a plumb-line dropped from the point of the shoulder should bisect all the limb bones and the hoof. The space between the front feet when the horse is standing square should

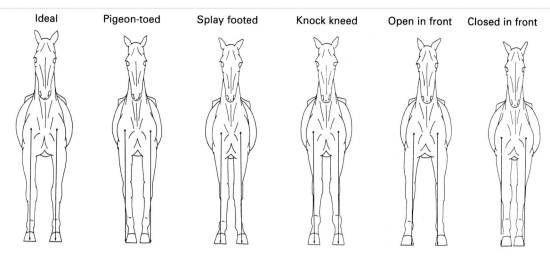

Ideal    Pigeon-toed    Splay footed    Knock kneed    Open in front    Closed in front

**Fig. 13.4** Forelimb from the front. (Courtesy of Goody, P.C. (1983) *Horse Anatomy*, J.A. Allen.)

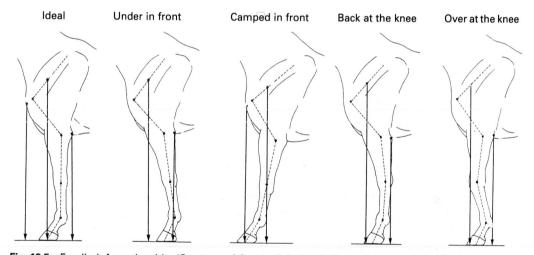

Ideal    Under in front    Camped in front    Back at the knee    Over at the knee

**Fig. 13.5** Forelimb from the side. (Courtesy of Goody, P.C. (1983) *Horse Anatomy*, J.A. Allen.)

be enough to fit in another hoof. This shows that the bones are arranged in a column, directly on top of each other, giving strength and ensuring that the concussive forces are spread equally up the limb. The knee should be flat and broad at the front with a good depth. Faults include:

- over at the knee when the horse stands as if the knee is slightly flexed;
- back at the knee when the back of the knee appears pushed back and the front of the leg concave;
- tied in below the knee when the circumference of bone is smaller just below the knee than it is further down the cannon bone;
- calf knees which are shallow from front to back;
- offset cannon bones where the bones are not placed directly on to of each other but displaced to one side. The toe does not turn in or out.

The fetlock joints should be well defined and bony rather than round and puffy.

## The feet (Fig. 13.6)

It is important that the feet should be a pair and a suitable size for the horse. The shape of the foot and the angles through the hoof and pastern should be as described for the balanced foot. The feet should not be boxy or flat, and the heel should be about half the height of the front of the foot. Always lift the horse's foot and examine the underneath when assessing the conformation and soundness; the wear on the shoe can tell you about the way the horse places his feet on the ground.

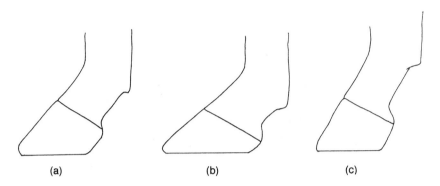

(a)                              (b)                              (c)

**Fig. 13.6** Examples of (a) normal, (b) sloping and (c) upright conformation with a straight hoof/ pastern angle.

## The back

The back should be strong, of adequate length and in proportion to the forehand and hindquarters. There is considerable variation in the 'normal' conformation of the horse's back; long-backed horses seem more prone to muscular injuries, while short-backed ones are more likely to suffer from the spines of the vertebrae rubbing together or impinging. The horse owner can judge whether their horse has a long or short back by using some well-proven measurements: first measure the horse's head from the bottom of its nostril to the poll, just behind the ears – this is known as the 'standard' and the rest of the horse's body should be in proportion to it (Fig. 13.7). (Obviously some horses have very large or indeed very small heads and here another measurement is used.) The length of the horse's back from just behind the shoulder blade to the point of the hip should be very similar to the standard. This measurement gives us some information about the weight-carrying ability of the horse; carrying weight for long periods of time causes stress, tires the horse and impairs performance. Remember that bending and rotation are minimal in front of the ninth thoracic vertebrae and maximal around the eleventh and twelfth, this is just beneath the saddle that you are sitting on, making this area very vulnerable! Stress to the joints in the back may manifest itself as problems in the feet and limbs due to the compensations that the horse is making trying to relieve the discomfort in its back. Think of some of the odd positions you assume to try and relieve backache!

If the back measurement is longer than the standard, stress will be put on the lumbosacral joint and the lumbar region. The lumbosacral joint is situated between the last loin vertebrae and the rump and the ability of the horse to move freely is dependent on the full function of this joint. The lumbosacral joint is part of the spine and acts to transmit the impulsion generated by the hindquarters to the forehand, its limited flexibility allows the pelvis and hindquarters to rotate forward when both hind legs move forwards, as when galloping and jumping. We must not confuse it with the sacro-

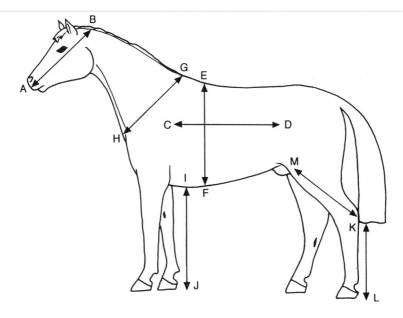

**Fig. 13.7** Using the head as the standard measurement.

iliac joint, which is the attachment of the sacrum to the pelvis. This area can be strengthened and supported with the correct muscle development.

### The hindquarters (Figs. 13.8 and 13.9)

The hindquarters are the powerhouse of the horse and vital to successful performance. The shape of the horse's quarters and the angulation of the joints can indicate the horse's potential for speed, jumping and athleticism. However, the bones are buried deep in the muscle of the quarters and it can be difficult to assess their position.

The hindquarters must be in proportion with good articulation of the hip, stifle and hock. Seen from the side the rump should be rounded with good length from the point

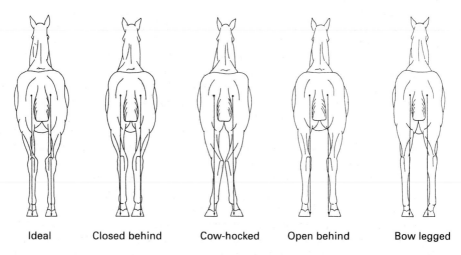

| Ideal | Closed behind | Cow-hocked | Open behind | Bow legged |

**Fig. 13.8** Hindquarters and leg from behind. (Courtesy of Goody, P.C. (1983) *Horse Anatomy*, J.A. Allen.)

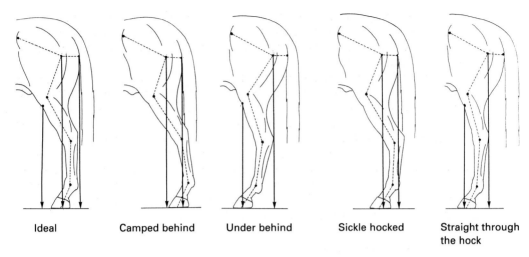

| Ideal | Camped behind | Under behind | Sickle hocked | Straight through the hock |

**Fig. 13.9** Hindquarters and leg from the side. (Courtesy of Goody, P.C. (1983) *Horse Anatomy*, J.A. Allen.)

of the hip to the point of the buttock and a well set on tail. From behind the points of the hip should be level with each other, set well apart and lower than the croup, making a roof shape. Many horses have one hip that is slightly dropped or uneven musculature that may indicate hind leg lameness.

The hock is one of the hardest working joints in the body and good conformation of the hind leg is essential for continued soundness. When a hind leg is well placed a vertical line could be drawn from the point of the buttock, down the back of the hock and lower leg to the fetlock. There should be plenty of length from the point of the hip to the hock: in which case the hocks are described as 'well let down'. The stifle joint should be close to the body but turned slightly outwards to allow free movement. The gaskin or second thigh should be well muscled. Viewed from behind, there should be enough room between the horse's hind feet to accommodate another foot and the feet should face straight forwards. A horse that is 'too close behind' is probably also narrow through the trunk with front feet that are too close together. This horse is much more likely to brush or speedicut, i.e. hit one leg with the other hoof either lower down (brushing) or higher up (speedicutting). Horses that are 'too open behind' tend to be stable, slow and powerful.

The hock should be wide when seen from the side and well defined, giving the appearance of bony strength, and they should not turn in or out. 'Cow hocks' turn in and are considered highly undesirable as the increased strain on the hock may lead to spavins. A 'bow-legged' horse has hocks that turn out and a rope-walking action that places stress down the outside of the leg.

A line dropped from the hip joint should pass through the tibia and the middle of the hoof. The distance from this to a line dropped from the patella and a third line dropped from the point of the buttock parallel to the cannon should be equal.

A horse is said to be camped behind when its hind leg appears to be too long for it. These animals may look sickle hocked if made to stand up square, but will naturally stand with the hind leg out behind them, lengthening the base of support. While stable this posture puts increased pressure on the muscles of the loins and back and the horse may become 'sway-backed'. Horses that are camped behind tend to be slower, less able to engage the hindquarters and prone to backwards slipping. A horse that is under itself behind has a shortened base of support and less stability, making it prone to forging and slipping. These two faults in conformation will both affect the efficiency of the stay apparatus which is dependent on a vertical line running down the cannon bone. The hock itself may not be displaced by very much, it tends to be the angulation of the joints that is at fault.

A sickle-hocked horse has curved conformation of the hind leg due to excess angulation of the hock. This tends to increase the wear and tear on the joint. The horse is described as straight through the hock when the tibia is more upright and the hock is placed in front of the vertical. This type of conformation tends to be quite common in flat race thoroughbreds bred to race on the flat and is said to impart speed.

Before assessing the details aspects of a horse's confirmation in a formal or examination situation the type, condition, sex, colour markings, height and age of the horse should all be stated. The horse should then be examined all over briefly, feeling all four legs for blemishes, heat or swelling. The conformation of the horse should then be described in a logical fashion (Table 13.1).

**Table 13.1** Description of conformation

| Feature | Comment |
| --- | --- |
| Type | Thoroughbred/hunter/cob/lightweight, etc. |
| Condition | Feel the horse to assess subcutaneous fat |
| Sex | |
| Colour and markings | |
| Height | |
| Age | |
| Head | In proportion |
| | Eye |
| | Room for flexion |
| | Outlook |
| Neck | Length |
| | Muscle |
| | Way set onto shoulder |
| | How will it affect the way the horse goes? |
| Withers | Height |
| | Length |
| Shoulder | Angle and length of scapula and humerus |
| Forearm | Length and muscle |
| Knee | Flatness and breadth |
| | Back at? Tied in? Over at the knee? |
| Cannon bone | Length |
| | Amount of bone |
| | Tendons? Splints? |
| Fetlocks | Bony or puffy |
| Hoof pastern angle | Unbroken |
| | Same as shoulder (50–55°) |
| Feet | Pair |
| | Symmetrical |
| | Adequate heel |
| | Open and circular |
| Forearm as a whole | Straight, not tied in, etc. |
| Chest | Adequate depth |
| | Straightness of limbs from in front |
| Ribcage | Depth |
| | Length |
| | 'Well sprung' |
| Lumbar region | Strength and length |

**Table 13.1**  Continued

| Feature | Comment |
| --- | --- |
| Hindquarters | Point of hip to point of buttock |
| | Croup high? |
| | Point of croup to hip |
| | Rounded |
| | Hocks well let down |
| | Tail well set on |
| | Adequate second thigh |
| | Plumb line from point of buttock to ground |
| Hocks | Strong and bony |
| | Turn in or out? Curb? Spavins? Thoroughpin? |
| Cannon bone | Length |
| | Amount of bone |
| Fetlocks | Bony or puffy |
| | Windgalls? |
| Hoof pastern angle | Unbroken |
| Feet | Pair |
| | Symmetrical |
| | Adequate heel |
| | Open |
| Hind leg as a whole | Plumb-line from hip joint |
| | Sickle or straight? |
| From behind | Level hip bones and even musculature |

If the horse's frame is in proportion his action will be balanced and he will lose less athletic ability when carrying his rider The more areas of poor conformation that compromise balance the more development work the horse will need to help him compensate. A careful assessment of conformation can make the rider aware of the weak areas so that a work programme can be designed that includes the necessary remedial work to develop the weak areas.

## Developing the ridden horse

The development of the abdominal muscles is important for the ridden horse. The abdominal muscles are attached to the pubic bone, sternum and ribs through to the spine. When they are strong enough to support the horse's gut, the base of the horse can shorten, allowing the pelvis to tilt correctly; the horse can then use its back, the quarters can engage and the spine will lift just behind the withers and the forehand will lighten. The horse's balance will improve and it will be able to carry itself and its rider without losing any athletic ability.

### Muscle problems

If a muscle becomes short and tight it cannot stretch; instead the forces are transferred to the tendons at the ends of the muscles which in turn are transferred to the joints and ligaments. Many horses are working with tense backs with no support from the abdominal muscles; as a result the limb joints take most of the stress and wear out prematurely. Tight backs pull on the lumbosacral area so the pelvis cannot rotate correctly and this puts strain on the hamstring muscles and the Achilles tendon which in turn affects the stifle and hock joints.

# Chapter 14
# Movement and Lameness

Studying the mechanics of movement, biomechanics, helps in the objective assessment of the way the horse moves and hence the diagnosis of lameness. Combined with a sound knowledge of anatomy and conformation, being able to assess the biomechanics of the horse can enable the training programme to be designed to prolong the horse's working life by strengthening the weak areas and avoiding problems.

## Centre of gravity

Unlike the greyhound, the horse has a large, bulky body and a relatively rigid spine; the horse is not a natural jumping animal. The centre of gravity is the point over which the horse's weight is balanced and altering the centre of gravity plays an essential part in effectively propelling the horse at speed. The centre of gravity varies with the individual horse and depends on conformation and weight. In a stationary horse the position of the centre of gravity can be judged by dropping a line from the highest point of the withers and crossing it by a line from the point of the shoulder to the point of the buttock (Fig. 14.1). This means that it lies nearer to the shoulder than the hips; this is why a standing horse can lift a hind foot off the ground and not lose its balance. The

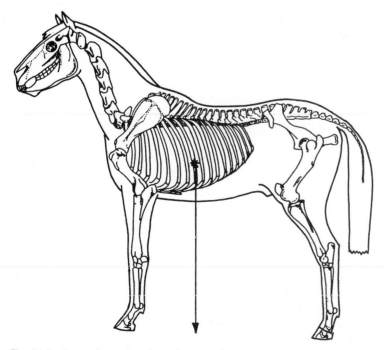

**Fig. 14.1** Approximate location of centre of mass (*) in the standing horse.

horse has a heavy head full of teeth, at the end of a long lever (the neck), and needs powerful muscles to support it. When the head is lifted the centre of gravity moves backwards, allowing the horse to lift its forehand off the ground; thus movement is preceded by a slight lifting of the head.

Unlike humans the horse does not have a collar bone; no firm, bony union exists between the ribcage and forelimbs, there is only muscle. The horse's body is slung in a cradle of muscle (serratus ventralis) between the two shoulder blades (Fig. 14.2). These muscles allow the horse's trunk to rise and fall or to lean a little to one side, and this enables the horse to keep its balance, particularly when cornering at speed – much like the suspension of a car.

The following points affect the way the horse moves:

- The forelimbs are attached to the trunk only by muscles and ligaments.
- The forelimbs bear most of the weight and the concussion involved with movement.
- The head and neck act as a balancing weight and the neck gives muscle attachment to the muscles which extend the forelimb.
- The spinal column has only slight sideways and up and down movement between the neck and tail. Thus the trunk is almost rigid and its role in movement is to transfer the power from the hindquarters forward.
- The hindlimb has a bony attachment to the spine to transfer the forces of movement directly to the spinal column.

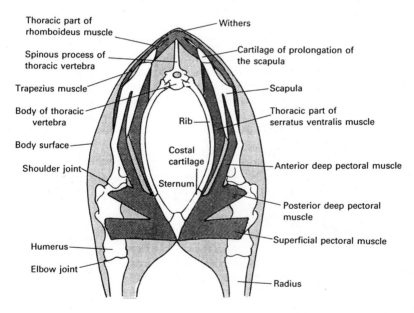

**Fig. 14.2**  Thoracic sling system. (Courtesy of Smythe and Goody (1993) *Horse Structure and Movement*, J.A. Allen.)

## The stay apparatus (Fig. 14.3)

Horses can rest for long periods of time in a standing position and this has the advantage of giving them a more distant horizon to spot the approach of predators and also allows a faster getaway should the predators surprise them. This is due to the stay apparatus – a system of muscles and ligaments that 'lock' the main joints into position, without expending a lot of energy so that the muscles do not get fatigued. The

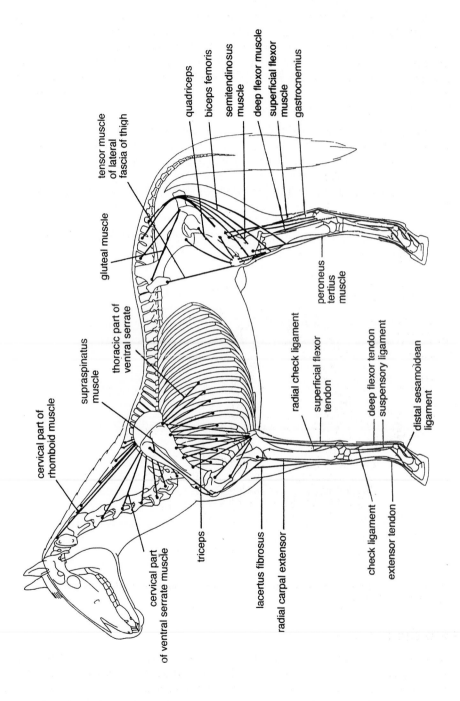

**Fig. 14.3** Stay apparatus of the forelimb and hindlimb. (Courtesy of Goody, P.C. (1983) *Horse Anatomy*, J.A. Allen.)

arrangement is much the same in the fore and hindlimbs; normally both the forelimbs are 'locked' but one hindlimb is relaxed or 'rested'.

The stay apparatus in the forelimbs is based on the suspensory apparatus including:

- the suspensory ligament;
- the deep digital flexor tendon with the deep digital flexor muscle, running from the elbow to the back of the pedal bone;
- the carpal check ligament which joints the DDFT to the cannon bone;
- The superficial digital flexor tendon and muscle from elbow to short pastern bone; and
- the radial check ligament.

The superficial digital flexor tendon of the forelimb has a check ligament which links to the radius of the forearm. The ligament stops the tendon being pulled too far down when the fetlock is weight-bearing and so helps prevent the fetlock collapsing onto the ground. The carpal check ligament of the deep flexor tendon links to the carpal bones of the knee. The suspensory ligament attaches to the top of the knee and runs down the back of the leg between the cannon bone and the flexor tendons. Just above the fetlock joint it divides into two; each branch attaches to one of the two sesamoid bones of the fetlock joint and then continues forward to join the extensor tendon at the front of the pastern. The suspensory ligament provides a link between the extensor and flexor systems, literally suspending the fetlock joint. As the body weight presses on the fetlock this joint moves down and the suspensory ligament tightens, followed by the superficial flexor and the deep flexor tendons. Higher in the forelimb the elbow is prevented from flexing, which in turn means that the biceps brachii, extending from the shoulder blade to the forearm, can stop the shoulder from flexing. The knee is prevented from buckling forwards by the lacertus fibrosus tendon.

The shoulder blade is balanced by two muscle groups:

- The ventral serrate (serratus ventralis) muscle acts horizontally with the thoracic and cervical parts supporting in opposite directions. The muscle is interspersed with fibrous tissue to help take the weight.
- The supraspinatus muscle, biceps and triceps acts vertically to balance the scapula with minimal fatigue.

The stay apparatus of the lower hindlimb is basically the same as that of the forelimb but the superficial flexor tendon does not have an equivalent to the radial check ligament. Higher up, however, the patella or stifle plays a vital role; this bone has a 'hook' which can lock over the inner trochlear ridge of the femur in order to fix the whole hindlimb rigid. If one joint of the leg is locked the others will not move readily so when the horse wants to move it contracts the tensor fascia muscle which attaches to the patella, so slightly lifting and freeing the bone. Thirdly, the stifle joint cannot be moved without moving the hock joint through the action of the gastrocnemius and the peroneus tertius. Finally the horse can 'sit' in a hammock of hamstrung muscles which run over the buttocks of the horse.

## Moving the front legs

Moving off begins with an almost imperceptible transfer of weight; two-thirds of the horse's weight is carried by its forelimbs, so that horse must shift its centre of gravity backwards to free the forehand. The front leg is moved forward by two main groups of muscles; some bend the elbow forwards, some actually pull the leg forward. The elbow-flexing muscles are the biceps (running from shoulder blade to radius) and the brachialis (humerus to radius). The limb is brought forwards by the action of the brachiocephalic and serratus ventralis muscle; the efficiency of this will depend on the position of the head and this is why a horse moves more freely in front when the neck is extended or carried high. Riding on a tight rein or fixing a horse's head with gadgets like a standing martingale can hamper movement. After the limb has moved forward sufficiently it is straightened again; the supraspinatus muscle straightens the shoulder joint, the triceps straightens the elbow and the carpet and digital extensors, the lower leg. Once the foot is on the ground it acts as a fixed fulcrum with the body turning above it.

Backward movement of the leg starts with contraction of the pectoral muscles which lie between the lower chest wall and the leg, and the latissimus dorsi which stretches from the withers to the forearm. This pulls the humerus back; at the same time various muscles pull the shoulder blade forward and the body rotates over the rigid leg. As the limb passes the vertical it no longer only supports weight but becomes a propulsive strut. The lower part of the leg is pulled backwards by the superficial and deep digital flexor muscles, acting on the foot via long tendons.

## Moving the hind legs

The muscles of a performance horse's hindquarters play an important role in generating power. The position of the superficial muscles can be traced through the skin; stretching down from the tuber coxae (hip bone) is the tensor fascia latae which attaches round the stifle, immediately above this is the superficial gluteal muscle. They both flex the hip joint, carrying the femur and a stifle forward. Behind the superficial gluteal is the biceps femoris, a curved muscle which appears to stretch from the spine to the stifle joint. This, with the semitentinosus at the back of the leg, extend the leg by moving the horse's body forward when the foot is fixed on the ground. They also push the leg out behind the horse when jumping and kicking.

The two muscles which can be seen at the front of the lower leg are the long digital extensor and the lateral digital extensor. Together with the tibialis anterior muscle these extend the leg forward. The muscles which flex the leg are not as evident as they lie under the muscle of the thigh; they are the superficial and deep digital flexor muscles and their tendons. There is also the powerful gastrocnemius muscle which ends in the Achilles tendon.

The forward propulsive thrust of the limbs is quite small so the speed of movement depends on the frequency with which the limbs operate; to move faster the hindlimbs must travel backwards faster than the speed at which the body is moving forwards at that moment. In order for a horse to gallop the muscles of the legs must pull the legs backwards as quickly as possible, even though they are bearing weight at the time; this calls for well-developed muscles. On the other hand, when the leg is pulled forwards it is not usually weight-bearing and so the muscles do not have to be so well developed, although they may still be quite sizable like the brachiocephalic.

## The diagnosis of lameness

Lameness is the abnormal placement or movement of the horse's limb due to pain and/or mechanical dysfunction. Sometimes horses are described as being 'unlevel' when their movement is uneven or there is an irregularity in the rhythm. This irregularity could be due to lack of balance, hurrying or finding a movement difficult. However, a horse that is persistently unlevel is probably suffering slight lameness and should be investigated further.

The lame horse needs to be systematically evaluated so that the source or sources of pain can be identified and hence the cause of lameness assessed and rational treatment given. Before even looking at the horse there are certain points to consider:

- Age – young horses can suffer from growth-related problems such as epiphysitis and are less likely to suffer problems associated with cumulative concussion.
- Breed – lightweight thoroughbred types and heavyweight and draught types tend to suffer from different types of lameness due to differences in conformation and occupation.
- Occupation – problems associated with galloping and jumping differ from those associated with power and endurance such as draught work.
- Fitness – a horse asked to perform beyond his present level of fitness is prone to sudden injury and hence lameness.
- Conformation – upright pasterns are subject to more jarring than sloping ones. However, horses with long, sloping pasterns put more strain on the tendons and ligaments of the lower limb.
- Shoeing – when and how the horse is shod is relevant.
- Gait abnormality – does the horse move in such a way that it is prone to brushing or over-reaching?
- Recent history – did the horse suddenly go lame or has the onset been insidious?

These points will all give clues as to the possible cause of lameness and can be used to piece together the picture. They should not, however, cloud judgement. Remember that most forelimb lameness is in the foot. The examination procedure consists of two stages:

- observation at rest in the stable or field
- observation during exercise, either in hand or ridden.

## Examining the horse at rest

If possible the horse should be observed while undisturbed and resting. This will include the position the horse finds most comfortable. It is normal for the horse to rest alternate hind legs intermittently, but it is unusual to rest a front leg or 'point a toe'. Some horses will rest a diagonal, i.e. a hind leg and the opposite front leg, particularly when tired or having worked on hard ground. If this persists, or the horse favours one diagonal, it may indicate slight lameness. The horse can then be stood up square on a flat level surface and assessed for:

- conformation;
- the symmetry of its bone structure and muscle development;
- temperament – has the horse started to refuse to jump or extend on hard ground?
- abnormal heat, pain and swelling. The neck and back should be felt as well as the limbs. If anything is detected it should always be compared to the other side or other limb;
- the size and shape of each foot and how and when it was shod or trimmed;
- each foot should be lifted, noting the range of movement of the joints, and the foot picked out, noting the wear on the shoes;
- hoof testers can be used to apply gentle pressure on the wall, soles and heels. Some horses will react to thumb pressure;
- the sole and hoof wall, particularly over each clench, can be gently tapped with a hammer.

Depending on the type of lameness it may be possible to identify the site and source of pain from this examination, without having to examine the horse while it is moving.

## Examining the horse during movement (Figs 14.4 and 14.5)

The horse must be properly restrained, particularly if it has been confined to the stable for some time. A bridle or a cavesson and lunge line are more suitable than a head collar, and the handler should have adequate protection, such as stout footwear, gloves and a hard hat. The horse should be led along a hard, level and flat surface and be allowed to move its head and neck freely. It should first be walked away, towards and then past the observer, handlers must turn the horse away from themselves and the turns should be watched carefully. The procedure can then be repeated in trot. As well as watching the horse it is important to listen for any irregularity of footfall.

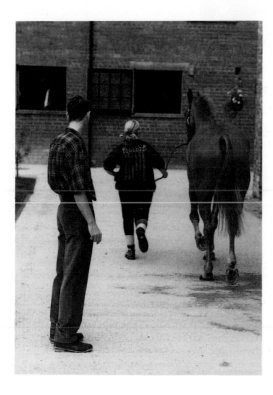

**Fig. 14.4** The horse is trotted away and allowed to move its head and neck freely. (Courtesy of Joanna Prestwich)

### In walk

It is important to spend some time looking at the horse in walk as it is easier to assess the way the horse moves because the limbs are moving more slowly. Initially an overall impression of the horse is generated by watching the whole animal, before concentrating on the front, each side, back, forelimbs and hindlimbs.

- The way in which the horse places its feet on the ground is important. Is each foot placed squarely? Does one side land first? Does the toe land first?
- The flight of the limb through the air should also be observed. Does the horse lift each foot the same height off the ground? Do the feet swing in or out? Does the horse brush or forge?

- Does each limb take the same length of stride? Is the stride length as would be expected for a horse of that type?
- Does each fetlock sink to the same degree as it takes the horse's weight?

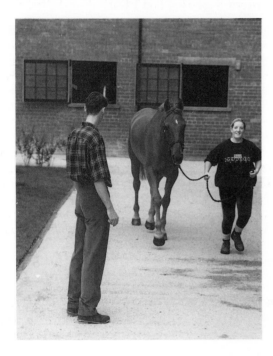

**Fig. 14.5** The horse is turned away from the handler and trotted back. (Courtesy of Joanna Prestwich)

**In trot**

Bearing in mind all the observations made in the stable and at walk, the horse can now be examined in trot, looking at the following points:

- The horse's head carriage should be watched carefully. The horse will 'nod' as the sound leg hits the ground because it is landing more heavily on this leg and 'favouring' the lame leg.
- The horse is said to be 'pottery' if it is taking a shorter stride than expected with both forelimbs, indicating that there is pain in both limbs.
- If hindlimb lameness is suspected the horse should be observed from the side and from behind. The lame leg may take a shorter stride and this irregularity may be heard. If the lameness is in the hock or above the horse may drag its toe and the shoe may show signs of abnormal wear. As it is impossible to flex the hock without flexing the stifle and hip joints it is hard to differentiate between lameness in these areas.
- The horse should be observed for asymmetrical movement of the hindquarters, with the quarter of the lame leg appearing to ride and fall more than the other side.
- The horse may nod as the forelimb on the same side as the lame hind leg hits the ground because the lame leg is non-weightbearing. This can lead to confusion.

**Small circles in walk**

If the lameness has not been pinpointed, the next step is to turn the horse in small circles. The handler should stand facing the horse's girth area and pull the horse round in nearly its own length. This assesses the flexibility of the horse's neck and back and its ability to move the outside legs away from the body and inside legs towards the body. It also puts more pressure on the inside limbs as they have to carry more weight. Any suspicion of lameness shown on the turns when trotting the horse up will be exaggerated by the small circles. At this stage the horse should also be asked to move backwards to assess if it is a 'shiverer'.

### Larger circles on the lunge

The horse can be lunged on hard ground to accentuate forelimb lameness when the affected leg is on the inside. If the horse has a pottery gait in a straight line, obvious lameness may appear on the circle. There are no rules for hindlimb lameness.

## Ridden exercise

Hindlimb lameness, particularly, may be exaggerated when the horse is ridden. This is sometimes most obvious when the rider is sitting on the diagonal of the affected leg. Some horses are 'bridle lame', unlevelness is only demonstrated when the horse is ridden. This may be due to several reasons including evasion, lack of forward movement, tension or unsteadiness of the rider's hands. If the horse is ridden forwards with a deep and round outline to engage the hindquarters the unlevelness should disappear.

## Flexion tests (Fig. 14.6)

Flexion tests are usually left to the veterinary surgeon, they are the subject of some controversy and it is useful to understand the procedure. Each joint is held partially flexed for 60 seconds, the horse is then immediately trotted away in a straight line.

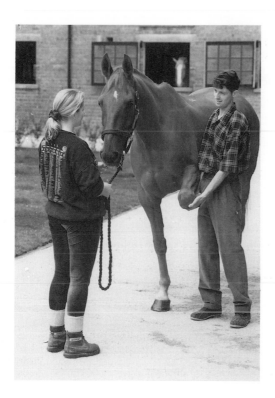

**Fig. 14.6**  Flexing the knee joint.
(Courtesy of Joanna Prestwich)

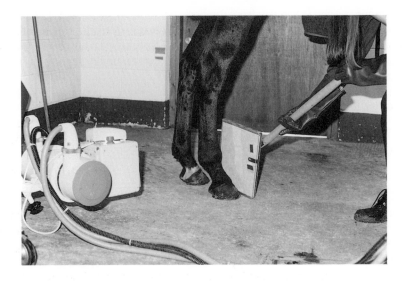

**Fig. 14.7** X-ray examination of the fetlock joint. (Courtesy of Joanna Prestwich)

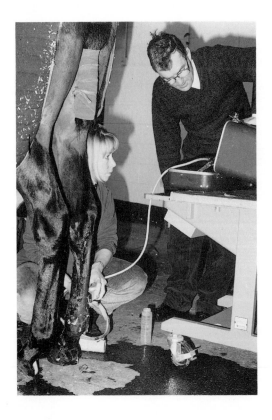

**Fig. 14.8** Ultrasound examination of the lower leg. (Courtesy of Joanna Prestwich)

This accentuates or produces lameness in the flexed joint. The knee should be flexed to eliminate the possibility of lameness in that joint, before flexing the fetlock as it is not possible to flex the fetlock without flexing the knee. It is impossible to flex the hock without flexing the stifle and hip joints.

## Identifying the exact source of pain

By now the lame limb or limbs should have been identified and the veterinary surgeon will identify the exact source of the pain. Local anaesthetic can be used to block specific nerves supplying the lower limb. It is a specialised technique requiring a detailed knowledge of anatomy and should only be used once the whole limb has been examined and the general area causing the problem has been identified. The idea is that if the pain originates in the desensitised area the horse should go sound. If the lameness is only improved, not eliminated, it indicates that there may be more than one problem. Other tools that the vet can use include X-ray (Fig. 14.7), bone scanning, ultrasound examination of tendons and ligaments (Fig. 14.8), blood tests and surgical examination.

In any examination it is important to keep an open mind. The small amount of heat discovered in the stable or the old tendon injury may not be the cause of the problem. It is always possible that the horse is suffering from more than one source of pain. No examination will be successful without a practical knowledge of the anatomy of the lower limb; it is no good mistaking the splint bone for the suspensory ligament.

# Chapter 15
# The Invaders

Throughout the horse's lifetime, it will be being continually challenged by disease-causing organisms of one sort or another. These are the invaders.

The invaders can be broadly categorised into one of two groups: micro-organisms and parasites. Parasites may live within the horse's body or on the surface. Many micro-organisms live quite happily within the horse's body without causing any problems (Table 15.1).

**Table 15.1**  Bacteria found in the horse's normal flora

| Site | Bacteria |
|------|----------|
| Digestive tract | Species of:<br>    Clostridium<br>    Enterobacter<br>    Escherichia coli<br>    Klebsiella<br>    Proteus<br>    Pseudomonas<br>    Corynebacterium<br>    Bacteroides<br>    Streptococcus faecalis<br>    Lactobacillus |
| Respiratory tract | Species of:<br>    Bacillus<br>    Streptococcus<br>    Acinetobacter<br>    Staphylococcus<br>    Micrococcus<br>    Moraxella<br>    Pasteurella<br>    Veillonella<br>    Fusobacterium |
| Genital tract | Species of:<br>    Micrococcus<br>    Staphylococcus<br>    Streptococcus |

An example of this is the millions of micro-organisms present in the horse's gut (see Chapter 11). In fact the horse could not digest its natural herbage diet without them. Another example would be the millions of bacteria which live naturally on the horse's skin without producing any effects of disease.

An infection results from the establishment of a colony of disease-causing micro-organisms such as bacteria, fungi or viruses. Disease-causing micro-organisms are known as pathogens. These organisms actively reproduce and cause damage to cells either directly or indirectly by the production of toxins. Infection should normally produce a response from the horse's immune system.

In some cases infection is spread throughout the horse's body and this is known as a systemic infection. Infection may also be localised within a particular area or tissue. The micro-organisms vary in their ability to invade and multiply and this capacity is known as virulence. Sometimes organisms may spread from a part of the body where they are normally harmless to another part where they become harmful. An example of this occurs when there is leakage from the horse's gut into the surrounding abdominal space resulting in infection of the gut lining, or peritoneum, known as peritonitis. Entry of micro-organisms from the soil into wounds or during surgery can introduce localised infection.

These disease-causing organisms fall into a number of well-defined groups which include not only viruses, bacteria and fungi but also rickettsiae, chlamydiae and mycoplasmas. All of these are relatively simple organisms which can multiply in the horse's tissues, particularly when the horse's defences are low. Other disease-causing organisms are the parasites. These include the single-celled parasites known as protozoa, worms, ascari and insects. Colonisation by worms, ascari and insects, however, tend to be called an infestation rather than an infection.

The horse's reaction to the presence of infection produces the symptoms of the disease. The symptoms are therefore caused in part by micro-organisms damaging cells and tissues, releasing toxins and drawing on the horse's nutrient supply. Symptoms are also caused by the horse's own defences which include the immune system whose job it is to destroy the offending micro-organisms. The outcome will depend on whether the micro-organisms or the horse's defence system gain the advantage. The strength of the horse's immune system, which is often a reflection of the general health and well-being of the horse, will strongly influence this outcome.

A higher temperature is often a feature in many infections.

Apart from diseases in which the symptoms and signs are easily recognisable, such as tetanus or strangles, diagnosis will often rely upon the isolation of the causative micro-organism. Testing may involve microscopic examination of a specimen of infected tissue or body fluid, by culture techniques or by detecting antibodies (proteins manufactured by the horse to defend against a particular organism) in a blood sample. A problem in detecting infectious diseases is that there is always a time gap between the entry of micro-organisms and the appearance of symptoms. This is known as the incubation period and may be as little as a few days or as long as several months. Furthermore, symptoms may never develop in some infected horses, but these horses nevertheless continue to carry the disease-causing organisms and unwittingly spread them to other horses.

As a result of this, an epidemic can be well established before it is recognised and before control measures can be introduced. Early recognition of symptoms is therefore important if treatment is going to be more effective.

Invasion of the horse's body may take place through one of several routes (Fig. 15.1). These possible entrance sites for micro-organisms include the eyes, mouth, nostrils, skin and genitals. All these areas have mechanisms to try and reduce the possibility of pathogenic micro-organisms taking hold. Horses may be susceptible to some micro-organisms but not to others. This is because many of the micro-organisms are species-specific. Horses, for example, cannot catch flu from humans. Some micro-organisms can cause severe reactions and symptoms and these cause acute infections. Others, on the other hand, may produce a slow reaction of the horse's defence

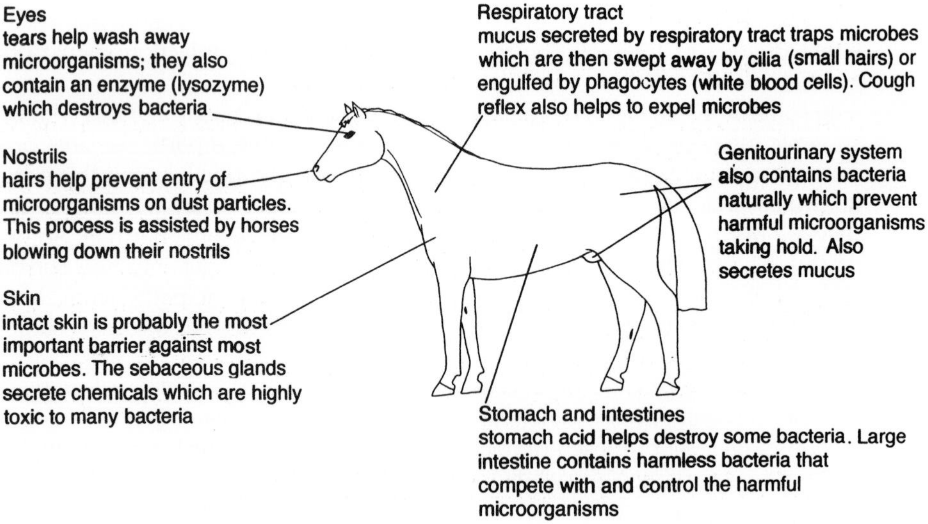

Eyes
tears help wash away
microorganisms; they also
contain an enzyme (lysozyme)
which destroys bacteria

Nostrils
hairs help prevent entry of
microorganisms on dust particles.
This process is assisted by horses
blowing down their nostrils

Skin
intact skin is probably the most
important barrier against most
microbes. The sebaceous glands
secrete chemicals which are highly
toxic to many bacteria

Respiratory tract
mucus secreted by respiratory tract traps microbes
which are then swept away by cilia (small hairs) or
engulfed by phagocytes (white blood cells). Cough
reflex also helps to expel microbes

Genitourinary system
also contains bacteria
naturally which prevent
harmful microorganisms
taking hold. Also
secretes mucus

Stomach and intestines
stomach acid helps destroy some bacteria. Large
intestine contains harmless bacteria that
compete with and control the harmful
microorganisms

**Fig. 15.1**  Summary of the physical and chemical barriers against harmful invaders.

mechanisms and the horse will be slow to overcome the chronic infection which has resulted.

## Bacteria

Bacteria are a group of single-celled micro-organisms which may cause disease. Their basic structure is shown in Fig. 15.2. Commonly known as 'germs', bacteria have been recognised as a cause of disease for over 100 years. Bacteria are naturally abundant in the air, soil and water and most of these are harmless to horses. When they harm horses they are called pathogenic.

Pathogenic bacteria can be classified on the basis of their shape into three main groups:

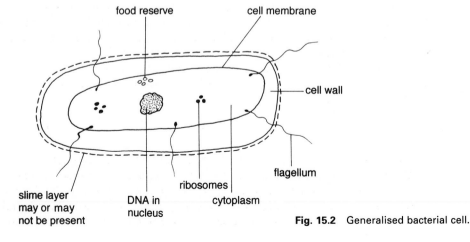

food reserve

cell membrane

cell wall

flagellum

slime layer
may or may
not be present

DNA in
nucleus

ribosomes

cytoplasm

**Fig. 15.2**  Generalised bacterial cell.

(1) cocci (spherical)
(2) bacilli (rod-shaped)
(3) spirochaetes or spirilla (spiral-shaped).

Diseases caused by the cocci include pneumonia and strangles. Tetanus and botulism are caused by bacilli.

The bacteria which invade the horse's body thrive in the warm, moist conditions. Some bacteria are described as aerobic, meaning that they require oxygen to grow and survive. They are therefore found in such places as the respiratory system or on the skin. Anaerobic bacteria, on the other hand, thrive in areas low in oxygen such as deep in wounds or tissues. Some bacteria which are associated with wounds and abscesses are shown in Table 15.2.

Many bacteria are naturally static and only move around the horse's body in currents of fluid or air. Others are very mobile and have filamentous tails to help them move.

**Table 15.2**  Bacteria species which may be found in wounds

Aerobes (require oxygen)
  *Escherichia coli*
  *Pseudomonas aeruginosa*
  *Staphylococcus aureus*
  *Streptococcus zooepidemicus*

Anaerobes (low or no oxygen)
  *Clostridium perfringens*
  *Clostridium tetani*
  *Clostridium septicum*

## Reproduction

Bacteria are able to reproduce by simply dividing into two cells, these in turn divide again and so on. Under ideal conditions this can take place every 20 minutes. After only six hours a single bacterium can have multiplied to form a colony of over 250 000 bacteria. Luckily these ideal conditions rarely occur within the horse's body due to action of the horse's own defence system in killing these bacteria.

As well as dividing, some bacteria can also produce spores. A spore is a single new bacterium which is protected by an extremely tough outer coat that can survive high temperatures, dry conditions and lack of nutrients. These spores can remain in this dormant state for many years. When conditions are right they will 'hatch' and invade body tissues. Spore-producing bacteria include clostridia responsible for tetanus and botulism. These spores are able to lie dormant within the soil for many years. When a horse has a wound (often very minor) the tetanus-causing bacteria (*Clostridium tetani*) can enter the body through this route. This is why it is so important to keep tetanus vaccinations up to date.

## Disease

Bacteria produce toxins or poisons which are harmful to the horse's cells. If they are present in sufficient numbers and the horse has not previously developed an immunity to them, disease will result (Table 15.3). Some bacteria release toxins known as endotoxins which can cause a high temperature, bleeding and shock. Others produce exotoxins which account for the major damage caused by bacteria such as tetanus.

**Table 15.3**   Some equine bacterial infectious diseases

| Disease | Bacterium |
| --- | --- |
| Tetanus | *Clostridium tetani* |
| Strangles | *Streptococcus equi* |
| Botulism | *Clostridium botulinum* |
| Rattles (summer penumonia) | *Rhodococcus equi (Corynebacterium equi)* |
| Leptospirosis | *Leptospira interrogans serovars* |
| Glanders | *Pseudomonas mallei* |
| Contagious equine metritis | *Taylorella equigenitalis* |
| Pseudomonas metritis | *Pseudomonas aeruginosa* |
| Salmonellosis | *Salmonella species* |

The horse's body will attempt to fight invading bacteria, and sometimes this is successful without treatment. In many cases though treatment is necessary, with the main form being given as antibiotics, either orally, in the feed or by injection.

Some antibiotics such as penicillin are bactericidal which means they kill invading bacteria. Others, such as tetracycline, are bacteriostatic, i.e. they stop the bacteria multiplying, enabling the body's defence to overcome them.

Some diseases such as tetanus are treated by the injection of an antiserum. This is a fluid taken from the blood of a horse who has been given a series of immunising injections and whose blood consequently contains antibodies against the *Clostridium tetani* organism.

Superficial inflammation and minor infected wounds can be treated with antiseptic solutions.

# Viruses

These are minute infectious agents which are much smaller than bacteria. They have a much simpler structure (Fig. 15.3) and a relatively uncomplicated method of multiplication.

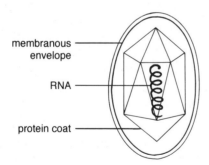

membranous envelope

RNA

protein coat

**Fig. 15.3**   An enveloped virus.

Viral infections vary from relatively minor problems such as warts to extremely serious diseases such as rabies. It is thought that some virus infections also lead to cancer. It is debatable whether a virus is a living organism as such or just a collection of nucleic material (deoxyribonucleic acid (DNA) or ribonucleic acid (RNA)) capable of replicating itself under specific, favourable conditions.

A viruses' sole aim is to invade the cells of other organisms which they then instruct to make more copies of themselves. Outside the living cell viruses are totally inactive. They are incapable of activities such as metabolism which we normally associate with living organisms. The number of different kinds of virus probably exceeds the number of types of all other organisms. Viruses are parasites and are known to be capable of parasitising all recognised life-forms. They do not always cause disease, however.

## Structure of viruses

A single virus particle is known as a virion and consists quite simply of a core of genetic material or nucleic acid. This is surrounded by a capsule or shell known as a capsid which is made of protein. These capsids may be surrounded by a viral envelope which again is made from protein and this envelope is usually lost when the virus invades the host cell. The central core of nucleic acid is known as the genome and consists of a string of genes that contain the code for making copies of that virus.

Depending upon the type of virus, the nucleic acid may be either DNA or RNA. The DNA consists of a double strand in a double-helix formation whereas the RNA is a single strand.

## Replication

Viruses do not reproduce in the usual way, instead they undergo a process known as replication (Fig. 15.4). Basically, the virus invades the host cell and begins the process of making copies of itself from materials within the host cell itself. Viruses often have elaborate methods of replicating themselves within the host cell. Some are straightforward, as previously described, whereas others invade the nucleus of the host cell and incorporate themselves in the cell's own genetic material before being able to replicate. Sometimes the viral genome may sit dormant within the host cell's nucleus, to become reactivated several months later.

The viral genome may also interfere with the cell's chromosomes, causing the transition of a healthy host cell to a tumour cell.

Viruses are grouped into families, some of which are shown in Table 15.4.

## Disease

Viruses can gain entry to the horse's body through all possible entrance routes. They may be inhaled in droplets or swallowed in food or water. They may be passed into the body through the saliva of biting insects such as equine infectious anaemia, or they may enter the horse's body during covering.

Many viruses, once they have entered the host's body, will begin to replicate near the site of entry. Others may enter the lymph vessels and spread to the lymph nodes (see Chapter 6) where many of them will be engulfed by white blood cells. Others may pass from the lymphatics to the blood from where they can invade every part of the horse. They tend to have target organs such as the brain (as in rabies) or the respiratory tract (as in equine influenza).

Viruses can cause disease in a number of ways. They can seriously upset the functioning of the host cells or even destroy them. This can cause serious disease if vital organs such as the brain or heart are affected in this way. Also, the horse's own immune system will respond to the viral infection and this response may lead to symptoms such as a high temperature and fatigue. Antibodies produced by the horse's own immune system may attach themselves to the viral particles and circulate as immune complexes within the blood. These antibodies may then be deposited in various parts of the horse's body causing inflammation and severe tissue damage.

Viruses may also cause cancer by taking over the host cell's DNA.

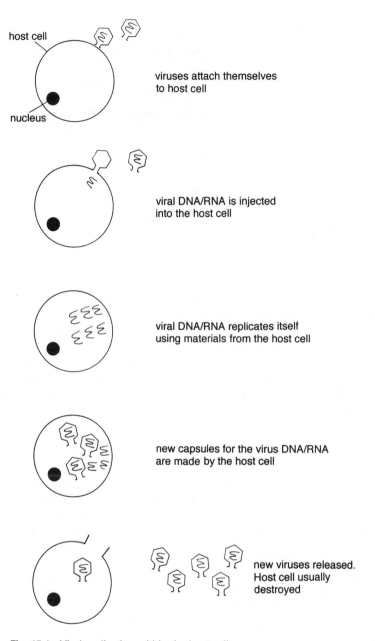

host cell

nucleus

viruses attach themselves
to host cell

viral DNA/RNA is injected
into the host cell

viral DNA/RNA replicates itself
using materials from the host cell

new capsules for the virus DNA/RNA
are made by the host cell

new viruses released.
Host cell usually
destroyed

**Fig. 15.4**   Viral replication within the host cell.

Fighting viral infections is very difficult because it is near impossible to design drugs which will 'kill' viruses without affecting the host cell in which the virus is situated. Some antiviral agents have been produced in human medicine, which prevent viruses from entering the host cells or by interfering with their replication within the cell.

Immunisation can be a much more effective method of eradicating or reducing the effects of viruses. Vaccination programmes are used widely for the control of equine influenza.

**Table 15.4** Common virus families

| Family | Example of diseases |
|---|---|
| Papovaviruses | Warts |
| Adenoviruses | Respiratory and eye infections |
| | Cold virus |
| Herpesviruses | Equine herpes virus 1 (EHV-1) and subtypes 1 (abortive strain) and 2 (respiratory strain) |
| | EHV 3 – coital exanthema |
| Togaviruses | Equine arteritis (pinkeye) |
| Picornaviruses | Equine rhinovirus 1, 2 and 3 and stable picornavirus |
| Rhabdoviruses | Rabies |
| Arboviruses | Viral encephalomyelitis |
| Orthomyxoviruses | Equine influenza |

# Fungi

Fungi are relatively simple parasites and include moulds, mildews, yeasts, mushrooms and toadstools. There are more than 100 000 species of fungi within the world. Most of these are actually harmless and may even be beneficial, for example some moulds are used to make antibiotics. Fungi are larger than bacteria.

Some fungi occur as colonies of individual cells such as the yeasts. Others form chains of tubes or filaments called hyphae which are formed into a complex network known as a mycelium. Many fungi form millions of tiny spores which can remain dormant until suitable conditions are available for them to grow (Fig. 15.5). Fungal spores are found mainly in the soil.

## Fungal diseases

Fungal spores can penetrate into the tissue of the host. An example of this is aspergillus causing infection of the mucus membranes and guttural pouch. Some of the yeasts which are present normally within the horse's gut may become a problem if the gut flora are upset or disrupted by the use of antibiotics. They can then overgrow the bacterial population because antibiotics destroy bacteria but have no effect on fungi.

Probably the most common fungal infection of the horse is ringworm. Both trichophyton and microsporum cause ringworm.

Fungi can also cause disease in other ways. Certain fungi that infect food crops produce dangerous toxins. A fungus which infects cereals, particularly rye, produces a toxin known as ergot. Whereas ergot is highly toxic to humans, horses given 500 g ergot showed only slight symptoms. More serious toxins are the aflatoxins. The horse seems more susceptible to aflatoxins than other domestic animals. Aflatoxins may be found in badly stored cereals or oil seeds. It has been suggested that grass sickness may also be caused by a fungal toxin. Ryegrass staggers is caused by a neurotoxin present in perennial ryegrass. Also, some spores of fungi, particularly those found in mouldy hay, can cause damage when inhaled by horses, causing persistent allergic reactions in the lungs or chronic obstructive pulmonary disease (COPD). The principal culprits are micropolyspora faeni and aspergillus fumigatus.

Antifungal drugs can be used to treat ringworm. These work by damaging the cell walls of the fungi, causing the eventual death of the fungal cells.

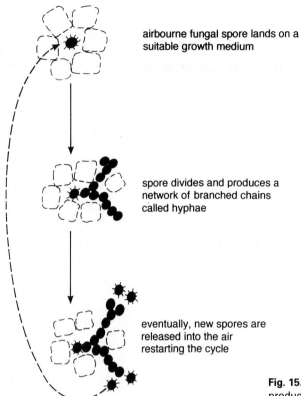

airbourne fungal spore lands on a
suitable growth medium

spore divides and produces a
network of branched chains
called hyphae

eventually, new spores are
released into the air
restarting the cycle

**Fig. 15.5**   Fungal growth and the
production of spores.

## Mycoplasma, rickettsia and chlamydia

These are neither bacteria nor viruses but are somewhere between the two.
Mycoplasma are the smallest free living organisms and because they do not have a
cell wall they are very susceptible to changes in their environment.

Mycoplasma have been isolated from the respiratory tracts of horses and it is
thought that they may be involved in mixed infections with other viruses or bacteria.
Rickettsia and chlamydia can only live and grow within the host's cells. Rickettsia are
associated with lice, ticks, fleas and mites which are responsible for their spread.
Chlamydia are pathogenic in humans but have not yet been associated with infective
disease in horses.

## Protozoa

These are simple, primitive single-celled animals. They are microscopic but larger than
bacteria. The more advanced types are capable of respiration, reproduction and
excretion. They move around by using a tail known as a flagellum. Some become
parasites as part of their life cycle.

A number of different protozoa affect horses. Babesia, trypanasomes, besnoitia and
sarcocystis are examples.

# The immune system

The immune system is a collection of cells and proteins which are able to protect the horse from potentially harmful infectious micro-organisms such as those mentioned above. The immune system is also responsible for allergic reactions and hypersensitivity.

Innate immunity is present from birth and is the first line of defence against disease. Acquired immunity is the second line of defence and develops either through exposure of the horse to the infectious organisms (after they have broken through the innate immune system) or through immunisation.

## Innate immunity

A newborn foal is to some extent protected against infection by innate immunity. This consists of the physical barriers such as skin and substances which are present in the mouth, urinary tract and eyes which kill bacteria, and also antibodies and immunoglobulins which have passed from the mare to the foal in the uterus and in her milk. This innate immunity does not guard the foal against all the disease-causing organisms. As the foal grows he will come across organisms which cause disease by overcoming these innate defences.

If micro-organisms are able to penetrate these first barriers, they will soon encounter white blood cells called phagocytes which can engulf them. Micro-organisms may also come across a group of blood proteins called the complement system which act to destroy invading bacteria.

If micro-organisms are still able to penetrate into the horse's body then the second line of defence known as the adaptive immune system comes into play.

## Adaptive immunity

This system as the name implies, adapts its response to specifically fight each invading type of organism. It also retains a memory of this organism so that it will be prepared should the same organism attack the horse again. The horse is then said to have acquired immunity to the infection.

This acquisition of immunity in response to infection may take a few days or weeks. In the interim period the foal or adult horse may become seriously ill and may even die. In the past many horses did die but now, due to better nutrition and vaccination, more horses survive.

The adaptive part of the immune system is extremely complex and is still not fully understood. Its main function is to produce specific defences against the vast array of micro-organisms which invade the horse's body. However, it must first recognise part of an invading micro-organism as an antigen, i.e. a foreign protein or particle that is different from any other body proteins. A response is then mounted against the antigen. This response may be humoral or cellular.

### Humoral immunity

This type of response is particularly important against bacteria. After a highly complex recognition process, the B-lymphocytes (a type of white blood cell) are stimulated to multiply (Fig. 15.6). These cells then begin to produce vast numbers of antibodies or immunoglobulins which are able to bind to the foreign antigens. Once this has occurred the organisms with the attached antibodies become easy prey to the

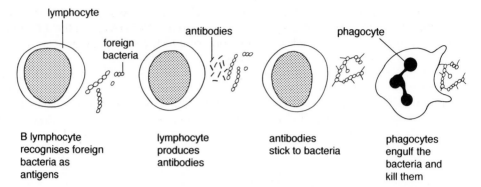

**Fig. 15.6** Role of white blood cells in overcoming bacteria.

phagocytic white blood cells which engulf them and break them down. Immunoglobulins also play a central role in allergies and hypersensitivity reactions (Fig. 15.7). In these cases they bind to antigens which are not necessarily a threat to the horse's health, and may provoke an inflammatory reaction. This can be severe, causing the horse to go into shock and even death.

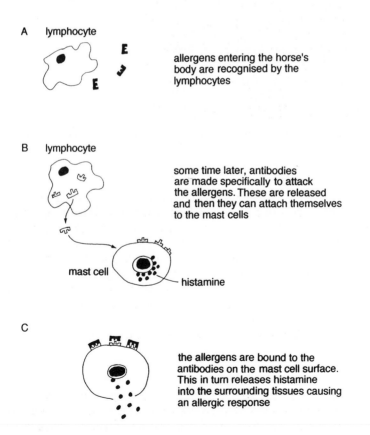

**Fig. 15.7** Origin of an allergy.

A very common allergic reactions, usually of a mild nature, occurs in the condition known as urticaria or nettle rash (Fig. 15.8).

There are five classes of immunoglobulins: IgA, IgD, IgE, IgG and IgM (Ig stands for immunoglobulin). Approximately 75% of the immunoglobulins are in the IgG group. The IgG molecule consists of two parts, one of which binds to the antigen and the other binds to phagocytes which then engulf the antigen.

This binding of antibody and antigen may also activate the complement system which increases the efficiency of the phagocytes. The complement system consists of a group of proteins or inactive enzymes found in the plasma. These become activated when an antibody binds to an antigen causing agglutination, neutralisation or inflammation to wall off the antigen.

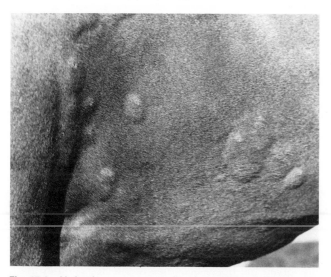

**Fig. 15.8**  Urticaria – a common allergic condition in horses. (Courtesy of Liverpool University Veterinary School)

## Cellular immunity

This is particularly important in the immune system's response to invading viruses and certain parasites which are able to hide within the horse's cells. This involves the T-lyphocytes (thymus lymphocytes) and there are two types which, for simplicity, are known as the helper cells and the killer cells. The helper cells play a role in the recognition of antigens. They are then able to activate the killer cells. Killer lymphocytes are able to lock onto cells which have been invaded by viruses or parasites and which have left recognisable antigens on the cell surface and then destroy these cells. The memory of the immune system which provides acquired immunity to certain diseases relies on the long-term survival of lymphocytes that were activated or sensitised to antigens when they were first encountered.

## Vaccination

Vaccination, also known as active immunisation, is a procedure which is used to stimulate the horse's immune system, whereby killed or weakened micro-organisms are introduced into the horse's body – usually by means of an injection. These micro-organisms then sensitise the immune system so that if they are encountered at a later date they will quickly be dealt with by the action of the antibodies which have now been primed to act. The antibodies may either kill the bug itself or neutralise the toxin it produces.

Most vaccinations are preparations which contain the organism or parts of it. These organisms are not able to cause disease. The term 'live attenuated organisms' refers to strains of organisms which have been treated to render them harmless to the horse. Attenuation is achieved by artificially altering their genes or by infecting laboratory animals first which reduces the ability of the organism to cause disease without reducing the ability to induce immunity. Other vaccines contain chemically modified bacterial toxins.

Vaccines are now available to protect the horse against a wide range of infectious diseases including influenza, tetanus, rhinopneumonitis (EHV-1), Eastern and Western encephalomyelitis, rabies and strangles.

Different vaccines have varying durations of effectiveness. Boosters are often required at intervals to maintain the immune status.

# Parasites of the horse

Both internal and external parasites infect the horse. The most common internal parasites of horses are worms. External parasites include lice, ticks, mites, and flies of several species.

## Internal parasites

Worms which live within the horse's body tissues are true parasites in that they use the horse as a source of nutrition and a protected environment. All horses have a degree of parasitic worm infestation, the adult worms laying up to 10 million eggs per day which are passed out in the horse's faeces to infect the pasture. Under suitable conditions the larvae within the eggs develop and become infective to the horses so that when the grazing horse ingests the larvae the horse becomes re-infected. Within the horse's body the larvae undergo further development before becoming adult egg-laying worms in the horse's gut to complete the cycle. Depending on the species of worm, the larvae migrate through the body tissues during their development, including blood vessels, the liver, lungs and the gut lining and may cause severe problems to the horse, particularly if the infestation is heavy. Foals and immature horses that have not yet developed any immunity to the worms are particularly vulnerable.

The degree of parasitic worm infestation can be determined using regular faecal worm egg counts to build up a picture of the events occurring in each horse. A small sample of dung is tested in the laboratory and a count made of the eggs present, giving an indication of the numbers of adult egg-laying worms in the horse's gut. However, the test does not indicate the number of immature larvae which may be migrating in the horse's body tissues so that false negative results can occur if the horse has recently been wormed. More useful diagnoses are made by supplementing with blood tests.

The most common worms which affect horses are shown in Table 15.5.

### Strongyles

These can be split into one of two groups depending on their structure, size and effect on the horse. The two groups are known as large and small strongyles.

#### *Large strongyles or redworms*

These are one of the most important parasites of horses, affecting horses of all ages.

**Table 15.5** The major parasitic worms that affect horses

| Migratory stages | | Adult forms |
| --- | --- | --- |
| Large strongyles or redworms | e.g. *St. vulgaris*, migrate through blood vessels. Damage may occur to blood vessels supplying the gut | Suck on plugs of bowel causing localised bleeding. May interfere with digestion |
| Small strongyles or cyathostomes | Enter gut wall and may lay dormant for up to two years within sealed nodules in the gut wall. These may interfere with nutrient absorption. Release of large numbers may lead to diarrhoea. | Interfere with digestion of nutrients |
| Roundworms or ascarids | Damage to lungs as larvae migrate through them, coughing, nasal discharge | Obstruct bowel and interfere with digestion |
| Tapeworms | No migratory stage | Erosion of ileo-caecal valve area. Irritation to large intestine. Loss of condition, occasional colic |
| Pinworms | No migratory stage | Interfere with digestion. Eggs deposited around anus cause irritation |
| Bot larvae | Eggs laid on hairs of forelegs and chest. Larvae migrate through tongue and mouth tissues. Painful mouth and reduced appetite | Pupa in soil for 1–3 months. Adult flies emerge in summer |

Large strongyles or redworms are round-shaped worms, 2–8 cm (1–3.5 in) long and coloured red from the blood that they suck. The most potentially dangerous of the redworms is *Strongylus vulgaris* because it migrates extensively through the body including the anterior mesenteric artery, which is responsible for supplying most of the gut with blood. This migration damages the artery walls (aneurysms) and causes blood clots; these clots may block smaller blood vessels and thus disrupt the blood supply to the gut, causing colic; indeed, redworm are thought to be the commonest cause of recurrent bouts of spasmodic colic. Eventually the mature larvae return to the wall of the large intestine before emerging into the gut where they become egg-laying adults five to nine months after infection (Fig. 15.9).

This prolonged migration may lead to 'false negative' faecal worm egg counts; there may be no adult egg-laying worms in the gut and thus a negative worm egg count will be recorded, even though the tissues may contain many larvae which are causing extensive damage and will eventually become adults in the gut. Both large and small strongyles can remain dormant in the gut wall so that when egg-laying adults are removed by worming, a new wave of larvae emerge to become egg-laying adults, this is known as larval cyathostomiasis and tends to be most obvious in the spring. Few wormers are active against these migrating larvae, although some are effective in high doses. It is therefore wise to give a larvicidal dose at intervals through the year to reduce the population of developing larvae.

Redworms can affect horses of all ages. Foals less than six-weeks-old will not

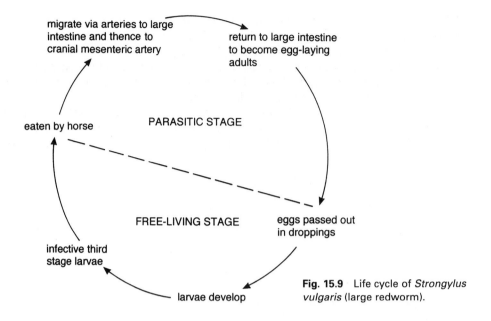

Fig. 15.9 Life cycle of *Strongylus vulgaris* (large redworm).

harbour any egg-laying adults but the larval stages will start to cause damage soon after being eaten.

### Small strongyles or cyathostomes

Otherwise known as cyathostomes, these are a sub-family of the strongyle group. As their name suggests they are much smaller than the large strongyles. These worms are damaging in that certain larval stages develop within the wall of the large intestine and can remain encysted for several months before emerging, sometimes in large numbers. This emergence can lead to severe diarrhoea and affected horses usually lose weight.

Cyathosomes may be killed with large, repeated doses of fenbendazole, but it is better to prevent their build up in the first place by adopting an efficient worming programme as recommended by the vet.

### Roundworms or ascarids

Roundworms (*Parascaris equorum*) are a parasite of young horses and can be fatal to foals, yearlings and horses under three years of age. Foals have little immunity to roundworms and may have up to 1000 adult roundworms in their gut, giving them a dull coat, pot-belly, loss of condition and slow growth. The worms will cause inflammation of the lining of the gut and in severe cases may actually block the small intestine, causing rupture, peritonitis and death. The migrating larvae can cause coughing and a snotty nose. After the age of two or three, horses develop resistance to ascarids and they do not cause problems in older horses.

The adults live in the small intestine and may grow to be 30 cm (12 in) long and be as thick as a pencil. An adult egg-laying female can lay 200 000 to 1 million eggs per day; the eggs have a tough sticky outer coat which makes them very resistant to disinfectants and the environment, allowing them to survive for up to three years outside the horse.

Infective larvae develop inside the egg and, when eaten by the foal, the larvae hatch in the foal's gut and burrow through the gut wall and migrate via the bloodstream to the liver and lungs. The larvae are coughed up, swallowed and undergo their final development to become egg-laying adults inside the small intestine. It takes eight to twelve weeks from infection (the foal eating the eggs) for the larvae to mature and for eggs to start being passed out in the foal's droppings and thus infect the pasture. From the eggs being passed out of the foal in the dung to the development of infective larvae takes about 30 days under optimal conditions (Fig. 15.10).

Very heavy contamination can occur on paddocks grazed every year by mares and foals; mares must be wormed regularly during pregnancy. Ideally foals would only be turned out on to pasture that had not been grazed by horses in the previous 12 months.

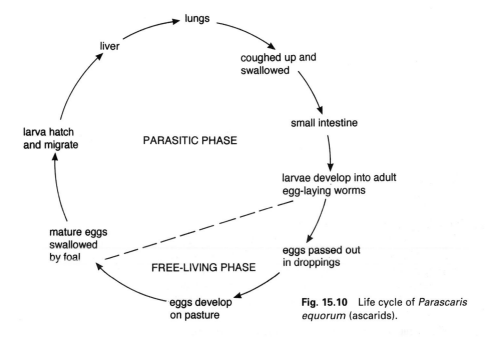

**Fig. 15.10**   Life cycle of *Parascaris equorum* (ascarids).

### Tapeworm

The adult tapeworm (*Anoplocephala perfoliata*) is found in the caecum and favours the ileocaecal junction, where the small intestine enters the caecum. The adult is segmented and about 8 cm (3.5 in) long and 8–14 mm (0.3–0.5 in) wide. It sheds segments containing eggs which are passed out in the dung, and eggs are eaten by an intermediate host, forage mites, where larval development takes place. The horse is infected by eating these mites while grazing and the larval form develops directly to the adult worm in the caecum, taking 6–10 weeks (Fig. 15.11). Although there is some debate as to the extent of tapeworm infection in horses, infection has been associated with colics, peritonitis and digestive upsets due to inflammation of the gut around the area of attachment.

### Worming

This is the administration of drugs to kill worms, and there are many available on the market. Some are shown in Table 15.6.

The ways in which the different drugs work are quite distinct from one another, but the benzimidazole group all act in the same way on the adult worm which feeds on the blood and tissues of the horse's gut. The drug is taken into the bloodstream of the

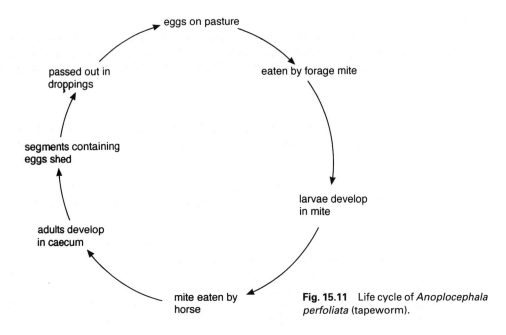

eggs on pasture

passed out in droppings

eaten by forage mite

segments containing eggs shed

larvae develop in mite

adults develop in caecum

mite eaten by horse

**Fig. 15.11**   Life cycle of *Anoplocephala perfoliata* (tapeworm).

**Table 15.6**   Wormers

| Trade name | Active ingredient |
| --- | --- |
| **Benzimidazole group** | |
| Panacur | Fenbendazole |
| Telmin | Mebendazole |
| Equizole | Thiabendazole |
| Equitac | Oxibendazole |
| Systamex | Oxfendazole |
| PanacurGuard | Fenbendazole (5 day dose) |
| **Other compounds** | |
| Pony & Foal Wormer | Piperazine |
| Strongid-P | Pyrantel embonate |
| Eqvalan | Ivermectin |
| **Organophosphorus compounds for worms** | |
| Equivurm | Haloxon |
| **Organophosphorus compounds for bots** | |
| Neguvon | Trichlorfon |
| Equiguard | Dichlorvos |

Availability of trade name wormers will vary from country to country.

horse and the feeding worm ingests it and eventually dies. Eqvalan is also absorbed into the horse's bloodstream and acts upon the worm's nervous system, causing paralysis. Eqvalan is the only wormer to date which acts upon the migrating redworm larvae when given at the normal dose.

Strongid-P is not taken into the bloodstream but stays in the horse's gut and paralyses the worms. Many horse owners like to rotate their wormers to prevent resistance, but care should be taken when choosing a brand. All the benzimidazoles work in the same way and rotating these brands will have no effect (Table 15.6).

## Resistance

There is little doubt that worms can and do develop resistance to anthelmintic drugs. Some worms have a genetic predisposition against certain classes of drugs, in particular the benzimidazoles. There has been no resistance shown to Eqvalan to date.

## Worming programme

Designing a worming programme is quite a difficult exercise as there are so many drugs available and some wormers seem more effective than others. Some factors need to be considered:

(1) Only a double dose of Strongid-P (pyrantel embonate) will kill tapeworm.
(2) Only Eqvalan (ivermectin) will also kill both larvae and migrating worm larvae as well as the adults.

Other products available include a five-day dose of fenbendazole known as Panacur Guard to remove encisted worm larvae from the gut wall.

Rotation of wormers can take place each year rather than at each worming. However, this is not recommended with the benzimidazole group.

A sample worming programme is given below. It is important to read the manufacturers' instructions carefully and to follow the doses suggested.

March – normal dose
April – normal dose
May
June – double dose of Strongid-P (if in high risk area for tapeworm)
July – normal dose
August
September – normal dose
October – double dose of Strongid-P (if in high risk area for tapeworm)
November – Eqvalan to remove bot larvae

The local veterinary school will be able to inform you of the prevalence of tapeworm in your area.

## Management methods to reduce the worm burden

The most effective method is the regular removal of droppings from the pasture. Care should also be taken when harrowing as this drags the worm eggs and larvae on to the horses' grazing areas (known as lawns) instead of leaving them in the dunging areas (known as roughs).

Harrowing should be done only in very hot dry conditions so that the larvae will be killed, or the pasture should be rested after harrowing and before horses graze or other livestock can be grazed as the worms do not complete their life cycle in other livestock. An example of a rotational grazing programme is shown in Fig. 15.12.

## External parasites

### Lice

Two species of louse parasitise horses: *Haematopinus asini*, the sucking louse and *Damalinia equi*, the biting louse (Fig. 15.13). The former feeds by sucking blood from

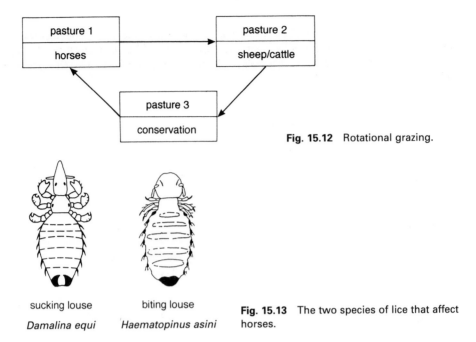

**Fig. 15.12**  Rotational grazing.

sucking louse             biting louse

*Damalina equi*      *Haematopinus asini*

**Fig. 15.13**  The two species of lice that affect horses.

the horse while the latter scavenges debris from the skin surface. Lice cause acute itching and the horse's coat rapidly becomes dull with bald and sore patches. Lice are grey in colour and 1.5–3 mm (0.06–0.12 in) long and infestation is usually identified by the presence of cream coloured eggs or nits, firmly attached to the hair and close to the roots. Lice are host specific and do not infect humans; their life cycle is completed in three weeks during which time they stay on the horse. Lice spread by contact between horses, thus all groups of horses should be treated simultaneously.

## Flies

Flies are not a true parasite of the horse but they are worthy of note as a health hazard. Flies spread disease and infection and can irritate horses to such an extent that they lose condition.

### House flies

House flies (*Musca domestica*) do not bite but they can cause intense irritation when they gather in large numbers on moist areas of the horse's body; for example, they can cause ulcerative dermatitis around the eyes.

### Stable flies

Stable flies (*Stomoxys calcitrans*) have a painful bite which may leave raised swellings on the horses skin due to an allergic reaction to the saliva of the flies. Stable flies breed in bedding and muck heaps and are found in large numbers in most stable environments.

### Horse flies

Horse flies (*Tabanus*) cause severe irritation and horses may be driven to galloping around to escape their particularly deep and painful bite. Horse flies transmit equine infectious anaemia.

### Bot flies *(Gasterophilus intestinalis)*

Bot flies lay their characteristic yellow eggs on the horse's front legs, chest and abdomen. Horses become quite distressed when these flies are around. The larvae attach themselves to the stomach wall after having been swallowed by the horse (Fig. 15.14).

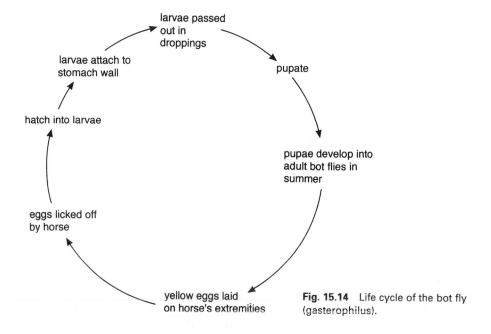

larvae passed out in droppings

larvae attach to stomach wall

hatch into larvae

eggs licked off by horse

pupate

pupae develop into adult bot flies in summer

yellow eggs laid on horse's extremities

**Fig. 15.14** Life cycle of the bot fly (gasterophilus).

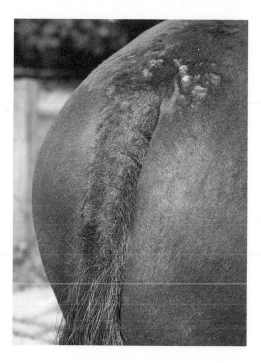

**Fig. 15.15** Sweet itch or seasonal recurrent dermatitis. (Courtesy of Joanna Prestwich)

### Midges

The biting midges (*Culicoides*) are very small (0.5–3 mm) (0.02–0.12 in), hence their name 'no see-ums'. Many species bite and annoy horses, but only some species cause the allergic reaction known as sweet itch or seasonal recurrent dermatitis (Fig. 15.15). Some horses have such severe reactions to the midges' saliva that they rub themselves raw on the mane and tail.

# Chapter 16
# Wounds and Wound Healing

There is no doubt that horses are particularly susceptible to injury. They are athletic animals capable of travelling at fast speeds and we ask them to jump over fences as well! When horses travel at speed they are more likely to cause themselves injury. Injuries are commonplace in all types of equestrian pursuits, but are particularly frequent in racing (both Flat and National Hunt), eventing and show-jumping. Horses are also susceptible to injury while in the field and often sustain such injuries as kicks and bites, as well as damages from fences. Barbed wire fencing is renowned for causing quite severe injuries to horses.

Whatever the source of the injury, all horse owners will have to apply first aid and should have a knowledge of how injuries repair themselves. This will help in the healing process and result in horses returning to work sooner. All horses will suffer from minor injuries during their lifetime but some seem to be particularly accident-prone.

The healing process of wounds in horses does to a large extent depend upon where they are. The wounds over the large muscle masses seem to heal remarkably well by wound contraction, leaving only a small scar, whereas wounds to the lower limb are notoriously difficult. Where wounds lie over joints, healing can also be difficult.

## Wound healing

Every injury has to be repaired for the horse to survive. All horses have the ability to repair damage tissues, but some tissues are better at regenerating than others. For example, horses can make new bone to repair a fracture, but not new cartilage, which is why arthritis is such a problem. New nerve fibres can be formed, but the cell bodies of the nerve cells cannot be replaced (see Chapter 6). The liver regenerates well, but slowly, whereas kidney and lung tissue, when damaged, can only increase the size of the undamaged area to compensate, a process known as compensatory hypertrophy.

Muscle regenerates poorly and any discontinuity is bridged by newly formed fibrous connective tissue which does not have the same contractile properties. This is why muscle loss in problems such as azoturia can have long-lasting detrimental effects. On the other hand, blood vessels and lymphatics, red and white blood cells, the epidermis of the skin and epithelia lining internal surfaces, are constantly dying and being replaced. Their life expectancy can be measured in days or weeks rather than years. The cells of the epidermis live for about 27 days and these tissues never grow old.

The reason for this is that these tissues have a reserve of embryonic type cells whose only function is to maintain the population of mature, working cells. Consequently they are all well placed to repair even major catastrophes by accelerating the process of normal day-to-day regeneration.

Whatever the injury the healing process follows the same stages and processes. Inflammation always takes place followed by repair and regeneration and finally remodelling. The most common type of injury to a horse is a skin wound and these can be superficial or extensive with severe damage to underlying tissues and not just the skin.

Regeneration and repair of wounds can occur by one of two methods:

(1) The first and preferred is known as first intention healing and this is where the edges of the wound are held together and quickly stick to each other. This type of healing takes place in surgical incisions, where the edges of the wound may be held together by stitches. First intention healing tends to occur when there is no tissue loss.

(2) The second type of wound healing is known as second intention healing. This takes much longer to repair and happens when there has been loss of tissue, excessive movement of the wound or infection and the edges of the wound cannot be held together. Healing has to wait until the wound has been filled with new tissue (granulation tissue) and only then can the new skin grow over the wound surface. There are often complications with proud flesh in these types of wounds.

As wounds to the skin are so common, a look at the skin structure in Chapter 8 is recommended.

## Skin

The epidermis of the skin covers the whole body surface in one form or another. It lies over the dermis of the skin, which houses the hair follicles, sebaceous and sweat glands and the blood capillaries and nerves. The epidermis is quite thin and consists of layers which are more flattened as they reach the epidermal surface. The cells at the base of the epidermis are plump and columnar in shape. The outermost epidermal cells have lost their nuclei and have been converted to thin, lifeless scales of keratin, the characteristic protein of the epidermis from which the hairs and hooves are made. These scales stick together to form a horny layer which waterproofs and protects the skin. The epidermis is geared to producing this layer continuously as the top layer is worn away. The epidermis forms a barrier to dirt and bacteria. Between the epidermis and dermis lies a thin membrane through which all nutrients required to nourish the epidermis must pass.

The dermis itself is richly supplied with blood capillaries and with sensory nerve endings. A layer of fat, which has an insulating and protective function, is situated between the dermis and the body wall. It varies in thickness between individuals.

Any injury will result in a process known as inflammation.

## The stages of wound healing

The first stage of wound repair is often known as the traumatic inflammatory phase.

### Stage 1 – the traumatic inflammatory phase (Fig. 16.1)

This is also known as the defensive stage. Inflammation is initiated immediately there is any damage to tissues. Chemical messengers flow from the damaged cells to the adjacent areas where they stimulate undamaged cells into activity. Certain chemicals, namely bradykinin and histamine (Fig. 16.2) cause the walls of small blood capillaries to become leaky and some plasma and white cells and platelets are able to leak into the damaged area and onto the wound surface, producing an exudate. If there has been extensive tissue damage, the blood capillaries may be over-stimulated causing excessive exudate, swelling (oedema) and pain.

The ends of severed blood capillaries are sealed by blood clotting which, through a

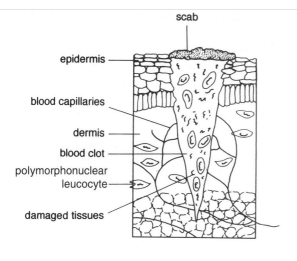

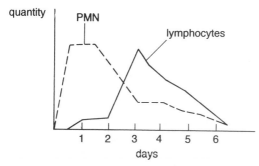

PMN = polymorphonuclear leucocytes

**Fig. 16.1**  Inflammatory phase of wound healing.

series of chemical reactions, brings about the formation of a mesh of fibrin fibres with trapped red blood cells stuck to them. Any blood that clots within the tissue spaces and lies between the wound surface and the tissue spaces must be broken down and removed at a later date as it will obstruct healing.

Within one hour, circulation of specialised white blood cells known as polymorpho-nuclear leucocytes or PMNs occur. These cells originate from the bone marrow and they are attracted by chemicals released by bacteria. The PMNs begin to stick to the inner surface of the capillary walls in the vicinity of the wound. They then squeeze their way through the leaky blood vessels by changing their shape to become flat, and move into the surrounding tissues.

Bacteria are always present in wounds. They live on the skin and in the atmosphere and even presurgical asepsis techniques cannot get rid of them all. So all wounds, be they surgical or accidental, will contain significant numbers of bacteria. In serious injuries it is sometimes preferable to control the amount of inflammation to prevent permanent swelling. This is often the case with tendon injuries where too much swelling can impair the healing process.

### Stage 2 – the destructive phase (0–3 days) (Fig. 16.3)

The second or destructive phase begins after about eight hours. The macrophages and

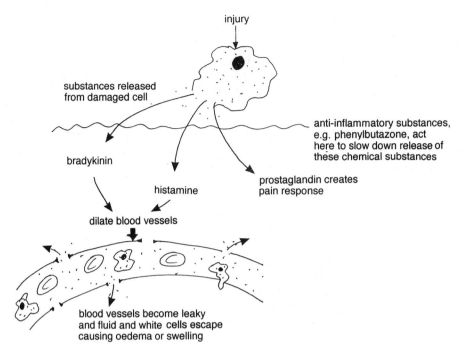

**Fig. 16.2**  Inflammatory response to injury at cellular level.

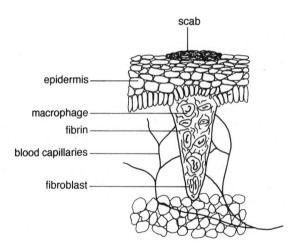

**Fig. 16.3**  Destructive phase of wound healing.

mononuclear cells are carried by the blood to the affected area. The macrophages, which are part of the reticulo-endothelial system, scavenge for dead cells and bacteria and clear away any blood and damaged tissue fibres. They will also try to remove any unwanted foreign material that has found its way into the wound and leave a clean pathway for the formation of new tissue which must follow, macrophages also stimulate the production of fibroblasts, the cells which make the body's principal structural protein, namely collagen. Collagen can be found in fresh wounds within 48 hours, new blood capillaries also start to grow into the wound from the edges and fibroblasts start to multiply. The fibroblasts make collagen in the form of cross-linked fibrils which form a network of fibrous bundles. Then remodelling begins at the start of the third phase known as the proliferative stage.

### Stage 3 – the proliferative phase (3–24 days) (Fig. 16.4)

Also known as the reconstructive phase, the fibroblasts start to make a collagen network behind the macrophages. Collagen is the main constituent of skin, tendons, ligaments, bones, cartilage and scar tissue. Early collagen is highly disorganised and its early formation depends to a large extent upon the blood supply to the injured area. Fibroblasts need stimulating to produce the vital collagen and one of the most important stimulators is vitamin C. Without vitamin C, collagen synthesis is inhibited. Since the horse's body cannot store vitamin C, the importance of good nutrition at this stage is apparent.

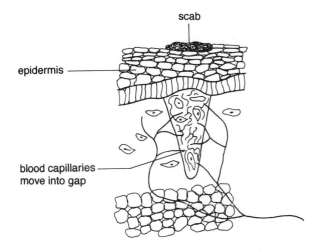

scab

epidermis

blood capillaries
move into gap

**Fig. 16.4** Proliferative phase of wound healing.

The considerable activity which occurs during this phase results in the formation of granulation tissue. This consists of newly formed and fragile capillary loops supported in a scaffold of collagen fibres. The amount of granulation tissue produced depends upon the amount of inflammation. As this proliferative phase continues, there is a rapid increase in the strength of the wound. Any excessive movement at this stage will result in impaired healing as the edges between the wound surface must be kept still. Usually, by about the fourteenth day, the wound has about one-quarter of the strength of the surrounding tissue.

Factors which may impair healing at this stage are age, the amount of oxygen available and zinc deficiency.

### Stage 4 – the maturation phase (24 days to 2 years)

During this stage, there is a progressive decrease in the vascularity of the scar, shrinkage of the fibroblasts, enlargement and reorientation of the collagen fibres and improved tissue strength. The dusky red colour of new, vascular granulation tissue changes to the pale, white, avascular (no blood capillaries) scar tissue. After the first six weeks only half of the normal strength of the wounded skin is achieved. Strength of the pre-injured tissue is rarely achieved in practice.

The scar then slowly reduces, causing flattening and softening of the scar. This may take up to a year.

## The speed of wound healing

The extent of the damage to the skin and underlying tissues will to a large extent determine the method and speed of healing, for example a shallow skin wound with some tissue loss, known as a partial thickness wound, will heal faster than traumatic injuries with extensive tissue loss (full thickness wound). This is because the hair follicles of the skin form most of the new surface epidermis when the skin is injured, with the sebaceous and sweat gland cells providing some also. Obviously, if the wound is extensive and much of the skin's dermis layer is missing, a different and much slower process occurs whereby the granulation tissue must fill the wound first before new epidermis can grow over the surface, a process known as epithelialisation. In these cases, the fat layer beneath the dermis produces the granulation tissue.

Often the granulation tissue overflows the wound so that new epidermis has to try and grow through this mass of pink flesh which is a very slow process. This overflowing granulation tissue is known as proud flesh and can often be seen bubbling out of wounds, particularly those on the lower leg of the horse (Fig. 16.5). The proud flesh also damages the new skin which has formed at the edges of the wound so that the injury tends to deteriorate rather than heal.

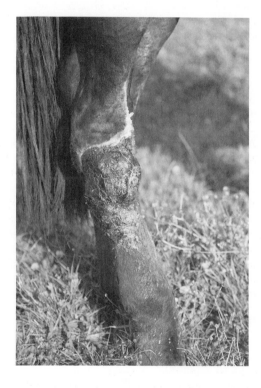

Fig. 16.5 Proud flesh or excess granulation tissue is common on wounds below the knee or hock. (Courtesy of Joanna Prestwich)

Proud flesh formation must be avoided. If it appears then veterinary advice should be sought, so that it can be removed by a process known as debridement to allow the epidermis to grow over the wound. Copper sulphate is often used to debride wounds, but it can damage the delicate cells on the wound edges so care should be taken when using it. These wounds can create real problems and may have to be continually debrided before being skin grafted.

Skin grafts may be required to help the epidermis to spread over the wound surface. This process involves the removal of small pieces of skin from the horse's neck, thigh or flank and they are embedded into the healthy granulation tissue at about 1 cm intervals. The majority of the grafts fail but each surviving piece stimulates the division of epidermal cells.

## Wound contraction

As granulation tissue grows it contracts, pulling on the skin at the edges of the wound and bringing them nearer together. This means that the wound area needing to be covered by new epidermis will be smaller. If the surrounding tissue is relatively loose and mobile, wound contraction will be very helpful in the healing process. The horse has a problem in that the blood supply to the lower limbs, from the hock and knee down, is relatively poor. This means that the chances of proud flesh forming are high and healing is generally slower. Wound contraction is minimal. If a horse has a wound extending from, say, above the knee to below the knee, there is often a difference in the speed of healing – the injury above the knee healing faster than the same injury that is below. Even small wounds of the lower limb can take a relatively long time to heal.

Foreign bodies which enter the wound, such as gravel, thorns, splinters all carry bacteria. If they are not removed they will be encapsulated by fibrous tissue with white blood cells trying to kill the bacteria. This results in the formation of an abscess. If small wounds will not heal a foreign body should be suspected. Sometimes these are brought to the surface as the body's defence system tries to remove it.

## Dressings

The wound surface beneath a scab is low in oxygen because the blood capillaries have been damaged and numerous inflammatory cells and bacteria mop up what little oxygen arrives at the site. This environment is far from ideal for epidermal wound healing. A better environment can be created by suitably designed dressings which absorb the majority of blood and exudate but prevent dehydration or drying out of the exposed dermis while allowing oxygen from the atmosphere to reach the wound. Under these conditions the epidermis is able to migrate in moist surroundings between the dressing and the wound surface about three times faster than under a scab and no secondary damage is done to the exposed dermis by drying out. The numerous white blood cells present in the exudate on the wound surface will be able to sterilise the wound. This is a better way to combat infection, by allowing the horse's body's own defence system to kill bacteria instead of using antibacterial chemicals.

## Factors which may delay wound healing

Delayed wound healing is often the result of an infection. The horse's body has a remarkable capacity to heal itself but often the inappropriate, though well-intentioned, efforts of horse owners can inhibit the natural healing mechanisms.

Factors that may delay wound healing include adverse local conditions at the wound site such as poor blood supply, necrotic (dead and dying) tissue, foreign bodies, dehydration and lack of oxygen.

Dried goat's dung, honey, urine, milk, soil, butter, oils and tars have all been applied to wounds at some time in history. It is not therefore surprising that until relatively recently the mortality from wounds was fairly high due to secondary wound infections. Today there is a wide range of topical agents (i.e. those applied to the wound surface) available for wound cleansing and treatment prior to any dressing being applied. The veterinary surgeon will know which product is the most appropriate to use. Because it has been shown that wounds heal better if moist, substances which dry out the wound such as sulphonamide powder may not always be appropriate. A product is available which forms a second skin over the wound surface, allowing the influx of oxygen to the wound but preventing the unwanted drying out of the exposed dermis.

Commonly used agents and their mode of action in the treatment of wounds are shown in Table 16.1.

**Table 16.1**   Topical agents most commonly applied to wounds

| Category | Mode of action | Commonly used agents | Advantages/ disadvantages |
|---|---|---|---|
| **Antibiotics** | Combat infection by killing micro-organisms or inhibiting their growth while being relatively harmless to the horse's tissues | Neomycin (Neostat) | Systemic antibiotics may be given by the vet where there are clear signs of infection. Topical use is controversial because it can cause allergy and microbial resistance may develop |
| **Antiseptics** | Antimicrobial agents. Used for cleansing and disinfection | Chlorhexidine (Hibitane) | Effective against a wide range of bacteria. Low toxicity but ineffective against spores, fungi, viruses and acid fast bacteria. Activity is reduced by blood and pus |
| | | Iodine (Pevidine) | Broad spectrum action, no resistant strains, causes staining of wound |
| | | Dermisol multicleanse | Recommended that the wound is cleansed with this product before the application of dermisol |
| **Debriding agents** | Designed to remove necrotic tissue and debris from the wound site which would otherwise delay wound healing and perhaps be a source for infection | Dermisol (also an antibacterial) | Concurrent use of disinfectants not advised as they will dilute the effect of dermisol. Dermisol multicleanse is recommended to be applied first. Also has an antibacterial action |

## Should the wound be stitched?

Many horse owners like to see their horses' wounds stitched as they assume this will prevent infection and improve the wound healing process. As mentioned previously, bacteria are always present in wounds – it is simply a matter of how many. Sometimes wounds have to be stitched to give them a chance to heal, but trying to pull the edges of the wound together, when too far apart, by stitches will inevitably lead to breakdown of the wound.

Large body wounds which involve the skin only will often heal well although they look horrific. If they are vertical they can be stitched (Fig. 16.6). Horizontal wounds on the shoulder, hip and thigh are often requested to be stitched, but they rarely heal by first intention due to the excessive tension on the stitches and the dead space behind the wound. Wounds of the chest and neck rely on wound contraction and effective drainage of the exudate and debris, but usually heal very well.

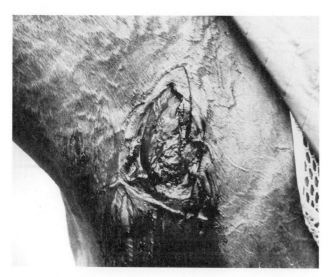

**Fig. 16.6** This nasty looking wound healed rapidly after the subcutaneous layers were sewn back together. (Courtesy of Liverpool University Veterinary School)

# Types of wound

Horses are very prone to injury through falls, kicks, bites, hitting jumps and getting tangled in fences. The wound sustained may be classified as open or closed; open wounds involve skin damage while closed wounds include bruises, sprains or ruptures.

Open wounds can be further classified as abrasions, incised wounds, lacerated wounds or tears, puncture wounds, penetrating wounds.

## Abrasions

These are very superficial skin wounds – for example saddle sores or grazes from falling.

## Incised wounds

These wounds have clean straight edges and often bleed freely. Usually there is little bruising and they normally heal quite quickly. Incised wounds are caused by surgical incisions or cuts by metal or glass.

## Lacerations and tears

These wounds have torn edges and an irregular shape, with some bruising. The amount of bleeding will be variable depending on the position of the wound.

Frequently there are torn flaps of skin which will probably die before the wound heals. Lacerated wounds are caused by wire, protruding nails and other hazards.

## Puncture wounds

These wounds tend to be more serious than they look; the skin opening may be small but the flesh can be penetrated to a varying depth. Puncture wounds are caused by bites, stakes and treading on nails and splinters, and bacteria are carried deep into the wound, leading to infection. The skin wound may be so small that it is overlooked. If you are not sure of the horse's vaccination status the horse should be given an anti-tetanus injection by the vet. The wound must be treated so that it heals from the inside out which usually involves poulticing the wound to draw out any infection.

## Penetrating wounds

These are wounds which occur when a horse stakes itself on a fence or a jump and the body cavity is penetrated. Such wounds are potentially very serious. The veterinary surgeon should be called immediately and the wound covered to contain the internal organs and prevent the entry of air.

## Closed wounds

These include injuries such as bruises, contusions, sprains, muscle damage and tendon strain. There is usually internal bleeding without breaking the skin, leading to swelling, heat and pain. The horse may need veterinary attention depending on the site and severity of the injury. Generally the area should be immobilised as much as possible (Fig. 16.7) and treated with cold hosing or ice packs. The horse may be given anti-inflammatory drugs. Once the heat has gone from the area heat treatments can be used to absorb excess fluid. Blood-filled swellings called haematomas may develop under the skin (following a kick on the chest, for example) and these may need draining by the vet after the bleeding has stopped.

# First aid

First aid is an important skill which all horse owners should be familiar with. Even the smallest of wounds should be given some attention. A first aid kit is a must for any yard as prompt attention will aid the healing process.

## First aid kit

- Bowl for antiseptic solution.
- Cloth upon which the kit can be laid.
- Antiseptics for cleaning wounds. A ready diluted antiseptic solution is useful in the travelling kit.
- Wound powder or spray for use if wound is left open. This prevents infection and dry wounds. In summer a fly-repellent powder is useful.
- Antiseptic ointment and a healing cream to put on the dressing before bandaging a wound.
- Clean crêpe bandages for support and slight pressure and adhesive bandages to hold dressings in place.
- Sterile non-adherent dressings to place over a wound before bandaging.

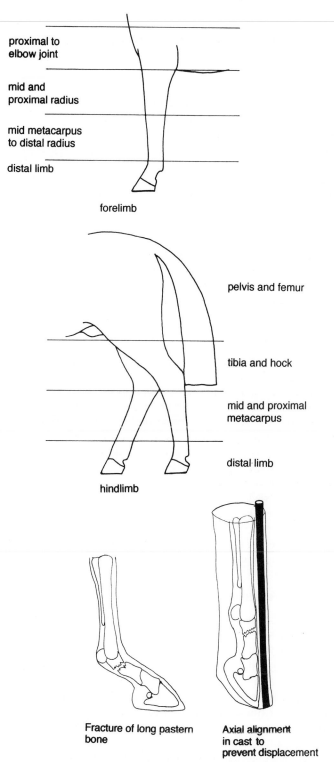

proximal to
elbow joint

mid and
proximal radius

mid metacarpus
to distal radius

distal limb

forelimb

pelvis and femur

tibia and hock

mid and proximal
metacarpus

distal limb

hindlimb

Fracture of long pastern
bone

Axial alignment
in cast to
prevent displacement

**Fig. 16.7** *Upper diagram:* division of the fore and hind limb before application of a splint. *Lower diagram:* immobilisation of a long pastern bone fracture to prevent displacement.

- Cotton wool – for cleaning wounds.
- Curved, blunt-ended scissors for cutting hair from wound and straight scissors for cutting tapes and bandages.
- Ready to use poultice in sealed pack.
- Veterinary thermometer and petroleum jelly.
- Forceps or tweezers to remove thorns and splinters from wounds.
- The travelling kit should also contain money for a telephone call.

Care should be taken if using purple spray, as it stains the wound dark purple and makes it very difficult to see. This can be very irritating for the veterinary surgeon if he has been called out to treat the wound.

The use of tourniquets to reduce excessive blood loss is now outdated and pressure on the area should be applied instead.

## First aid procedure

The success with which a wound heals in the long-term is greatly influenced by the immediate first aid that the wound receives. The following action should be taken.

- Control the bleeding by applying pressure to the wound. A clean dressing can be pressed firmly to the wound or, if the wound is on the horse's leg a pressure bandage can be applied over several layers of gamgee. Care must be taken that the bandage does not act as a tourniquet and cut off the blood supply. The bandage should be removed as soon as the bleeding stops.
- Call the veterinary surgeon if the horse is distressed or if the wound is bleeding profusely and requires stitching. If any doubt exists the vet should be called.
- Clean the wound using cooled boiled water or sterile saline solution. Once the wound is superficially clean the hair around the wound can be carefully cut away and the wound examined more closely and any foreign object carefully removed. Deep wounds can be thoroughly irrigated using a sterile syringe while superficial wounds can be bathed with an antibacterial wash and dressed with a suitable ointment.
- Reassess the cleaned wound and call the vet if necessary.
- Dress the wound using a healing cream covered with a non-adherent dressing, bandaged in place if possible. Deep wounds or puncture wounds where infection is suspected should be poulticed.
- The horse should be confined to the stable and walked out in hand if it is sound and the exercise will not disturb the wound.

# The use of lasers in the treatment of wounds

Laser treatment stimulates the production of collagen and thus stimulates wound healing. Lasers have an antibacterial effect and they are becoming increasingly useful in the treatment of open wounds, but should always be used alongside the conventional methods of wound treatment. If treatment with laser is started within 24 hours of the injury occurring, the appearance of unwanted proud flesh can be halted. Wounds which have been treated with lasers tend to have little scarring and normal hair growth. This can be very important for horses which are being shown.

Laser treatment is thought to reduce inflammation and thereby reduce pain and reduce infection. It should not, however, be used on wounds which are already infected, or in conjunction with steroids as it stimulates natural cortisone production.

# Chapter 17
# Fitness and Feeding

The aim of a fitness programme is to produce a horse that is 'fit', in other words in a state suitable for carrying out the work required without excessive stress. The level of fitness required is dictated by the intensity of the effort the horse has to perform.

Getting a horse fit is a mixture of correct work and a balanced, adequate diet. One without the other will not produce a horse capable of performing at his best. The basis of any fitness programme is to increase the horse's ability to tolerate work by gradually increasing his workload and energy intake. This slow, steady progression is fundamental to the physical and mental well-being of the horse, building confidence and security in his own ability.

The traditional methods of getting horses fit have developed from getting hunters fit from grass. Traditionally, hunters are brought up from grass at the beginning of August, allowing three months to get them hunting fit – equivalent to one-day event fitness or 20 mile distance ride fitness. This three month period can be split into three four-week blocks: preliminary walking and trotting work, development work and fast work.

## Preliminary work

The preliminary work is designed to exercise the horse slowly for increasing lengths of time to tone up the muscles, tendons and ligaments and to harden the soft horse's skin. The importance of the initial walking and trotting work cannot be over-emphasised – fitness is a pyramid, the broader the base, the higher the peak that can be reached. Ideally, the horse should be walked on the roads for up to two hours a day for four weeks and never less than two weeks – the longer the holiday the more roadwork is needed. If the horse has been walked two or three times a week from the field, another two weeks on top should suffice once the horse has come in.

After the initial walking work trot can be introduced; the trotting can be alternated between the roads and grass or in the arena; a certain amount of trotting on the road helps the horse cope with hard ground but too much causes concussion and jarring. Initially, the trot should only be for a couple of minutes at a time, building up over the next couple of weeks to 15 minutes in total, split into three or four periods.

## Development work

The horse should now be ready to progress to the next stage of training, with the introduction of canter work and suppling exercises. Development work will vary according to the discipline the horse is being prepared for but the principle is to begin to work the horse harder so that the heart and lungs become accustomed to exercise, building up the horse's stamina while the muscles continue to strengthen and adapt to the work the horse is being given.

# Fast work

The third period of the fitness programme is even more specialised; the power and athleticism of the dressage horse and show jumper are developed further, while the racehorse and the event horse have fast work. Some horses, for example ridden show horses, never embark on this third stage but would continue to build up body, skin and coat condition and become more highly trained.

# Interval training

Interval training was originally developed to train middle-and long-distance runners and swimmers, and has been used successfully in human athletics for over 20 years. Interval training has been adapted for event horses and successfully used by top British and American event riders.

## What is interval training?

Interval training consists of giving a horse a period of specific work (canter) followed by a brief interval of semi-rest (walk) during which the horse is allowed to partially recover before being asked to work again.

## The aims of interval training

The aim is to increase the horse's capacity for using oxygen and performing aerobic work; the point at which anaerobic work starts is delayed as much as possible so that the resultant lactic acid build-up is also postponed. This results in the horse being able to work for longer before fatigue sets in. The periods of work given during interval training develop and extend the horse's capacity for intensive work as the programme progresses, without a build-up of lactic acid. Lactic acid is a major factor contributing to fatigue; the walking periods between canters allow the blood to remove any lactic acid that may be building up in the muscle. Interval training increases the horse's tolerance to stress and the measurement of pulse, respiration and recovery rates means that the horse's reaction to the training programme can be closely monitored.

## Monitoring interval training

An essential part of the interval training regime is monitoring the horse's temperature, pulse and respiration (TPR). The horse cannot tell the rider how he feels, the rider must learn to read the signs of stress. To obtain 'normal' values each of these measurements should be taken while the horse is calm and at rest, for example between feeding and the daily exercise. These values are then used as a baseline against which the values after exercise can be compared.

## Before starting

Interval training cannot cut corners and the following factors must be considered before starting a programme:

• The horse should be capable of 90 minutes walk and trot over rolling terrain without distress. If conditioned slowly and carefully, the horse will stay in peak condition longer than one pushed too fast in the early stages.

- It is essential to keep a notebook with a running record of the horse's response to work, allowing the programme to be adjusted accordingly. As well as TPR the weather, type of work and how the horse 'feels' should also be noted. The weather can have a profound effect on how quickly the horse recovers from work – during hot and humid weather the horse will continue breathing fast for longer than expected because more rapid breathing is necessary to reduce body heat; so even though the pulse rate may drop to normal, the horse's breathing may still be fast. Pulse is a more reliable gauge of the horse's recovery and how fit he is, and is the most important reading to take.
- As in any form of training the rider must be alert to any change in the horse's attitude, appetite, coat, dropping, appearance, muscle tone, etc.
- The breeding, condition and previous training must also be considered; stuffy horses may need to work up to a different end point so that they are fitter than the more athletic thoroughbred type.

## How to use interval training

During interval training the horse is cantered at a predetermined speed for a certain time. After this piece of work the horse is pulled up and the pulse and/or respiration rates recorded immediately, the horse is walked for a set time and the rates recorded again. The difference between the two readings is the 'recovery rate' of the horse. The horse repeats these work-outs every four days and the pulse and respiration rates are recorded at the same points; as the horse gets fitter, he will recover faster from the work. The horse's pulse and respiration values will rarely return to the resting values obtained in the stable due to excitement and the fact that he is recovering in walk, so a value for the horse's warmed up pulse and respiration should be obtained and used as baseline values.

Fitness is gradually built up by slowly increasing the amount of work the horse is asked to do by increasing the speed and/or length of the work-out or using more demanding terrain. If the recovery rate is not good enough after a work-out, the work is adjusted so the horse is never over-stressed. This system is markedly different from the more traditional methods where horses are trotted and cantered for long distances with short sharp gallops later in the training programme and no repetition of fast work in each work-out.

During the first canter work-out the horse can be cantered for three minutes at 400 mpm (metres per minute). This is followed by one minute in trot and a recovery period in walk of three to five minutes. This is repeated twice, after which the horse is cooled down in walk for at least 20 minutes. The heart rate should be no more than 150 beats per minute at the end of each canter and no more than 100 bpm before the next canter commences. If the heart rate takes more than five minutes to drop below 100 bpm, then either the canter was too long, the terrain too steep, the speed too fast or the initial work was not carried out correctly.

The canter work is gradually built up until the horse has reached the desired fitness. The flexibility of interval training means that it can be used to fitten horses as diverse as event horses and long-distance horses very effectively.

## Points to remember

- Interval training must be monitored by pulse and respiration rate, not by time alone. It is the pulse rate immediately after the work that shows how much stress the horse has been subjected to, and the recovery rate that shows how fit he is. Without these records interval training is meaningless and can actually be harmful.

- If the horse is required to work anaerobically the pulse rate should exceed 200 beats per minute; this can be estimated by looking at the pulse one minute after pulling up. If the horse has been beneficially stressed his pulse will lie between 120 and 150 beats per minute one minute after stopping work. If greater than 150 bpm he has been overstressed, below 120 bpm he has not worked hard enough. This guide should only be used well on into the programme or the horse may be over-worked.
- If the pulse and respiration have not returned to normal within 20 minutes of completing the work-out the horse has been over-worked and the programme should be adapted accordingly.
- The respiration rate should not exceed the pulse rate. If it does, stop work and ask what has caused this – lack of fitness, environmental conditions or a problem with the horse's respiratory tract?
- Never finish the work if the horse is distressed.
- On the other hand, the horse must be stressed enough to stimulate the body systems to become better adapted to exercise. The heart rate must be raised above 100 beats per minute after work.
- Always warm up and cool down thoroughly before cantering, particularly if the horse has to travel in a lorry or trailer to the work area.

## The effects of training on the horse's body

### The respiratory system

In order to perform effectively the horse must be 'right in its wind' and much of a training programme aims to improve the horse's ability to get oxygen into the bloodstream. A fit horse will be able to do more work than an unfit horse before it starts to blow and the respiration will also return to normal more quickly. An effective fitness programme results in the following changes to the horse's respiratory system:

- Alveolar recruitment – during periods of inactivity some of the tiny air sacs in the lungs become blocked by mucus and debris. Exercise clears this debris out of the lungs, increasing the horse's lung capacity. Unfit horses may be described as 'thick in the wind' and may discharge mucus from the nostrils when first brought into faster work.
- Pulmonary capillarisation – the tiny blood vessels that surround each alveolus respond to the increased oxygen demands of the exercising horse by increasing in number. This, combined with having a greater lung capacity, means that the horse can get more oxygen from the lungs into the bloodstream and hence the muscles.
- Muscular development – the muscles of the diaphragm and chest may become stronger with exercise.

### The muscles

Muscle is able to adapt during training to the varying demands placed upon it. There is unlikely to be a significant change in the proportion of slow twitch to fast twitch fibres. The main effects of training are on the metabolism of the fibres; stamina training can increase the oxygen-using capacity of fast twitch fibres and thus enhance the ability of the horse to utilise oxygen.

A muscle fibre can only adapt if it is given suitable stimuli, thus the training programme must include work of similar intensity and type to that involved in competition. If speed is required, sufficient sprinting should be included to recruit the muscle fibres involved with power and acceleration, i.e. fast twitch low oxidative fibres. If the competition involves endurance work at varying speeds, prolonged exercise at similar levels is needed to increase the oxygen-using capacity of the muscle, i.e. fast twitch high oxidative fibres and slow twitch fibres. This means that the onset of fatigue due to lactic acid build-up will be delayed.

Training also increases fuel availability to muscle fibres by encouraging more mitochondria and higher levels of enzymes for the breakdown of glycogen and free fatty acids. The blood capillaries supplying the muscle also proliferate, increasing the oxygen supply and the muscle develops a greater ability to store a glycogen. Fit horses are better able to use free fatty acids as an energy source, this 'glycogen sparing' effect delays fatigue.

# The circulatory system

The horse's resting heart rate normally lies between 36 and 42 beats per minute, but may be as low as 26 beats per minute in a fit horse, reaching a maximum of 240 beats per minute when galloping. The heart responds to training by:

- increased heart size – as any other muscle, the heart responds to work by increasing in size, enabling the heart to pump more blood round the body;
- capillarisation – training increases the number of capillaries supplying the muscle, increasing the oxygen supply to the muscle (Fig. 17.1).

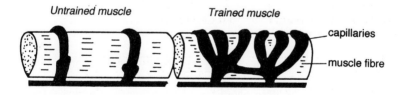

**Fig. 17.1**  Training causes capillaries to multiply around the muscle fibres.

The effect of training on the blood are that:

- both the red blood cell count and packed cell volume increase with training, improving the ability of the blood to carry oxygen;
- the red blood cell turnover increases – red blood cells have a limited life span and the horse works harder, the cells 'wear out' more quickly and the turnover increases so that the average age of a red blood cell decreases. Younger cells have a better oxygen carrying capacity and also increase the ability of the blood to carry oxygen.

These internal changes to the respiratory and circulatory systems manifest as:

- a slower resting heart rate;
- a less dramatic rise in heart and respiration rates for a given piece of exercise;
- a better recovery rate.

## Getting the Novice one-day event horse fit

A period of three months should be allowed to prepare for the first event of the season, bearing in mind that show-jumping, dressage and cross-country competitions may be part of the build-up. To achieve basic fitness the programme outlined earlier should be used – two weeks of walking work, followed by two weeks of walking and trotting with canter introduced in weeks five and six.

By the end of week six interval training can start. Canter work is repeated every fourth day, building the sessions up minute by minute. The day after a canter session should be a rest or just a hack for one-and-a-half to two hours. Over the next two weeks the sessions are built up so that the horse can do three lots of five minute canters at 400 mpm, with three minutes walking in between.

The first horse trial can be planned for week 12; in the final two weeks the road work, schooling and jump training continue as usual. After a couple of these work sessions, the last minute of the last canter can be increased to a speed of 500 mpm. The canter work is shown in Table 17.1.

**Table 17.1** Interval training to Novice one-day event fitness

20 minutes warm-up
*Canter 1:*   5 minutes @ 400 mpm
              trot 30 seconds
              walk 3 minutes
*Canter 2:*   4 minutes @ 400 mpm
              1 minute @ 500 mpm
              trot 30 seconds to 1 minute
              walk 3 minutes
*Canter 3:*   4 minutes @ 400 mpm
              1 minute @ 500 mpm building up to 550 mpm
              trot 1 to 2 minutes
              walk at least 20 minutes.

The heart rate after the third canter should drop below 100 bpm after 10 minutes walking.

The idea of interval training is to allow the horse to work aerobically for longer periods, but at some stage during the cross-country or steeplechase the horse will work anaerobically. Increasing the speed at the end of the last two canter sessions makes the horse work anaerobically; the trotting afterwards helps disperse the lactic acid and thus the heart rate recovers more quickly. It cannot be over-emphasised that all horses are individuals and must be treated as such, tables are merely a guideline and do not allow for lost shoes, heavy going or lazy horses. The real skill in training lies in the ability to design programmes for individual horses and to recognise the need to adapt the programme without hindering the horse's progress.

## Interval training to Advanced levels

The demands made upon horses competing in three-day events require that the horse is at peak physical fitness and condition. The rider and trainer must be aware of the rigorous task that they are training the horse for. The aim of the training programme is for the horse to complete this severe test at the required speed without fatigue in the latter stages which could lead to an error and a fall. The horse must also be fit enough to pass the veterinary inspection the next day and to show jump accurately.

The horse trained to Advanced one-day event fitness should be able to work aerobically during canters of up to 500 mp. Cantering for longer times does not actually increase the horse's ability to cope with the demands of the faster speeds in Advanced horse trials and three-day events. This means that the speed and/or hill work must be used to train horses at these levels; this is particularly true for part-bred horses. Before a rider attempts to get a horse to this level of fitness, he needs to know the horse intimately and have a thorough knowledge of his requirements, capabilities and limitations. The breeding or type of horse, his present condition and previous fitness must all be considered when devising the horse's training programme. The first six weeks would be much as outlined for the Novice horse, the next four to six weeks would see the work being stepped up to get the horse Advanced one-day event fit as shown in Table 17.2.

**Table 17.2**   Interval training to Advanced one-day event fitness

| | |
|---|---|
| 20 minutes warm-up | |
| *Canter 1:* | 6 minutes @ 450 mpm |
| | trot 30 seconds |
| | walk 3 minutes |
| *Canter 2:* | 4 minutes @ 450 mpm |
| | 3 minutes @ 500 mpm |
| | trot 30 seconds to 1 minute |
| | walk 3 minutes |
| *Canter 3:* | 4 minutes @ 450 mpm |
| | 3 minutes @ 500 mpm building up to 600 mpm |
| | trot 1 to 2 minutes |
| | walk at least 20 minutes. |

For the four to six weeks prior to a 4-star three-day event such as Badminton or Burghley, the speed and length of the fast work would be gradually increased so that the last minute was performed at steeplechase speed (690 mpm), preparing the horse to go the required distance at that speed. The length of the gallop is thus kept down to 690 m (less than half-a-mile) so that the horse is not over-stressed but the body systems are primed to cope with anaerobic work.

The final levels that riders work up to vary, for example:

- Three repetitions of 9 minute canters at 550 mpm, 2 minutes walking between each, with the last minute of the final two canters at 690 mpm.
- Three repetitions of 10 minute canters at 550 mpm, 3 minutes walking between each, with one full-speed 800 m gallop at the end.
- Some riders believe that three repetitions of 8 minute canters are adequate and that increasing to 10 minutes does not significantly increase fitness, providing the canters are fast enough.

The short sprints develop speed and strength while the long, slower canters develop rhythm and staying power. During racing and three-day eventing maximum muscle contraction is demanded and lactic acid will accumulate in the muscles. The horse's body must learn to cope with and dissipate these high lactate levels so it is important that these levels of exercise are experienced in training – hence the importance of the short gallop at the end of the canter work-out.

# Feeding the competition horse

An essential ingredient of any training programme is correct feeding; no matter how well trained the horse, without good nutrition he will not be able to perform at his best. Feeding must ensure that the horse's demand for vital nutrients is met by a balanced, palatable ration.

## What to feed

Feeds can be divided into two categories – concentrates and forage. Concentrates are energy feeds and traditionally cereals have been the principal source of energy for horses in hard work. Cereal grains contain 12–16 MJ DE/kg (megajoules of digestible energy per kilogram) of dry matter compared with about 8.5 MJ/kg in average grass hay. In other words, 1 kg of cereals can replace up to 2 kg of hay in the ration – hence the name concentrate. As a higher energy output is demanded from the horse it must be fed more concentrated energy sources in order to keep the ration within appetite; this also reduces the horse's natural grass belly to give a trim athletic outline. However, it is important that adequate levels of forage are fed to maintain healthy gut function and to prevent the horse becoming bored. Ideally the ration of the horse in hard work is at least half forage with the levels never falling below 40% of the ration, even if the horse is in fast work.

Cereals also contain proteins but these are not as nutritionally valuable as animal protein and oil-seed protein because they are relatively deficient in the essential amino acids lysine and methionine. All cereal grains are very low in calcium, containing less than 1.5 g/kg, but they contain three to five times as much phosphorus. The phosphorus is principally in the form of phytate salts which reduce the availability of calcium and zinc, further increasing the horse's need for a calcium supplement.

**Table 17.3**  Typical nutrient values of commonly fed concentrate feeds

|  | Crude protein % | Oil % | MAD fibre g/kg | Ca g/kg | P g/kg | DE MK/kg |
|---|---|---|---|---|---|---|
| Oats | 9.6 | 4.5 | 17.0 | 0.7 | 3.0 | 12.0 |
| Naked oats | 13.5 | 9.7 | 3.2 | 0.2 | 0.4 | 16.0 |
| Barley | 9.5 | 1.8 | 7.0 | 0.6 | 3.3 | 13.0 |
| Maize | 8.5 | 3.8 | 3.0 | 0.2 | 3.0 | 14.0 |
| Linseed | 22.0 | 32.0 | 7.6 | 2.4 | 5.2 | 18.5 |
| Extruded soyabean meal | 44.0 | 1.0 | 10.0 | 2.4 | 6.3 | 13.3 |
| Wheatbran | 15.5 | 3.0 | 12.0 | 1.0 | 12.0 | 11.0 |
| Sugarbeet pulp | 7.0 | 1.0 | 34.0 | 10.0 | 11.0 | 10.5 |

## The 'heating' effect of grain

Grain is often said to be 'heating', meaning that it results in a horse being over-excited and difficult to control. This heating effect stems from two sources:

- Overfeeding energy – many 'hot' horses are simply getting too much energy for the job they are doing and a reduction in the concentrate ration and an increase in the roughage will solve many problems.
- Fermentation – any grain passing through into the large intestine is rapidly fermented by the intestinal micro-organisms. There is an increase in the acidity of the caecum which may lead to discomfort, and the products of digestion pass very quickly into the bloodstream. There is a rise in blood levels of glucose and

volatile fatty acids which stimulate the metabolic rate, thus 'heating' the horse both literally and mentally. Processing cereals increases the amount of digestion in the small intestine, reduces caecal fermentation and keeps the horse's metabolism more stable.

## Compound feeds

Compound feeds are convenience feeds for horses and have several advantages:

- convenience
- standardised diets for specific purposes
- constant quality
- good shelf-life
- dust-free
- palatable
- uniform weight and size, making the feeding routine more convenient
- economy of labour, transportation and storage
- no wastage

**Table 17.4**  Typical nutrient values of compound feeds

|  | Crude oil % | Crude fibre % | Crude protein % | DE MJ/kg | Total ash % |
|---|---|---|---|---|---|
| Horse and pony cubes | 3.0 | 14–15 | 10.0 | 9.0 | 9–10 |
| Performance cubes | 3.5–4 | 8.5 | 12–13 | 12.0 | 8–10 |
| Stud cubes | 3.0 | 9–10 | 13–15 | 11.0 | 8–10 |
| Creep feed | 4–4.5 | 6.5–7.5 | 17–18 | 13.0 | 7–9 |
| Yearling cubes | 3–3.5 | 8.5 | 15–16 | 11.0 | 7–9 |

## Rationing

The ration of a performance horse is decided after three important factors have been assessed:

- size
- condition
- work done.

### Size

The amount of food a horse needs to keep him alive and to maintain his bodyweight is called the maintenance ration. Horses will eat about 2.5% of their bodyweight a day. Thus a 500 kg (1100 lb) horse, a 16 hands middleweight, will eat 12.5 kg (28 lb) of food a day. Table 17.5 illustrates approximately bodyweight and appetites for different horses and ponies.

### Condition

If the horse is thin then the nutrient requirement for energy will be higher to enable it to put on condition. Assessment of condition is very subjective and care must be taken to look at the whole picture because while a show horse would look fat in a racing yard, a racehorse would look very lean in a showing yard.

### Work done

One of the old established rules of feeding is to feed the horse for the amount and

**Table 17.5** The relationship between height, girth, bodyweight and appetite

| Height (hands) | Girth (cm) | Bodyweight (kg) | Appetite (kg dry matter) |
|---|---|---|---|
| 11 | 135–145 | 200–260 | 4.5–6 |
| 12 | 140–150 | 230–290 | 5–7 |
| 13 | 150–160 | 290–350 | 6.5–8 |
| 14 | 160–170 | 350–420 | 8–9.5 |
| 15 | 170–185 | 420–520 | 10–12.5 |
| 16 | 185–195 | 500–600 | 12–14 |
| 17 | 195–210 | 600–725 | 13–18 |

The values in this table are averages and only approximate

intensity of the work it is doing. It is important for the horse's health, for your safety and your joint success not to overfeed or underfeed your horse for his degree of fitness.

## The ratio of forage to concentrates

In the practical situation when a new horse arrives on the yard you have to decide what to put on the feedboard immediately, there is no time to get our your calculator! A rule of thumb that has been used for many years to help us decide what to ration horses has been a simple table, relating the intensity of the horse's work to the ratio of forage to concentrates fed, as shown in Table 17.6. Modern thinking is that, in order to stay healthy, even horses in hard and fast work should not receive more than half of his ration as concentrates. If top quality forage is not available more concentrates may have to be fed to supply the energy demands of the horse. This means that a 500 kg (1100 lb) horse in medium work is fed 40% concentrates and 60% forage, resulting in a ration of 5 kg (11 lb) of concentrates and 7.5 kg (16 lb) hay.

**Table 17.6** Ratios of forage to concentrate

| Work level | Hay | Concentrates |
|---|---|---|
| Resting | 100 | 0 |
| Light | 75 | 25 |
| Medium | 60 | 40 |
| Hard | 50 | 50 |
| Fast | 40 | 60 |

It is best to feed a horse slightly below appetite so that he is always eager for his next concentrate feed and has always finished his haynet when you come to fill it again. If you feed a weighted ration of hay and concentrates within the horse's appetite, he should always eat up; if he does not eat all his hay and concentrates it may indicate that the quality of the feed is not up to scratch or that the horse is off-colour.

## The energy requirements for work

The horse's energy requirements for work depend on many factors including:

- speed of the work
- duration of the work
- terrain
- incline

- the weight of the horse
- the horse's fitness
- rider/driver ability
- environmental temperature and humidity
- the horse's soundness and conformation.

**Table 17.7**  Rations for 15.2–16 hh, 500 kg horse at different work levels

| Work level | DE required (MJ DE/kg) | Crude protein required (%) | Ratio of hay to concentrates | Ration Hay (8 MJ DE/kg) kg | lb | Concentrate kg | lb | Comments |
|---|---|---|---|---|---|---|---|---|
| Maintenance | 9 | 7.5 | 90:10 | 9.5 | 21 | 1 | 2 | Horse and pony cubes (10 MJ DE/kg) |
| Light (getting fit) | 9.5 | 8 | 80:20 | 8.5 | 19 | 2 | 4.5 | As above |
| Light to medium (Novice horse trials) | 10 | 8.5 | 70:30 | 7.5 | 16 | 3.5 | 8 | Event cubes (11 MJ DE/kg) |
| Medium (Intermediate horse trials) | 11 | 9 | 60:40* | 6.5 | 14 | 5 | 11 | As above |
| Hard (Advanced horse trials) | 12 | 9.5 | 50:50* | 6.0 | 13 | 6.0 | 13 | As above |
| Fast (Racing) | 13.5 | 10–11 | 50:50* | 6.0 | 13.0 | 6.0 | 13 | Racehorse cubes (14 MJ DE/kg) or oats plus protein concentrate |

* If good quality forage is available.

At one extreme a sprint race of 6 furlongs (1200 m) theoretically increases a horse's daily energy requirements by a mere 4%, while a day's hunting would more than double the day's energy requirement. In sprint races the majority of the energy for muscle contraction is obtained by the anaerobic breakdown of glucose, whereas long-distance horses like eventers, hunters and endurance horses use a combination of anaerobic and aerobic energy production, where glucose is burnt up in the presence of oxygen to produce the energy for prolonged muscle contraction.

Training involves priming the horse's body systems so that the horse can do the work demanded of it with maximum efficiency and minimum fatigue.

## The protein requirements for work

The horse's dietary requirement for protein is not greatly increased by work; the loss of protein in sweat and the protein incorporated into the greater muscle mass of the fit horse are reflected by an increase of about 2% in the diet. As the horse works the energy requirement increases substantially and the concentrate ration fed to sustain this energy requirement very often increases the protein component of the ration sufficiently to meet the extra protein demand. Horses with high energy requirements do not need to be fed high protein feeds unless they are being fed poor hay, with a protein content of below 6%. The feeding of excess protein may, in fact, be

**Table 17.8**   The protein needed for different types of work

| Work level | Crude protein in the ration (%) |
| --- | --- |
| Light | 7.5–8 |
| Medium | 7.5–8 |
| Hard | 9.5–10 |
| Fast | 9.5–10 |

detrimental to performance with horses not racing as fast and sweating and blowing more heavily.

The exception to these statements are the two-and three-year-old racehorses in training, which are still growing and consequently have a higher protein requirement. The quality of the protein in terms of its amino acid make-up is an important consideration.

## The utilisation of nutrients during exercise

Energy is the major nutrient requirement of the adult performance horse; the chemical energy in feed is converted into energy for muscle contraction so that the horse can do the work we demand of him. At one extreme this work may be a sprint over 6 furlongs (1200 m), at the other 160 km (100 miles) at an average speed of 13 km per hour (8 mph). The physiological body processes that produce energy for either speed or endurance are quite different; theoretically a short flat race barely increases the horse's daily energy requirements while a 100 mile ride would increase energy requirements five or sixfold.

The way food and nutrients are used in the horse's body is affected by several factors:

- the horse's health
- the horse's fitness and type of training
- the environmental temperature
- the diet
- the amount of nutrients stored in the horse's body.

Feeding and training must work together in harmony to produce the truly fit equine athlete.

## Training and energy expenditure

The aim of getting horses fit is to alter the metabolism of the horse so that it functions at maximum efficiency with minimum fatigue. The amount of energy used will vary depending on the type of work and the size of the horse (Table 17.9). Horsemen have known this for years and summarised it in one of the 'rules of feeding' – *feed according to work done.*

Walking, which is generally accepted to be an extremely good form of exercise for toning muscles, tendons and ligaments, barely increases the horse's daily energy requirement above maintenance. Strenuous or extended effort increases the horse's requirement to such an extent that the horse physically cannot eat that much energy in one day. Combined with the fact that hard work often reduces the horse's appetite means that recovery from hard work requires several days for the horse's energy reserves to be replenished.

**Table 17.9** Digestible energy (DE) demands of maintenance and work

|  | Bodyweight (kg) | | |
| --- | --- | --- | --- |
|  | 200 | 400 | 600 |
| Maintenance requirement/day (MJ DE) | 35 | 58 | 79 |
| Additional energy requirement for work (MJ DE/day) | | | |
| 1 hour walking | 0.4 | 0.8 | 1.3 |
| 1 hour slow trotting, some cantering | 4.2 | 8.4 | 12.5 |
| 1 hour fast trotting, cantering, some jumping | 10.5 | 20.9 | 31 |
| Cantering, galloping and jumping | 25 | 50 | 75 |
| Strenuous effort, racing, polo | 42.0 | 85 | 127 |
| Endurance work, 100 km in 10.5 hours | 43.5 | 87 | 130.5 |

Experiments on horses and ponies working on treadmills with an incline show that working uphill increases the energy requirement 17 times! Work over uneven and hilly ground is much more arduous than on flat terrain.

Even though during hard work a horse will use up more energy than he can consume during the day, he should not be fed to fortify himself for future events, because any energy supplied over and above immediate needs will be stored as fat and fatness will impair performance. Overfeeding can also lead to problems such as filled legs, laminitis, colic, azoturia and excitability.

## Sources of energy to the muscles

The two major sources of energy for the horse are carbohydrates and fats; except during starvation, proteins are of little importance. The energy for muscle contraction is derived from high energy phosphate compounds (ATP and creatine phosphate) which in turn comes from glucose, free fatty acids and volatile fatty acids which result from the break-down of food in the horse's gut. The glycolytic pathway converts glucose to pyruvic acid with the release of ATP. This process transfers some of the chemical energy of glucose to ATP in the absence of oxygen. In the presence of oxygen glucose is broken down completely to carbon dioxide and water. This takes place in the mitochondria of the cell and results in further ATP production. During digestion fat is broken down to fatty acids and glycerol; fatty acids are converted to acetyl-CoA and enters the Krebs or TCA cycle to be broken down to carbon dioxide and water with the transfer of energy to ATP. The break-down of fat leads to the synthesis of about three times as much energy per gram as the breakdown of glucose.

Glucose is absorbed into the bloodstream and blood glucose is a readily available source of energy. Excess glucose is stored as glycogen in the liver and muscles, ready for mobilisation and energy production when necessary. If the horse is overfed further glucose is stored as body fat.

The liver has a role in regulating blood glucose levels by breaking down glycogen to glucose to top-up blood sugar when needed during exercise and by storing blood sugar as glycogen after a meal.

Glucose is broken down in the muscle cells to create ATP; maximum energy is released when there is an adequate supply of oxygen arriving in the blood. Immediate and rapid release of energy can take place in the absence of oxygen in a process known as anaerobic respiration; the resulting chemical compound, pyruvate, can only be completely broken down to carbon dioxide and water in the presence of oxygen. Anaerobic respiration results in the production of lactic acid, which eventually needs oxygen to be broken down to harmless substances in the liver. The more anaerobic respiration (sprinting) the horse undergoes the more lactic acid builds up and the more oxygen will eventually be required to break it down. This is called the 'oxygen debt' and is being repaid when the sprinter blows after his race. Anaerobic respiration yields less energy than aerobic respiration.

During extended work the healthy, fit horse easily breaks down fatty acids to carbon dioxide because there is enough oxygen being breathed in to cope with the energy demand.

The changing demands of the horse for energy are monitored by the secretion of a number of hormones; as the racehorse leaves the starting stalls his nervous system sends rapid messages to the appropriate gland, which in turn causes essential changes in the body systems involved with exercise, e.g. the heart and blood vessels. Some hormones affect the enzymes that regulate the chemical reactions involved in energy production; other hormones such as insulin influence the permeability of cell membranes, thus the cells can take up more glucose and blood sugar levels fall.

Resting blood sugar levels tend to be higher in horses trained for sprinting. This is caused by stimulation of the systems which form glucose and which spare glucose by encouraging the use of fatty acids during exercise. Blood glucose also fluctuates during day and night; it peaks 3–8 hours after feeding, the height of the peak depending on the type of diet. Rations containing more grain and less roughage lead to higher peaks after feeding and lower troughs when the horse is hungry. Horses on a roughage-based diet become better at making glucose from other absorbed nutrients, so that they can resist a fall in blood glucose more easily. When hungry, however, they are not able to meet the high glucose demands of exertion. There are also breed differences; thoroughbreds have a high insulin sensitivity and consequently their blood sugar levels vary more than those of a pony on the same diet. This could partially explain the more volatile temperament of the thoroughbred.

As the intensity of training increases, the demand for energy released by particular metabolic pathways also increases, as does the need for the appropriate enzymes to help the reactions along. Sprinting is primarily anaerobic and training increases the horse's ability to break down glucose in the cytoplasm of the cell, with the enzymes that help prevent a build-up of lactic acid being present at nearly twice the untrained level. Longer periods of fast work involve aerobic processes, consequently the training of these horses results in an in increase in the numbers of 'powerhouses' or mitochondria present in the cell. The mitochondria house the enzymes needed for the aerobic production of energy. Enzymes need substances called co-factors in order to function properly, as the concentration of enzymes increases so the need for these co-factors is increased. Co-factors include the minerals, magnesium and zinc along with several B complex vitamins and this may indicate that horses in training require a dietary supplement of these micro-nutrients.

## Feeding for performance

The eventual performance of a horse is dependent on many factors but, no matter how well-trained the horse, if he is not fed properly he will not perform at his best. The difference in the metabolic processes by which energy is produced for sprinting work and endurance work means that long-distance and endurance horses have to make effective use of body fat reserves to provide energy and to conserve glucose sources. Studies have shown that horses can digest oil well and that oil can be used to replace some of the cereal ration. Fat in the diet also slows down the fall in blood glucose during endurance rides, due to its 'glycogen-sparing' effect. In other words, oil provides an alternative energy source for horses doing long, slow work. Levels of oil as high as 8–10% of the total ration have been suggested; in practical terms this amounts to 1–1.5 litres every day for a 500 kg horse. Adding 500 ml of oil to your horse's feed will enable you to reduce his concentrate by 1–1.5 kg of oats, depending on the quality of the oats.

It has been suggested that endurance or long-distance horses should have their concentrate ration built up by 1 kg per day for the two days preceding the ride, with the roughage being reduced by 2 kg. This is to ensure that the horse has adequate energy stores for the strenuous work ahead of him. On the day of the ride the horse may have a small concentrate feed and free access to water but hay should not be given.

Racehorses may actually benefit from a small concentrate feed 3–4 hours before their race as this will coincide with peak blood glucose levels, ensuring that adequate 'instant' energy is available. In practical terms this may not be possible, depending on how far the horse has to travel to the racecourse.

Whatever the discipline, work should always be kept ahead of feed, so that concentrate intake is increased as the intensity of work increases. In all cases make sure that hard feed is dramatically reduced – by at least half. If the horse has a rest day, the hay ration should be increased so that the horse does not go hungry. If the rest is enforced through energy or illness and is likely to be of a long duration, it may be wise to knock back the concentrates even more than this. A little loss of condition is preferable to azoturia.

# Index